Catfish

and Mandala

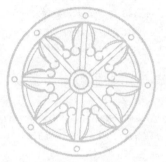

A Two-Wheeled Voyage through
the Landscape and Memory of Vietnam

A N D R E W   X .   P H A M

FARRAR, STRAUS AND GIROUX / *New York*

Farrar, Straus and Giroux
19 Union Square West, New York 10003

Copyright © 1999 by Andrew X. Pham
All rights reserved
Distributed in Canada by Douglas & McIntyre Ltd.
Printed in the United States of America
Designed by Abby Kagan
First edition, 1999

Library of Congress Cataloging-in-Publication Data
Pham, Andrew X., 1967–
    Catfish and Mandala : a two-wheeled voyage through the landscape
and memory of Vietnam / Andrew X. Pham. — 1st ed.
        p.   cm.
    ISBN 0-374-11978-3 (alk. paper)
    1. Pham, Andrew X., 1967–   .   2. Vietnamese Americans Biography.
3. Pham, Andrew X., 1967–   —Journeys.   I. Title.
E184.V53P455   1999
915.9704'44—dc21
    [B]   99-22711

Catfish

and Mandala

To the memory of my sister

C h i ,

my brother

M i n h ,

one and the same . . .

if only I had learned to see

without looking.

What is the proper number of kisses

For a man to leave this world?

The average depth of melancholy?

The approximate wetness of hope?

— M a x   G a r l a n d

Catfish

and Mandala

Prologue

Grandmother told me it had been written in my sister Chi's fortune penned by a Vietnamese Buddhist monk on the day of her birth, in the year of the Tiger: suicide at thirty-two. We were sitting on Grandmother's bed in the very room where Chi had hung herself. The rope was gone, but there was incense ash in the carpet, its fragrant prayers locked in. Grandmother closed her hands over mine and asked me quietly if I wanted to read my birth fortune. It was from the hand of the same monk, written twenty-seven years earlier. She pressed into my chest a yellowed fortune-scroll, crushed and tattered, its secret bound by an umbilical cord of red twine. I looked at this relic from a distant world, dreading its power. I said no, quit my job, and bicycled into the Mexican desert.

Exile-Pilgrim

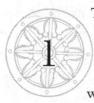

1   The first thing I notice about Tyle is that he can squat on his haunches Third World–style, indefinitely. He is a giant, an anachronistic Thor in rasta drag, bare-chested, barefoot, desert-baked golden. A month of wandering the Mexican wasteland has tumbled me into his lone camp warded by cacti. Rising from the makeshift pavilion staked against the camper top of his pickup, he moves to meet me with an idle power I envy. I see the wind has carved leathery lines into his legend-hewn face of fjords and right angles.

In a dry, earthen voice, he asks me, "Looking for the hot spring?"

"Yeah, Agua Caliente. Am I even close?"

"Sure. This is the place. Up the way a couple hundred yards."

"Amazing! I found it!"

He smiles, suddenly very charismatic, and shakes his head of long matty blond hair. "How you got here on that bike is *amazing*."

I had been pedaling and pushing through the forlorn land, roaming the foreign coast on disused roads and dirt tracks. When I was hungry or thirsty, I stopped at ranches and farms and begged the owners for water from their wells and tried to buy tortillas, eggs, goat cheese, and fruit. Every place gave me nourishment; men and women plucked grapefruits and tangerines from their family gardens, bagged food from their pantries, and accepted not one peso in return. Why, I asked them. *Señor,* they explained in the patient tone reserved for those convalescing, you are riding a bicycle, so you are poor. You are in the desert going nowhere, so you are crazy. Taking money from a poor and crazy man brings bad luck. All the extras, they confided, were because I wasn't a *gringo.* A crew of Mexican ranchers said they liked me because I was a *bueno hermano*—good brother—a *Vietnamito,* and my little Vietnam had *golpea* big America back in '75. *But I'm American, Vietnamese American,* I shouted at them. They grinned—*Sí, sí, Señor*—and grilled me a slab of beef.

Tyle says, "So, where are you from?"

"Bay Area, California."

"No. Where are you from? Originally."

I have always hated this question and resent him for asking. I hide my distaste because it is un-American. Perhaps I will lie. I often do when someone corners me. Sometimes, my prepared invention slips out before I realize it: I'm Japanese–Korean–Chinese–mixed-race Asian. No, sir, can't speak any language but good old American English.

This time, I turn the question: "Where do you think?"

"Korea."

Something about him makes me dance around the truth. I chuckle, painfully aware that "I'm an American" carries little weight with him. It no doubt resonates truer in his voice.

The blond giant holds me with his green eyes, making me feel small, crooked. So I reply, "We *nips* all look alike."

But it isn't enough. He looks the question at me again, and, by a darkness on his face, I know I owe him.

"I'm from Vietnam."

A flinch in the corner of his eye. He grunts, a sound deep from his diaphragm. Verdict passed. He turns his back to me and heaves into the cactus forest.

I stand, a trespasser in his camp, hearing echoes—Chink, gook, Jap, Charlie, GO HOME, SLANT-EYES!—words that, I believe, must have razored my sister Chi down dark alleys, hounded her in the cold after she had fled home, a sixteen-year-old runaway, an illegal alien without her green card. What vicious clicking sounds did they make in her Vietnamese ears, wholly new to English? And, within their boundaries, which America did she find?

A man once revealed something which disturbed me too much to be discounted. He said, "Your sister died because she became too American."

Later in the night, from the thick of the brush, Tyle ghosts into the orange light of my campfire. He nods at me and folds himself cross-legged before the popping flames, uncorks a fresh tequila bottle, takes a swig, and hands it to me. We sit on the ground far apart enough that with outstretched arms we still have to lean to relay the bottle.

I grip the warm sand between my tocs and loll the tart tequila on my tongue. A bottom-heavy moon teeters on the treetops. Stars balm the night. We seem content in our unspoken truce.

When the bottle is half empty, Tyle begins to talk. At first, he talks about the soothing solitude of the Mexican desert. Life is simple here, food cheap, liquor plentiful. He earns most of his money from selling his handicrafts—bracelets, woven bands, beads, leather trinkets—to tourists. When times are tough, there are always a few Mexicans who will hire him for English lessons or translations. And the border isn't too far if he needs to work up a large chunk of cash. Between the mundane details, his real life comes out obliquely. Tyle has a wife and two boys. He has been away from them nine years. I am the first Vietnamese he has seen since he fled to Mexico seven years ago.

When four fingers of tequila slosh at the bottom of the bottle, he asks me, "Have you been back to Vietnam?"

"No. But someday I'll go back . . . *to visit.*"

Many Vietnamese Americans "have been back." For some of us, by returning as tourists we prove to ourselves that we are no longer Vietnamese but Vietnamese Americans. We return, with our hearts in our throats, to taunt the Communist regime, to show through our material success that we, the once pitiful exiles, are now the victors. No longer the poverty-stricken refugees clinging to fishing boats, spilling out of cargo planes onto American soil, a mess of open-mouthed terror, wide-eyed awe, hungry and howling for salvation. Time has veiled the days when America fished us out of the ocean like drowning cockroaches and fed us and clothed us—we, the onus of their tragedy. We return and, in our personal silence, we gloat at our conquerors, who now seem like obnoxious monkeys cheating over baubles, our baggage, which mean little to us. Mostly, we return because we are lost.

Tyle says, "I was in Nam."

I have guessed as much. Not knowing what to say, I nod. Vets—acquaintances and strangers—have said variations of this to me since I was a kid and didn't know what or where Nam was. The contraction was lost on a boy struggling to learn English. But the note, the way these men said it, told me it was important, someplace I ought to know. With the years, this statement took on new meanings, each flavored by the tone of the speaker. There was bitterness, and there was bewilderment. There was loss and rage and every shade of emotion in between. I heard declarations, accusations, boasts, demands, obligations, challenges, and curses in the four words: *I was in Nam*. No matter how they said it, an ache welled up in me until an urge to make some sort of reparation slicked my palms with sweat. Some gesture of conciliation. Remorse. A word of apology.

He must have seen me wince for he says it again, more gently.

At that, I do something I've never done before. I bow to him like a respected colleague. It is a bow of acknowledgment, a bow of humility, the only way I can tell him I know of his loss, his sufferings.

Looking into the fire, he says softly, "Forgive me. Forgive me for what I have done to your people."

The night buckles around me. "What, Tyle?"

"I'm sorry, man. I'm really sorry," he whispers. The blond giant begins to cry, a tired, sobless weeping, tears falling away untouched.

My mouth forms the words, but I cannot utter them. No. No, Tyle. How can I forgive you? What have you done to my people? But who are my people? I don't know them. Are you my people? How can you be my people? All my life, I've looked at you sideways, wondering if you were wondering if my brothers had killed your brothers in the war that made no sense except for the one act of sowing me here—my gain—in your bed, this strange rich-poor, generous-cruel land. I move through your world, a careful visitor, respectful and mindful, hoping for but not believing in the day when I become native. I am the rootless one, yet still the beneficiary of all of your and all of their sufferings. Then why, of us two, am I the savior, and you the sinner?

"Please forgive me."

I deny him with my silence.

His Viking face mashes up, twisting like a child's just before the first bawl. It doesn't come. Instead words cascade out, disjointed sentences, sputtering incoherence that at the initial rush sound like a drunk's ravings. Nameless faces. Places. Killings. He bleeds it out, airs it into the flames, pours it on me. And all I can do is gasp *Oh, God* at him over and over, knowing I will carry his secrets all my days.

He asks my pardon yet again, his open hand outstretched to me. This time the quiet turns and I give him the absolution that is not mine to give. And, in my fraudulence, I know I have embarked on something greater than myself.

"When you go to Vietnam," he says, stating it as a fact, "tell them about me. Tell them about my life, the way I'm living. Tell them about the family I've lost. Tell them I'm sorry."

I give Tyle the most honored gift, the singular gift we Vietnamese give best, the gift into which one can cast all one's sorrow like trash into an abyss, only sometimes the abyss lies inside the giver. I give him silence.

Catfish - Dawn

2 I am a Vietnamese-American man. In my work boots, I am of average height, of medium build, and not too ghastly of face. I like going to the movies and reading novels in cafés. If I had to choose one cuisine to eat for the rest of my life, I'd take Italian without hesitation, though I do harbor secret cravings for hickory-smoked baby-back ribs and New Orleans gumbo. And I like buying cookbooks more than cooking. I enjoy tennis, basketball, baseball, football, and, lately, yes, hockey—from the bleachers or in my La-Z-Boy. My choice daily wear is a pair of five-year-old Levi's and a mock turtleneck (I have a drawerful, all the same size, same brand, different colors). I don't wear yellow, red, orange, or anything bright: they complicate the laundry process. No G-string underwear. Socks, plain white or black only.

My family arrived in America on September 17, 1977. I was ten. Of the Vietnam War I knew little, recalling only vignettes and images. Too young to know about its politics until I was about to enter American middle school. Fifth grade, Mr. Jenkin's class, I raised my voice against a teacher for the first time. Eighteen months in America, that much English learned. He was lecturing on the history of the Vietnam War. Something he said must have set me off because I shouted at him, summoning forth adults' drunken words I'd picked up eavesdropping: America left Vietnam. America not finish war. One more day bombing, Viet Cong die. One more day! No. America go home! America chicken! Mr. Jenkin colored, a tomato-flush rising from his buttoned collar to his feathery blond hair. I could tell he wanted to strike me, but I knew they didn't do that in America so I didn't say I was sorry. Chopping the air with his hand, he screamed, No! No! Wrong! And five minutes of English I couldn't understand.

Much later, I realized with some guilt that perhaps his brother had died in the War, and if it had gone on, he might have lost another. I wish I could tell him now that what I really meant was that my father was in prison because of the War. I was shouting about our imprisonment, about the dark wet cells, the whippings, the shootings, the biting rats, and the fists of dirty rice we ate. These things I remember unfogged by the intervening years. Somehow terribly vivid, irreducible.

I was there. After Saigon fell on April 30, 1975, our family fled deeper south, hoping to find a boat that would take us to Thailand. Outside of Rach Gia, a port city, the Viet Cong had set up a road barricade and caught us along with some three hundred people heading toward the coast to flee the country. Women and children were locked, fifty to a room, in a wing separate from the men. We took turns sleeping on wet concrete, side by side. After a month, the women and children were released with permission to go home. The men were either executed or trucked off to the jungle to work.

My mother and I regularly visited my father at the Minh Luong Prison and Labor Camp. We lodged with peasant families and stayed for weeks near the compound so she could watch him working in the field under guard. Hiding behind bushes, I watched him whenever I could find him. Like her, I felt that if I kept my eyes on him, stayed vigilant enough, bad things wouldn't happen. Some nights, she lay awake until dawn after hearing gunshots snap in the nearby woods, where they executed prisoners.

Two decades have thundered by since his imprisonment. Although we rarely talk beyond the safe grounds of current events, education, investment, and work, he has frequently shared his tales about the Viet Cong reeducation camp with me. The adventure stories he had told me as a boy on his knee were replaced by his death-camp saga. I believe it had something to do with my being his first son, with my having been there at the prison watching over him, witnessing what he thought were his death rites. In the years of telling, they became almost as much my stories as his. And this was strange, since my father and I have never shared much, never done father-and-son things, no camping trips, no fishing excursions; no ball games, no hot dogs in the park; no beers and Super Bowl on the tube. Still, the stories passed back and forth between us even when I had grown and moved away. My father, Pham Van Thong, was bequeathing his rarest pearls of wisdom, imparting a sense of value for life.

Of his last days in the death camp, Thong remembers the silence most. It was a thick creature that sat on his chest and lodged its fists in his throat. In the Viet Cong prison hut, he heard only his heart. Above, an indigo sky spilled light into the room, dyeing the gaunt faces of his fellows squatting on the dirt floor, fifty-four prisoners waiting for the execution call.

It came twice every week over the loudspeakers. Sometimes days passed between the calls, sometimes the calls came back-to-back.

Every evening just after they had scraped the last of the rice and the broth from their tins, silence fell as crickets wooed the coming night. The hut stank with fear and the food in their belly soured. Always, someone vomited.

He waded through his swamp of emotions. As the end neared when the indigo was deepest, two feelings remained. Sorrow for his wife, his children. Regret for a thousand things not done, a thousand things not said, a thousand things taken for granted.

His best friend in prison, Tuan, a helicopter pilot, edged close to him. Sitting on his hams, Tuan leaned over and whispered in his ear, "Thong, promise me."

He squeezed Tuan's shoulder. It was December 17, 1975. If they called his name tonight, Tuan would die and his promise would be worthless. Tuan believed the VC would release Thong in a few years. He would carry Tuan's last words to his wife and son. Thong didn't tell Tuan he believed that death was the only way out of Minh Luong Prison.

"Promise me!"

"Tuan . . ."

"You'll get out soon. Your wife's uncle is a VC colonel—a war hero."

"The bribes didn't work, Tuan. We're broke. Anh borrowed and sold everything we owned."

"No, she'll find a way. Anh is smart." Tuan had never met her.

The gloom obscured his friend's face, but Thong could pick out the hollow cheeks and the wild vacant eyes. Before Vietnam fell, Tuan was a handsome young officer with all the promise of a good military career. He was only twenty-eight. He was married to his high school sweetheart and they had a son. On nights when it was very cold and the prisoners huddled together for warmth, he would speak of her, the way she moved and intimate things. Things not meant for the ears of others, but in this place it was all he had. All that kept him going.

Tuan's quivering voice was rife with self-reproach. "I shouldn't have confessed that I was a pilot. I was scared. When they said the penalty for lying on the confession essay was execution, I lost my mind. I wrote down everything. I confessed everything. Everything I could remember."

Thong didn't.

"Thanh said I was honest. That's why she loves me. I shouldn't have written about my service in the air force."

He wanted to tell Tuan they wouldn't call tonight, wouldn't come for him, wouldn't punish him. But he didn't. It would have been a lie. He wanted to hear Tuan's voice because it might be the last time they talked. A dying man had the right to talk, Thong said, and they were all dying. If the executioner didn't kill them tonight, jungle diseases would kill them soon enough. Then there were the minefields, the hundreds of land mines they were forced to unearth and defuse with shovels. Death always came round, one way or another.

"You'll be all right," Tuan said, reassuring his friend even through his fear. "You're just a teacher. They don't punish teachers."

Tuan didn't know his secret. No one in the prison did.

"They'll let you go soon. You only violated martial law."

Tuan murmured himself to silence. There were nervous movements in the hut. Someone in the far corner retched. The loudspeakers crackled and screeched to life, whipping a charge of adrenaline through the room.

"Bastards!" someone hissed in the dark. "Why at night? Why do they only call at night?"

Silence answered him.

"If they are going to kill me, I want to die in the sun," the man said, his voice rising on a false note of courage. "Why do they only come at night?"

A voice replied from across the darkness. "They are afraid of what they do. It is easier to kill in the dark."

Someone else said, "No laws, no reasons, no mercy."

"It is the way of the Viet Cong. I know them," an old voice said. It was Khuong, the fisherman. He was in his sixties. He had given fifteen years to the Nationalist Army.

The first man shouted out the window, "Cowards!"

"Shut up!" a new voice trilled.

"Yes, shut up. It'll go hard for us if you don't."

The murmurs of consent angered the first speaker. His voice, tinged with fear, became a shout. "You're all cowards. You wait like chickens—they kill you like chickens. When they kill me, I'm not going to kneel. No shooting in the back of the head. I'll look at the eyes of the man who pulls the trigger."

Khuong replied, "You won't. It is dark. The night hides everything."

The loudspeakers blared. "Stand outside your hut when your name is called." Without preamble it rattled off names like a shopping list. "Nguyen Van Tung, Do Nhan Anh, Tran Truc Dang . . ."

A wail pierced the hut. A man across the room convulsed on the ground. The loudspeakers boomed, "Vo Ba Sang." Oh, God. Not the auto mechanic.

"Le Tin Khuong." The village fisherman. "Dinh Yen Than." The pig farmer. "Vu Tan Khai." The town storekeeper. They were killing all the locals linked to the Nationalists. People were turning in their own neighbors.

Thong stared at his friend. Tuan's family had lived in this province for generations. They both heard it: "Phuoc Tri Tuan."

Then it was over: thirteen names, six from their hut. Tuan retched on his mat and curled up in it shaking. Thong held him. Sang, the mechanic, took his place at the door, seemingly at peace with his lot.

The guards came in with oil lamps. Thong saw the fear, the ugly fear of the spared, and knew his face mirrored it. He saw the terror of the condemned and the way the tallowy light danced wicked shadows on their twisted features. The VC took the fisherman, the farmer, the storekeeper, and another man.

They dragged Tuan away by his ankles. He did not resist and he did not speak. Tuan gave Thong no final look and no parting words. It was so quick and simple how the VC had taken him and plunged them back into darkness.

Thong sat on his mat in a vile mixture of grief and relief. He had learned to block out the VC's "trials" broadcast over the loudspeakers. They invariably followed the same script: an account of offenses against the country, a conviction, and a death sentence—never a defense or a last rite. Occasionally, a few men were not tried. Tuan was the fourth one tried and his crimes were the same as those before and after him.

A long, long silence followed. Then eleven sharp pistol reports, distance-softened. It was over. They never knew what happened to the remaining two men.

Thong woke three hours before dawn. He heard some other early risers moving in the dark and hurried to be the first out of the hut. The smart ones woke early to use the latrine before the morning rush. Not all could go before the guards came to take them out to work.

The bloat-bellied moon sagged low on the horizon and silhouetted the guard tower just beyond the barbed-wire fence. The night sounds of the jungle hummed and the earth was cold and rough beneath his bare feet. Outside the compound, the sentries shadowed the perimeter on their watch, ignoring him.

The latrine was a wooden structure overhanging the edge of a shallow pond inside the prison fence. He snagged handfuls of grass and climbed up the five-stepped ladder. The latrine reminded him of a hangman's platform, the kind in the American Western movies his wife was so fond of. Only this one did not have a hanging post and in place of the trap door was a circular hole situated over the water. The surface beneath the latrine began to churn, roiling with catfish. He squatted over the opening and proceeded. The catfish fought wildly for their meal, leaping out of the water. He shifted to avoid the splashes. And so it went—the fish leaping and him shifting—until the business was concluded and the soiled grass discarded.

As he made his way back to the hut, others strayed out one by one to the pond. The clouds had swallowed the stars on the horizon. He crawled back to his bed and, before he remembered, he moved to huddle against Tuan for warmth. Tuan's straw mat was still there, reeking of the sourness of vomit and the cloying sweetness of urine.

Thong curled up and wound himself tightly in his blanket and Tuan's. The wind snaked through the thatched wall and ran cold tendrils over his scalp. He rolled onto his other side and bumped against Danh, a prison mate who lay perfectly still. Danh could have been dead. Thong could not tell and he did not wake him. If Danh were dead or dying, there was nothing Thong could do and nothing the VC would do besides tossing Danh into the mass grave in the woods and covering him with a thin layer of dirt.

Thong often daydreamed of the time before his world became undone. His Saigon in April of 1975 was another life. A good life that he didn't think could end even in the final days. He was a teacher, three years retired from the military. His wife, Anh, was a tailor in her own shop with three workers. They had made their fortune before the Americans pulled out in 1972 and they had to shut down their business. Comfortably well-off, they continued to work because it was in their nature. They lived in a three-story house and had five children, one girl, four boys. A shining member of Vietnam's tiny middle class.

It had been very different at the beginning. His family were impoverished refugees, fleeing south in 1946 when the Viet Minh took over North Vietnam. Hers were Southerners scratching out a living amid civil unrest. They married without the blessings of either family. Under a leaky roof, they scraped, worked hard, and saved prodigiously. Somehow, they got by on love and rice. Then came the *thing*—the *thing* that catapulted them out of poverty—that which he would forever keep behind doors closed to his children.

When the army drafted him, they gave him an officer's commission because he was a college graduate at a time when South Vietnam's annual crop of college graduates was fifty. His fluency in French and English yielded a translator post. In 1967, his education landed him the office of Assistant Chief of Phan Thiet Province, a coastal city-state of central Vietnam. It was a paramilitary post that dealt in psychological warfare. He was only a lieutenant, but under his proctorship were two thousand men. They wrote literature, broadcast Nationalist ideology, pro-American sentiments, and anti–Viet Cong messages. They accused, ridiculed, blamed, and generally vilified the Viet Cong, their actions, their theories, and everything they stood for. His men patrolled the countryside and played Good Samaritans, lending the peasants a hand to win their favor, their loyalty.

They swayed the peasants who did not care which side won the war because they were so hungry and poor. It was difficult for simple farmers and fisherfolk to understand how one regime could be worse than another. They paid the poor to spy on the VC movement in the countryside. They kept many from openly joining the VC. They found men to replenish the South Army.

The VC hated propagandists more than they hated the American GIs. They hated propagandists more than they hated the Nationalist Army. More than the Nationalist Air Force. And Thong was the director.

"Get up!" cried the guard from the doorway. It was Hong, the local hoodlum turned VC. He was seventeen, mean as a fighting cock, taut as a bamboo switch. He leaned on the door frame and sucked a cigarette, the tip flaring an evil eye in the half light. "Fuck! Fuckin' lout!" He kicked the closest man, who was old enough to be his father.

They filed out of the hut into the ashen dawn, and marched across the compound, going down the row of barracks, five corrugated steel buildings wallowing in mud and overgrown grass, the sidings riddled with bullet holes and bleeding rust, the glass windows cracked and furred with dust. They slowed as they came upon the VC mess hall, where the air was fat with aromas of coffee and fried eggs. They marched out of the garrison and onto the dirt road that cut through the rice paddies to the jungle beyond. They left the road at the edge of the jungle and began to work beside it, clearing undergrowth and cutting down trees to prepare the land for farming. The trees and grass were burned in a great bonfire. Black smoke curled skyward. The sky turned a steel-gray and the sun baked the air through the clouds.

Midmorning, rain came down heavily. Warm tears slapped the broad green leaves of the jungle canopy and killed the bonfire. They pounded Thong's back and they pounded the brown earth on the road. The water gushed down, steady and thick, from a gray sky. The dirt road that bandaged the jungle to the rice paddies—but parted both—was reduced to an endless series of large gray-brown puddles: grayed by the sky, browned by the rich soil. There was no wind, no peals of thunder, no ruptured flashes of lightning, no crackling gunshots in the distance, no muffled booms of artillery fire from the horizon. It was just another rain like those of his youth.

He looked to the road where the rice paddies met the forest. A boy in faded black shorts stood, feet apart, in a fighting stance, ankle-deep in a puddle. Tanned skin a shade lighter than the soil molded around his slim muscles, defining the thinness of his body. One raised arm held a long bamboo stick like a javelin with the sharpened end canted at an angle to the ground. Water plastered straight black hair against his sharp face, young but all edges without a hint of softness. Slanted black eyes riveted on the ground blinking away the water streaming down his face. He stood frozen. At his feet, the rain pockmarked the puddle like pebbles.

A flash of motion, the bamboo stick speared into the water. He thrust his face at the torrential sky and barked a cry of victory. An impaled frog jerked its death throes on the spear tip. He taunted the sky with his prize before stashing it in the burlap pouch at his waist. Thong felt a brief rush of joy, a touch of pride at the boy's success, remembering the simple pleasures of his youth, remembering his first son.

The boy looked at Thong looking at him, then turned away and left the road in long, limber, barefoot strides, heading toward the rice paddies. The curtain of rain closed over the boy and all was silent save sky-water drumming the earth and old men hacking the jungle.

A revolution—everything shifted and nothing changed. Thong flailed at the weeds, a boy speared frogs barefoot in the rain.

When the rain stopped, they ate lunch, two fists of rice in a tin of vegetable broth. Because the cut trees were drenched and would not burn, they were marched back to the garrison to clear land mines.

The prison had been a Nationalist garrison during the war, a country outpost far behind the fighting front. It was deep in South Vietnam, but it was viciously fortified. A hundred yards of no-man's-land ringed the garrison, thoroughly infested with land mines, studded with claymore mine posts, laced with miles of barbed wire, and scarred with concentric trenches, all cloaked in thick grass, vines, and small brush.

Given shovels which they dared not use, the prisoners began from the sandbagged walls and worked their way outward. They had already cleared the mines and trimmed the vegetation of the first twenty yards, but everyone still treaded lightly to the outer markers. The VC waited behind the walls with their guns trained on the prison crew. No one spoke save the VC, who wagered on the outcome of today's session.

Thong was to clear a straight path for the log team. He hunched down low and began parting the grass one cluster at a time, searching for the black trigger rods of the canister and ball mines. He probed the ground with his fingers, praying to the gods he didn't believe existed that there were no pan mines in his path. These were completely buried and nearly impossible to find without metal detectors. The soft earth played tricks on his mind, giving under his knees.

He found two canister mines and marked two parallel paths, fifteen yards apart, with ropes. It was the loggers' turn. Everyone else took cover.

Six men pulled on two ropes tied to opposite ends of a log. The team divided and walked on the parallel paths, dragging the log on the ground between them. Eyes quivering on the edge of hysteria, the loggers trembled, looking like overworked nags strung out by the scent of slaughterhouse blood. One young man in his early twenties cried as he put his back to the task.

Thong lay flat on the ground, shielding his head, listening. The log rustled the grass. Loggers traded nervous words. An explosion rent the air.

Screams. A man clutched a raw gash in his thigh. Blood spewed out, reminding Thong of a butchered pig—making him hungry. Dirt and wood splinters filtered down. A bitter piquancy of gunpowder. Another man sat on the ground, childlike surprise on his face, holding his red squirting wrist, hand blown off.

The VC replaced them with two others and a new log. The work went on until sunset.

Back in the compound, the murky pond captured the clouds fleeing from a crimson waning of light. Prisoners bathed and washed their clothes at the far end of the shimmering water, across from the latrine.

Dinner was rice and catfish soup. They fed the catfish at dawn and ate them at dusk. Then the indigo light fell and silence crept in.

The loudspeakers crackled to life. A smothering stillness glassed them off from the world.

"Stand outside your hut when your name is called. Pham Van Thong . . ."

They came with their oil lamps and dragged Thong out into the dark.

The next day, Thong climbed off the back of an army truck at an unmarked crossroads. The truck spat blue exhaust at him and rumbled back on the dirt track. He stood barefoot and penniless under the blazing sky, looking down the forked roads before him.

Fallen-Leaves

Winter of 1961 in Phan Thiet, Vietnam, came in wet and cold, a damp cloth over the fisherfolk's heads, mildew in their lungs. Along that scraped-up seacoast, ill winds scoured villages like bold ravens, reaching through thatched walls and clawing around crevices with impunity, pilfering the souls of the weak and the unsuspecting.

Thong and Anh lived in a one-room shack, nailed together in a back alley of the fishing town. They were young, in love, and strong, but their hands were like old people's, seasonally water-crinkled from mopping the concrete floor and tending the leaky roof. A baby girl, their first child, slept peacefully in her crib—a cardboard box on their bed. They were cheerful about their meager lot, joking that the heavens were so generous to their rainwater cisterns, they hadn't had to visit the village well in a month.

They were vulnerable, though they did not know it. Their happiness was an unshielded beacon. Those who eloped did not have the protection of their dead ancestors.

One gray day, an ill wind slipped through their curtain-door and wrapped its wings around their first child. The baby girl took sick and became as red as chili-pickled cabbage, then as pale as ivory. She was feverish, then cold. They rubbed her with heat-oil, but the heat did not come back into her tiny chest, which was hardly bigger than a loaf of bread. No money for medicine. No silver coin to scrape the ill wind from their baby girl. They fretted and they summoned the midwife, but she could do little. No money for Western doctor, Western medicine. The baby coughed. She cried, would not suckle her milk. Another morning, she was cold. Died during the night, not yet a year old.

Clan - Rift

Four months ago, I emerged from Mexico and returned to the Bay Area, jobless and homeless. I did something unthinkable in America: I moved home to my parents. It was the perfect Vietnamese thing to do, fall back into the folds of the clan. Free food, free shelter while you lick your wounds and plot your resurrection. My non-Asian friends pitied me. My Vietnamese-American friends wondered why I hadn't lived at home in the first place; a good son doesn't leave home until he is married.

It doesn't matter to me. I have to accumulate funds and settle my affairs. I tie up loose ends, freelance all sorts of work for the extra cash, do it all in silence, the whole time wondering if the flash of desert inspiration was only a fluke. No one, not my brothers or my best friends, knows about my plan to bicycle to Vietnam. They say, Andrew is finding himself. He's trying to get his life in order. He's still getting over Trieu. She really devastated him, cheating on him and leaving him like that. When I finally tell them, I lie. Going up the coast, I say. Just going to ride my bicycle up toward Seattle, maybe British Columbia. It's safe. Once-in-a-lifetime thing. It'll do me good. I don't tell them I might not be coming back.

On the dawn of my departure from San Jose, California, I wake groggy from a night of tossing in wistfulness. I fetal beneath my blanket, a jumble of nerves, high with adrenaline, sick with uncertainties, knotted with fear. I could be camping on the road already if it weren't for my mother.

"BAD! Bad day to go on a trip!" she pecked at me day before yesterday, flapping her Chinese calendar in my face, chasing me from the bathroom to the kitchen.

"Look, Mom, I don't believe in your Chinese calendar," I told her delicately.

She made angry egg-eyes, scolding me in front of the family altar atop the refrigerator, her favorite place to win arguments. "I know these things. I picked our escape date from Vietnam, didn't I?" She regularly pulled proof of her sixth sense. How she had seen a ghost in her dream and begged it not to take the soul of her youngest son, who was deathly ill. How she had predicted which job my father would land. How she had fathomed the good spirits residing in each house they had ever rented or bought. She knew she could spook me.

I caved in. "Yes, Mom. You're right, Mom."

"Good. Because if you go this day, you will get hurt. Many omens. You wait two more days, the chart is okay, suitable for a Horse-sign like you. Next week is even better."

"I'll wait two days."

"Next week better."

"Two days."

"No patience, that's you."

Patience I have aplenty. Courage is what I need. If I don't leave now, I never will. In the face of parental opposition, my determination wanes by the day.

My father has said "Good" to me twice in my life. This time is not one of them. The first "Good" was for making Phi Beta Kappa during my senior year in Aerospace Engineering at UCLA. I showed him the glowing congratulatory letter from the national honor society, then threw it away, too poor to afford the initiation banquet and too proud to request a fee waiver.

He awarded me the second "Good" for landing a cushy engineering post at a major airline. That job was doomed from the start. I graduated out of college and right into a recession. Desperately hungry for work after mailing out a hundred résumés, I hooked one interview. During the office tour, my would-be boss, a turtle-chinned, red-faced thirty-five-year-old-timer, Paul, waxed on about the company's expansion overseas and his getting an M.B.A. in international business to keep abreast of it all.

"I like you," Paul said, walking round behind me and putting a hand on my shoulder, which I didn't like. "I like you people. Orientals are good workers. Good students, too. Great in math, the engineering stuff." He smiled at me, reassuring, beaming. "Oh, I think you'll do just fine here. We won't have any trouble at all."

When I finally resigned, I was no longer a "good Oriental." I even left behind in my desk three files titled "Stuff Paul Rejected Because He Doesn't Know Any Better," "Stuff Paul Rejected Because He Didn't Want to Jeopardize His Promotion," and "Stuff Paul Rejected Because They Didn't Originate from Engineers but from Mechanics Who Have More Practical Experience on the Subject." I heard later that the files were discovered. Eventually, after a few more escapades with the mechanics, supervisor-bossman Paul was moved "laterally" into a cubicle labeled "independent contributor" on the third floor, where they put troublemakers out to pasture.

Giving up this job and burning my bridges, my father believed, were the undoing of me, and nothing I had done since elicited a "Good" from him. "You don't do that. You do job best you can. You get promotion. You get new job. You say, 'Thank you very much, sir' and you go. Think about future. You are Asian man in America. All your bosses will be white. Learn to work."

Yes, Father. Okay, Father. I will, Father.

I can't be his Vietnamese American. I see their groveling humility, concessions given before quarters are asked. I hate their slitty-measuring eyes. The quick gestures of humor, bobbing of heads, forever congenial, eager to please. Yet I know I am as vulnerable as they before the big-boned, fair-skinned white Americans. The cream-colored giants who make them and me look tribal, diminutive, dark, wanting.

So, what the hell, I have to do something unethnic. I have to go. Make my pilgrimage. I roll out of bed and pull on my cycling shorts, T-shirt, and windbreaker. I throw my panniers into the trunk of the car and mount the bike on the rack. Kay, my sister, the youngest in the family and the only one born on American soil, watches me as I gather up my few worldly possessions.

"You're not going to be using your car," she points out, smiling mischievously.

"You can borrow my car."

A high school junior, she is the youngest and prettiest of our clan. Her skin glows like a pale rose and her eyes shine with an unlikely hazel. She was born in Shreveport, Louisiana, a month after our arrival in the States. When the nurse handed her to my parents, they insisted that she had made a mistake. This child wasn't theirs. Why, it looked like an American baby! The nurse showed them the only other baby born that day: an African-American child.

Kay grew up to look just like the rest of us, her father's face and her mother's nose. She is a Pham with the exception of her leggy height, brownish hair, light whitish-pink skin, and strange hazel eyes. Her gift is her flawless English, a smooth, clean California-American, middle-class burb. Our English, even Hien's, is only an imperfect prototype. My parents think it has something to do with her having been born on American soil. "American food, American air," said my mother.

Kay is the final hope of our dysfunctional Vietnamese-American family. I have found myself casually examining her for the wounds we have inadvertently inflicted. *It is your responsibility,* Father always says to us, *to set a good example for your younger siblings.* I abandoned my career in favor of a dream. Tien, an exceptional student, couldn't make up his mind about the trajectory of his education. Huy and Hien are gay. And not one of us breathed a word of Chi's existence to Kay in all these years. She never knew she had a runaway sister. To Kay, Chi came home in a shroud of mystery and died a self-inflicted death within arm's reach of her family, who should have seen it coming—should have prevented it with love.

"An, are you going to be gone long? Can I move into your room?"

"Sure, go ahead."

She is referring to the guest house I built in the backyard of my parents' house. Although I rarely use it, my mother insists that it remain untouched. The same applies to the rooms belonging to Hien, who is down in San Diego pursuing a bio-engineering degree and medical school, and Huy, who holes up in Berkeley slaving for his law degree. Neither comes home much, each trying to hide his homosexuality from our parents. Empty rooms are Mom's way of keeping us home.

Mom comes from the old world, where mothers are lifelong housewives who expect to be near their children all their lives. Senior homes, retirement communities don't exist in their vocabulary. When her friends explained the concepts of children leaving home at eighteen and parents going into rest homes in their "golden years," Mom's eyes went wide with disbelief. *That is so cruel. Strange, strange country.*

The last few years, I think my father, who is more culturally savvy, has been talking to her because she has started saying things to us in Vietnamese like *"We'll be all right when we retire. Your father is working a few more years so we'll be financially secure. We're in America; if we live with you, no girl will marry you. And no girl will let you support us. We know it's different here."*

She tries so hard I ache for her, this simple woman who takes pleasure nickeling the grocers for bargains, deals for the family. This woman who lets in every Mormon that comes by the house with pamphlets. This woman who makes egg rolls for cosmetic girls at the department store who give her free makeovers. This woman who eats cold leftovers standing in the kitchen alone because lunch in her American household is too lonely. This woman whom we've shortchanged.

Tien comes out and helps me with the bike. "Mister An," he says, using the funny form of address we picked up as immigrant kids who didn't know that Mister was followed by a last and not a first name. "Are you ready?"

"Mister Tien. That's it. Let's go."

Mom steps down from the porch to say good-bye. She places her hand on my arm and I on hers so that we're both touching each other's forearm. Between telling me to be careful and asking me if I'd like her to pack some fried rice to go, she squeezes the back of my arm. Some oranges, then? She touches my hand. It is awkward, for we have never learned to embrace and we don't throw our arms around each other so easily. But I like the way her fingers dance on my arms fluttering over my shoulders, touching my back. Saying all that she cannot in words.

I want to hug Kay, but I can't. Don't know how. So I smile and say, "Bye, Kay. Have a good time. Take care of yourself."

"You too. Bye, An." She waves that teenage wave, elbow at her side, hesitant fingers rising to chest sketching tiny arcs.

Mom hugs me then. Clumsy, quick.

I feel sick and hot around the eyes.

Father went to work earlier, I heard him leave. He didn't say much about my trip, but last week, I caught him peeking at me through the living room window as I tinkered with my bicycle. To him, this trip and the last one to Mexico are a waste of time. He has plenty to say about it, but he hasn't. He has given me his gift of silence, knowing that at least I am free to construe my own truths about his feelings. It's generous.

He started being generous with me when I told him I wasn't following in his footsteps, no longer a man of the mind, a first-rate engineer. I started freelancing as a technical writer and editor. After I had published a few articles, people sought me out for various assignments, some small, some large. Just enough to keep food on the table. I decided to pursue a career as a freelance writer. Do the American thing, chase your dream, follow your heart. I showed him some of my best published works.

My father said, *Oh, you're just a freelancer.* I heard only the *just,* the diminishing qualifier. *Yes, I'm just a freelancer. Yeah, that's me.* Hitching words together, like boxcars making a train, for a quarter apiece. Sometimes more. I wrote anything. Pen for hire. Words for sale, words I don't own, someone else's birthright. Technical jargon. Differential calculus. Euclidean geometry in easy English. Love ballads. Naturalization applications. Obituaries. Résumés. Letters of recommendation. Business plans. Articles. Interviews. Book reviews. Your view. My view. Whatever you wanted, I wrote, a quarter a word, no byline required. But I wasn't a credentialed writer, so, in his eyes, I was forever the impostor, the slick fraud called in on midnight contracts and sent out on guerrilla forays. In and out and paid before anyone was the wiser.

Tien and I bucket up to San Francisco, winding on the long I-280 scenic route. I hand him the pink slip to my car with instructions to sell it in a few months. My finances are dismal. My account balance says I'll be traveling on a disintegrating shoestring budget even though I have liquidated nearly everything I own and canceled my health insurance. Aspirin and chicken soup will have to suffice from here on out.

I splurged on two bike racks with panniers and packed them with my old camping gear. My vehicle is a rickety 18-speed hybrid. I didn't know the first thing about bike touring and was lucky to survive the Mexican desert. I'd gone into it with a backpack and a bike, and wound up pushing the bike through sand as often as riding it. This time I am prepared. I have maps, touring gear, and a dime-store handbook on bicycle repair.

It appeals to me. Riding out my front door on a bicycle for the defining event of my life. It is so American, pioneering, courageous, romantic, self-indulgent. I'd read *Miles from Nowhere* by Barbara Savage, who had ridden her bike around the world with her husband, Larry. It is so simple. All I need I learned in grade school.

Tien wants to come with me, but he can't tear himself from his fil-ial obligations. Besides, I tell him, it is something I have to do by myself. Deep down, I believe he knows why I am leaving, the reasons I need to find before I can mend the mess that is my life. As the third son, Tien carries his parents' failed hopes for the family's first son, me. He is the only one in the family with whom I can talk about my sister Chi. Her death left a silent, dark hole in our family like an extinguished hearth no one could relight. We talk around her history, unknowingly lacing her secret and our shameful failures deeper into ourselves.

Tien parks us in the tourist lot at the San Francisco end of the Golden Gate Bridge. He snaps a few pictures of me leaning on my old bike and my brand-new, untested gear, the bridge looming in the backdrop. Then he hands me a bag of PowerBars, the very stuff I avoid religiously.

"Good luck," he says, and shakes my hand.

I mount my bike and pedal shakily across the bridge. It is the first time I've ridden the bike fully loaded.

Thin strokes of clouds score a sky as blue as a blessing. A brisk wind washes across the bridge. I wobble through the throngs of pedestrians and cyclists with a ready grin for everyone I pass. A lightheadedness buoys me as if ambrosia courses in my veins. I am intoxicated with a feeling of rightness, a psychological snapping together of mating parts, a lucid moment of geometrical perfection. A liberating bliss.

"Yes!" I shout over and over as I race away from San Francisco.

The euphoria lasts until I crank up the cliffs of Highway 1. I'm not a cyclist. The bike is heavy. My precious enthusiasm dissipates with every incline. My map shows an inland road meandering some way from the coast rejoining Highway 1 at Stinson Beach. Confident that it will spare me grueling coastal hills, I huff up the grade, too exhausted to venture a guess why this stretch of blacktop was named Panoramic Road. It steadily gets steeper without a sign of leveling out. I inch up the mountain, pulling over to breathe at every half mile.

At one turn, I look up and the peak of Mount Tam rears over me. *Good God, I have been climbing the road to the highest peak in the area on my first day! Stupid! Stupid!*

That evening, I squeak into Pan Toll State Campground drenched in sweat, shaking with fatigue. My knee bleeds from a fall I'd taken a couple of miles back, when the road was too steep and I couldn't uncleat my feet from the pedals fast enough. My odometer reaches 18.7 miles. That leaves, oh, about 4,000 miles to go . . . Whoopee . . . Great . . . Somewhere out there ahead of me are Portland, Seattle, Tokyo, Fuji, Kyoto, Saigon, and Hanoi.

Fallen-Leaves

Anh's aunt took pity on her and gave her two wedding presents, both heirloom secrets, mere words in the ear.

Anh put the first gift to work in her kitchen. With pennies for market scraps, she cooked small but tasty meals for her husband, who worked very hard. He was taking on a double teaching load at the high school and doing extra academic jobs on the side, working the elbows of his shirt and the knees of his pants as thin as rice paper. Despite Anh's savory food, he grew thin, and his gauntness and fierce determination made his students fear him, the rigid academic. Every day he woke to a breakfast of the previous night's leftovers. For lunch he ate cold rice balls Anh wrapped in leaves with shreds of dried meat. Although each morsel she served him was exquisitely flavored and he adored every dish she cooked, there simply wasn't enough rice to put meat on his bones, not with the way he was working.

She put the second gift to work in her washtubs, taking in her landlord's wash to reduce the rent. Then she took in her neighbors' laundry to bring in a little more money for groceries. She was young so she was strong. Many times each day, she carried water, ten gallons a haul, from the village well to her house, where she perched on a block of wood to do the wash. Using her aunt's homemaker secret, she scrubbed, stomped, pounded, wrung each piece of clothing until her fingers ached and her palms were raw. She hung the laundry in *her patch of alley-sun and kept a close watch for thieves. Then she pressed shirts and pants with a coal iron, folded and delivered them to their owners.*

Anh worked through spring, summer, fall, and winter. One more year passed, and she gave birth to another baby girl. And she continued to work, six days a week, year after year. People heard about her, the woman who could remove difficult stains from any shirt and iron such hard creases that they were as good as sewn into the pants. They sought her out and gave her the grime they could not banish and the pleats they could not set straight.

Coming home after each long day of work, Thong felt a squeezing tremble of love in his chest when he saw his wife hunched over great tubs of wash. He told her she was working too hard. She must think of the baby. Look at the way her great belly was practically dragging on the floor. No, no, she told him. The child was strong. Look at the way he clung so high in her ribs, surely this must be a boy, their first son.

They had buried two coffee cans full of money beneath their bed. Soon there would be another. And the country was changing with the War. Opportunity was in the air. Thong said the Nationalists had drafted him, but he stood a fair chance of rising in the bureaucratic ranks because of his education. Thong and Anh were happy. They talked of buying that little tavern way out in the countryside near the American army base.

Headwind-Tailspin

I remember Tien asking me if I thought someday I could take my own life as Chi had done. Could you do it, Andrew, if everyone you loved had forsaken you—no hope left, nothing to live for? Maybe, I told him, I don't know but I always think I have one last ticket, one last hand to gamble. What would you do then before you die? I'd walk out the door to destinations unknown, spending the sum of my breaths in one extravagant gesture.

Since the day Chi ran away, I have wondered how utterly alone she felt. I have wanted to run away the way she did. In the years it took me to become an American, I haven't been able to answer the one question that remained framed in my mind from the day she left: How did America treat Chi, one vulnerable yellow in a sea of white faces? At my age "running away" requires a measure of innocence I've lost. Riding out my front door with a pocketful of twenties is the best I can do.

Touring solo on a bicycle, I discover, is an act of stupidity or an act of divine belief. It is intense stretches of isolation punctuated with flashes of pure terror and indelible moments of friendship. Mostly, it is dirty work particularly suitable for the stubborn masochist. I was suckered into the adventure, the elegant simplicity of its execution, and, yes, even the glory of its agony.

Along the Pacific Coast, I meet cyclists who lick their chops at the challenge of a six-percent grade or an eighty-mile ride. I am a distracted rider, the sort that thrives on flat roads without wind. I haven't encountered a mountain I like—from the front side. The only mountains I like are the ones I've summited. And there are no mountains finer than the ones I'm coasting down. On the road, I find myself vacillating between elation and abject misery, my senses narrowed to the hundred yards immediately before me. Beyond this, I am solely concerned with my next meal and my next campsite.

I learn it all the hard way. From San Francisco, I curse my way up the California coast. Every fiber in my body balks against the strain of propelling two hundred pounds uphill mile after mile. The second day out, I keel over again, this time halfway up another mountain. My loaded bike topples like a wildebeest felled by one well-aimed bullet. I crawl out from under the bike and try to stand, but my legs give out. I roll onto my belly, my legs locked rigid—a pair of two-by-fours jackknifed by a stampede of charley horses. I bite my knuckles, tears welling in my eyes. High school kids in a red Jeep roar by, laughing. I begin to suspect the authors I'd read weren't entirely forthcoming about the physical ordeals of bicycle adventures. The next three days, I learn that saddle sore is a euphemism for self-inflicted torture. My crotch is raw. Hitting a pothole feels like jabbing hot coals into the seat of my pants. Every muscle groans and complains with each movement. My back aches. I am so stiff I can barely tie my shoelaces. What am I thinking? My Baja trip could hardly be called cycling: I had dragged that bike through the desert like a crucifix.

A woman I meet at a convenience store says the California wine country is beautiful, so I ride over the mountain to Sonoma Valley. I spend my second night camping illegally at a PG&E power plant. The third night I am at an abandoned train station, the fourth in one of Buena Vista's vineyards, the fifth at the Carmelite Monastery in Oakville. The grounds-keeping monk tells me that the monastery was originally a haunted estate: the owner had hung himself. Sleep on the road is fitful at best. I sleep with a knife under my pillow of dirty laundry and wake repeatedly at the sounds of broken twigs. One night when my tent collapses, I fight my way out, roaring, a drawn knife in hand, stalking my would-be attackers in my briefs. It is the wind tittering.

I work my way back out to the coast again, up through Mendocino, Fort Bragg, Leggett, the Avenue of Giants, Eureka, Crescent City, and right into Oregon, heading ever northward against head wind and prevailing wisdom. The mornings are chilly, the afternoons blistering hot, the evenings swamped with mosquitoes. The days seem filled with new friends and engaging meals with strangers. Thousands of bicyclists tour the Pacific Coast from Seattle to San Francisco every summer, so it isn't difficult for a soloist heading in the wrong direction to find a cheerful campfire nightly. The day my odometer registers 500 miles, just before coming into Eureka, I feel invincible. I've fixed plenty of flat tires, warped rims, loose brakes, and broken spokes. Somehow through the torment, I have developed a taste for bicycle touring. Every time I top a big mountain, I dismount and dance a little victory jig around the bike, not caring who might see me. The coast is gorgeous. I cannot swallow, breathe, soak it in fast enough. At least once a day, there is a moment of absolute perfection when my muscles sing with power, full of vigor, raw and very alive— the air sweet with grass and pine, the whirling chain and the humming tires but extensions of me.

I find myself on the outskirts of Corvallis, Oregon. I am on my way to Portland to visit Patty, a free-spirited traveler whom I'd met in Mexico. A few days earlier, I phoned Patty and she suggested I spend the night with Ronnie, a friend of hers in the area. Ronnie sees me coming from the window of her second-story apartment and starts braying, Hey! You! You're Patty's friend, aren't you? It's dark. I jump at the fusillade of words and look up at the gesticulating scarecrow haloed in the light spilling from her window.

As soon as I cross the threshold, Ronnie slams the door, barring it with her back and turning the full wattage of her green eyes on me. Glaring from beneath a blond Einstein-fuzz, she leans close and growls, "Patty told you, didn't she?"

"Uh, told me what?"

"About me."

"You're her friend."

"AAAAAAhahahahahahahahahaha!" Her shrill laugh ices my spine. I grin, hoping to get in on the punch line.

"What's so funny?"

"You know, I was in *there.*"

"There where?"

"There," she hisses, as though I am woefully dense. "Institutionalized! They put me in *there* for three years."

"Oh."

"Don't worry. I'm okay now."

I want to ask her how long ago that was, and how "okay" she is, but I've learned my lesson: Don't look a gift horse in the mouth. It might bite. I wish I had camped out on the sod farms. Hoping to provide her some positive reinforcement, I say, "I'm not worried. You look fine to me."

Ronnie radiates an angel's goodwill as she tours me through her home. After my shower I join Ronnie, who is making dinner in the six-by-six-foot kitchen. I try to help, but there isn't enough room for two people around the stove of her suburban hovel. She stirs me a cup of instant tea with tap water and sits me at the kitchen table, which at one time might have been a schoolroom desk.

Crazy Ronnie is into astrology, karma, chakras, energy lodes of the universe, and the wheel of time. She is "a minor goddess" sent to earth to even out the balance between the forces of light and the forces of darkness. I, on the other hand, she confirms, am "a technician—like a worker ant." I ask her if she is sure. She is. Not even a minor deputy god? Nope, she assures me, no such luck.

"You've been working very hard the last millennium," she explains patiently, "ever since you were put on earth, so on this cycle, you are done with work. You're out exploring the world, having a good time."

I agree that I am having a good time on my bike tour. Crazy Ronnie takes that as evidence of my grubby worker-ant status. Despite our celestial disparity, I think her vastly interesting. She gets very excited talking about the true nature of the universe, the Wyrm of the World, voids, angels, and other dimensions. She shrieks, she shouts. She bounces off walls, her arms pinwheeling, a chopping knife in hand.

She stops mid-rambling, turns, and points the blade at me. "Are you a vegetarian?"

Oh, dear. My mind zips to infinity and back. Duh. Truth? Lie? Can this minor goddess tell the difference? I blurt, "Yes! Yes, I am. But I'm not a very good one . . . I . . . I have my weak moments."

"Hmm." Her green orbs roam my face for duplicity. "Well," she grunts, "we all make mistakes now and then. But we gotta be strong. You gotta try harder."

"I will. I really will."

We chomp on a dinner of veggie-burgers and garden salad. I rabbit into the burnt faux-burger patty, banishing all thoughts of juicy red steaks. It would have been a decent night if she hadn't told me about the devil rascaling in her apartment. She found *him* endearing. As I wash the dishes, she roots violently around the apartment, banging drawers and kicking furniture out of her way until she finds a small wooden box. She opens it and pulls out a mishmash ball of twine, thread, and yarn, multicolored, a little psychedelic.

"*He* did this!" She puts the furry thing under my nose, expecting me to smell traces of the devil. "I save the threads and look what he did to them."

I don't sleep much that night. When I do, my dreams are variations of murder. Goddess Ronnie wielding a sword and coming after me, the lowly worker ant. Crazy Ronnie sacrificing me to her devil, tying me up in her ball of psychedelic twine. Vegetarian Ronnie slathering me with mustard and making a sandwich. In the morning, my mind is tangled with a hundred things Crazy Ronnie said. Some outright ludicrous, others oddly insightful. I know she probably told me something important but I don't know what. I am just jolly to leave her den in one piece.

The next day, a logging truck slows and pulls alongside me. "Hey, Jap!" a man in the passenger seat shouts. Still chugging onward, I look and fluid gushes out the cab's window and gets me full in the face. I have a sick sensation in the pit of my stomach. Urine? Soda? A paper cup follows the water. They laugh when it bounces off my helmet. The passenger sticks his head out the window and pushes up the corners of his eyes, making "Chinese eyes" at me. They roar off, hooting their horn, laughing, whooping: "Yeah! Right on the head!"

I stand on the side of the road, drenched. The water is no big deal. I've had plenty of trash and pennies thrown at me from cars. I usually console myself that it is just one downside of bicycle touring, and that some people throw trash because I am a bicyclist and not because of the slant of my eyes.

Ten miles down the road, I catch up to my antagonists at a truck stop. The empty rig is parked outside the bar. I stand in the parking lot, fuming for ten minutes. Part of me wants to go inside and confront the truckers. Part of me wants to slash their tires. I want to feel my fists smacking into their fleshy red faces. Giving them the full force of my righteous fury. Realizing how badly I want to hurt them, I am glad I don't have the gun my brother Huy and his boyfriend had offered to loan me.

Before I left, Huy and his Vietnamese-American lover, Sean, took me to Sean's San Francisco flat to give me safety advice. Even in gay-friendly San Francisco, they never ventured out without a canister of pepper spray, clipping it on their belts like a pager. Sean laid out his arsenal on the coffee table and told me I could have my pick: a stun gun, a semiautomatic 9mm, a snub-nosed .38 revolver, or a .45 Dirty Harry. I said I already had a canister of pepper spray, similar to the ones that mailmen carry. In Mexico, I'd given more than one rabid dog sneezing fits.

"You're crazy, man," Sean said, shaking his head. "Forget about it. You know how many rednecks there are between here and Seattle? You're Asian and who knows what sort of bigots you're going to come across. They might give you a beating for fun."

He truly believed it. For him, a gay Asian male, his America was outlined by the boundaries of San Francisco and Berkeley. He grew up in San Francisco and having Asian faces around him had become an integral part of life. Like most Vietnamese who have settled in the

Bay Area or in Orange County, California, he couldn't imagine living in the Midwest or the South, anywhere impoverished of Asian faces. No, to a minority, any white face could be a face of violence—a quiet fear we live with.

Once, when my brother Tien and I were driving through Arizona, a pickup drew alongside us. The scene played out as it had countless times before, the driver and his passenger gave us the one-finger salute: "Go home!"

This time, Tien replied, "To California?"

The day after the trucker incident, I roll into Portland to see Patty. My visit coincides with the birthday of one of her friends. Patty and I cross town to pick up the birthday girl, Pocahontas, a spunky eighty-three-year-old wit-hollering, wine-guzzling, cigar-smoking, poetry-spewing artist. She lives in one of those nasty slum apartments they dole out to seniors a couple of breaths shy of croaking. Except Pocahontas isn't a geezer by a long shot. As soon as we pull up curbside, Pocahontas descends from her seventh-floor digs in as many seconds.

A dozen souls of the fringe congregate in the flat Patty shares with five women. We are all dirt poor. The three things we have, we have in plenty: wine, bread, and vegan spaghetti. I bring a jug of cheap wine from Oregon's Willamette Valley. A Merlot of some bad year. Several others show up with wines as well. All reds, and fairly nasty. By some psychic agreement it seems. We have Merlot, Cabernet, Chianti, and Sangiovese. It is a loud meal. Pocahontas starts a noodle-slurping contest and by the time it is over, everyone is splattered with marinara sauce.

Someone lights a hot dog of a joint and passes the homegrown bud around. The giggling starts and lasts all night. Patty uncorks a home-made batch of Irish creme, brews a pot of coffee, and we go nuts with it. Virginia, a flaming-redheaded guitarist who has bicycled through Europe, uncases her guitar and plays. Pierre, a gay French dancer, pirouettes around the room for us, scooping up Pocahontas for a whirl. We drink liters of cheap wine. I recite snatches of poetry.

John and Debbie perform a comedic skit. Suddenly, everyone is banging on pots and pans, singing along with Virginia and Bryan. The night crashes on for a long time, and because we are in a great Portland neighborhood on the southeast side, no one calls the cops.

Bryan sings "Blue Moon" and nearly makes me cry. When the revelry comes to a close, and those of us who haven't gone home already are staring at the ceiling in a hazy bliss, Bryan, who has so very little and could not contribute much to the feast, goes around the room to each person with a gift—a foot massage. I am at once honored and disturbed by his open humility. I fall asleep on the dirty living-room carpet, thinking I belong here. I haven't talked to an Asian person in weeks. Tonight I forget I am Asian.

Three days later it rains and I know it is time to leave. Fall is on the way. Bryan and Patty see me off.

"You know," Bryan says, "when it's all over, you'll realize that the answer is already within you."

"It's almost a cliché, isn't it?" I say, although I don't know what the answer is. "When I find it, I still need the rigor of proof."

They laugh with me. "The road is a wondrous place. Go with an open heart," says gray-haired Bryan, who has been on the road most of his life.

And they bid me the one true farewell I have come to love: "So long, we'll see you when we see you."

As I pedal away with a light heart, I think that perhaps, inside, I am really an aging hippie.

I ride up to Olympia, Washington, then tour the eastern side of the Olympic Peninsula. A more magnificent land I never did see. Then I ferry over to Seattle. I stay in the Emerald City for weeks as a guest of Sasha Kaufman, a woman I met a month earlier at a gas station in a place called Trinity. I spend my time pounding the pavement looking for steerage passage on cargo ships. It is a defunct form of travel rumored to still be in practice on a few ships where a few penniless hopefuls are allowed to work off their passage and board, mostly by tending to filthy chores the crew avoids. I hang out at seamen's bars and drop queries at various sailors' and longshoremen's associations. I even go down to the docks and try to talk to the ships' officers. No dice. At marinas and yacht clubs, I post ads looking for a crew position on any yacht heading across the Pacific. There aren't any. It is too late in the season. I wait and wait for calls without any success. The rain begins to roll into Seattle. At last, with my funds dwindling, I give up and buy a one-way plane ticket to Vietnam with a forty-five-day layover in Japan.

Japan-Dream

Mom used to whisper to me when I was a kid that there was Japanese blood in my veins, a fanciful notion, unproven. She never said it in front of my father because it made him angry. No one wanted to be reminded of the Japanese occupation during World War II, especially Dad, who witnessed the atrocities of the Japanese army.

"Pinch it, like this," Mom told me, grabbing the ridge of my nose between her thumb and index finger, "and pull. It'll make your nose longer, thinner, and better looking."

She prided herself on the lightness of our skin. "Don't play in the sun in the middle of the day! You'll be dark like a peasant's kid. And don't forget to pull on your nose three times a day."

The Vietnamese harbor a grudging hate-admiration for the Japanese. They cannot forget how the Japanese defiled their country, yet they cannot help feeling a sense of pride that an Asian nation ranks among the world's industrial powers. And I have heard my elders say Vietnam dreamed about America, but it pragmatically yearned to be Japan. To Vietnam, Japan didn't embody success, it *was* success. I wanted to see for myself the third link of this love triangle.

My plane lands in Tokyo's Narita International Airport on a rainy night. Sleep-deprived, I grumble my way through immigration, drag the boxed bicycle out to the bus loading zone, and reassemble my vehicle at the airport terminal amid swarms of Japanese. I have no idea how to get out of the airport, much less find affordable lodging for the night. Besides a few phrases I've gleaned from a *Learn Japanese* cassette tape, I don't speak Japanese. Streets signs, in kanji, are useless.

The people at the information booth can't help me either. According to one supervisor, foreigners have been seen toting touring bicycles out of baggage claim but no one has tried to ride out directly from the airport. I am about to be the first fool to try—at 9 p.m. in the rain. I pace the terminal, frustrated and unsure of what to do. Even if there is room on the bus, I doubt they will let me board with a bike. My funds are a little lean. Besides, I figure, if I am to tour Japan, I might as well start now. Except the only road out is choked with cars and buses. Is it legal to ride in the street? Where in the hell is the sidewalk?

I sit on a bench, dumbstruck and lonely. Maybe this is how my sister felt on the streets of San Francisco, poor, hungry, cold. Grasping the tails of an incomprehensible language. Wishing for a place to sleep. Looking at pedestrians, wondering why no one stopped to offer a helping hand.

I am soaked in self-pity. Then it rains and I begin to shiver. Cornered, I do what I always do in absolute desperation: I bite my lip and plunge into the street. Pedaling like a racer, I try to keep up with the traffic, maneuvering between autos traveling on the *wrong* side of the road. I edge into a narrow lane and barely avoid entering the free-way on-ramp. A bus swerves away from me, brakes screeching. I turn my head and its headlights stab my eyes. Blinded, I hit a bump in the road, sideways. My tires skitter across the rain-slicked asphalt. I carom off a retaining wall. Somehow, I don't go down. The bus would have flattened me.

Shaking, I coast into a parking lot and spot an old man on a bicy-cle. No time to gather my wits. I chase after him, shouting questions in my bad Japanese: *How do I get out of this airport? Where can I find inexpensive lodging? Where's the public rest room?*

He looks at me the way people look at dogs foaming at the mouth. He pedals harder to get away. I tail him like a shadow. There is no way the old man is going to get away from me. Biking up the Pacific Coast has given me muscles, so I feel powerful. I chase him as easily as a cat toys with a mouse. The sight of me swooping down on him must be terrifying because he pumps standing, as though his life depends on it. I should feel a twinge of guilt, but I don't. It is late: he must be going home. And home couldn't be in the airport. I am feeling nasty and have no desire to sleep on an airport bench.

"*Gomen nasai!*"—Pardon me—I shout, but he ignores me.

After a few blocks, his strength fizzles and he paces himself, realizing that he can't get away from the lunatic screaming incomprehensible Japanese. I tell myself I can ignore him as well. Just shadow him. Sooner or later, he's bound to lead me out of the airport. The rain runs down my face, misting my glasses as I gloat at my brilliance, my prey unwittingly guiding me out of the airport and meandering me through guarded checkpoints and a maze of construction-project detours.

In the second it takes me to swipe water from my glasses, he shifts into hyperdrive and runs a red light. I skid to a stop, the cross traffic separating us. I feel bad, good, guilty, tired-sick. That old guy is one slippery noodle. It is a daring escape, very gutsy and well timed. I explode with laughter, roaring my appreciation to the wet sky. A sharp sensation of being alive suffuses me, tickling, tingling. I'm not miserable anymore. The rain comes down hard, soaking me, and through my foggy glasses I see him glancing back as he swings the corner. I wave farewell. A magnificent night. Everything forgivable.

I wander for half an hour and stumble on an empty lot next to a bamboo grove—the perfect place to steal some pillow time. I am so relieved to get out of the airport that nothing bothers me. Within four hours of setting foot in Japan, I have already harassed a citizen and trespassed on private property, courting trouble with the law at every turn. I don't care. I could always plead ignorance.

The last time I was here, my family was passing through on our way to America. We changed planes and never left the airport. My mother had always dreamed of visiting Japan. I remember telling her that someday when I was bigger, rich, and famous in America, I would come back to tour Japan. Never in twenty years had I thought I would find myself in Japan camping in an empty lot like a hobo.

I pitch the tent under a large oak out of the downpour and in a cloud of bloodthirsty mosquitoes. I strip to my underwear, crawl into my sleeping bag, and reward myself with a candy bar. As I close my eyes, a whining, screaming metallic thunder startles me into a cold sweat. I peep outside, a jumbo jet booms overhead. The lot is at the end of the airfield. Oh, gee. I wish I had pocketed a few mini-bottles of scotch on the plane.

At 2 a.m., I wake to bright lights and what feels like a small earth-quake or a landing jumbo jet. An emergency runway? I bolt out of the tent and stop dead in my tracks. Bright-eyed monsters coming at me. Naked save for a pair of cotton briefs, I quiver in the flood of headlights from a battalion of tractors. They are coming for me. Gonna run me over. OH-SHIT! My tent! My bike! My passport! My *pants!* They growl forward. Coming. Metal screeching. They grind to a halt. A million incandescent watts pin me where I stand. I am camp-ing on a parking lot for construction vehicles and earth-moving equipment. The drivers look at me. I look at them. They don't say a word. How very Japanese. Maybe they think I am Japanese. I grin, wave hello, then burrow into my tent. They cut the engines and the lights. I go back to sleep.

Morning brings a drizzle as fine as fish bones. In convenience-store parking lots, workers slurp instant noodles from Styrofoam bowls, fog-ging up their car windows, making small conspiracies of their meager privacy. Japanese are on their way to work, grim faces looking out windshields, truck drivers with white cotton gloves, office dwellers in dark suits. Villages are emptying. Children walk to school, quietly obe-dient in navy-blue uniforms. The populace ambles dispassionately toward duties, so little said in these early hours. People move in com-plete silence, their shoes louder than their breathing. Long electric worms hiss into concrete stations, swallow the people, and hiss away.

I ride oceanward, planning to go north along the Pacific Coast. Daybreak in Chiba Province is beautiful with fields of sleeping grass and lakes enshrouded in mists. The days are shortening, the chill hinting a fading fall. Persimmons polka-dot the roadsides like windfallen roses, ravished by drunken clouds of fruit flies. I stop at a wall with a laden tree branch nodding over the top. Juicy persimmons hang no more than two steps and a leap away. I am rationalizing minor theft when an old Japanese woman comes out the gate. Blushing, I bow. She smiles and asks a question in Japanese, gesturing at the tree. Beautiful, I reply, taking money out of my wallet. May I buy some? She shakes her head at the cash, disappears inside, then comes back with a woven basket of four ripe lovelies. Present, present, she says in English. She watches me eat. I bite off the point, then suck the flesh out, savoring each tender lip. Nectar, food of angels, this is how sugar should taste. Orange-red mush covers my face. She tells me I should go south to a more moderate climate. I take this as a sign and turn around toward Tokyo.

Into the megalopolis, I merge myself with the great masses of Japanese. It takes me fourteen hours to go seventy miles. I stagger in and out of crushes of people, hemmed in on every side by cars, trucks, bicyclists, and pedestrians. Up and down ramps, under bridges and over freeways, I carry my loaded bike. I accept the vague state of being constantly lost. The streets make no sense, laid in the feudal days when roads were designed to confuse invading armies. They go in spirals, circles, radiate from some center, come together in acute wedges, making comedies or marvels of buildings.

I lodge for a week at a hostel and meander all over the city, gasping at the dark undercarriage of Tokyo, its industry, its strata of life, its one-mindedness, its fascination with America. A hacking cough develops in my lungs. When I blow my nose, snot comes out black. My eyes are bloodshot from the air pollution. My throat is scratchy from car fumes. I wash it with can after can of Coca-Cola. Eventually, I get on my bike and swear never to return, in any case not with mere pocket change.

Too cheap to buy a map, I fail to escape Tokyo in a day. As the afternoon fades, I take refuge on the bank of a river that divides Tokyo and Yokohama. Sitting on a boulder next to the swamp of river reeds, I eat an early supper of rice balls wrapped in seaweed. Steamy runoffs from manufacturing plants crack the river white. The sun sets in apocalyptic colors as though the air itself is burning, turning the smog gold, the clouds molten, dangerous. Smokestacks poison the sky. The skyline of bridges and skyscrapers folds behind even more skylines of the same. Everything is smeared in this bizarre glow, even my hands. I think I can feel it on my face. Magnificent colors, a fine death, glorious, defiant. A despairing beauty. A consummation. Abruptly, the taste of rice and nori is precious on my tongue. In my nostrils, a heaviness of diesel exhaust.

The moment might have fragmented me if it weren't for Michiko-san and Tanaka-san. Something needy in my face must have stopped them short as they emerged from the grass. Smiling kindly, they lead me back to their home of plywood and appliance boxes wired together in the tall reeds. We sit on homemade stools, drinking green tea and exchanging phrases in two languages. Boys play baseball in the field beyond. Shouts in bright lights. Above us night is slowly hardening.

In the morning, when I leave them, I wish I don't have to. I lower my head and pedal to Mount Fuji. The tourists have followed summer down the mountains. I want to talk but there is no one. I wander the lakeshores, watching the snow line creeping down the volcano. Silence distills the days into one long continuous moment. I drift onward. I talk to myself, hum favorite tunes in my head for hours on end. Solo touring provides too much time for contemplation, self-doubt. These are times I would trade two mountain ranges for one new friend. In America, you can make friends with a good joke—even one borrowed from a book. Stand on a street corner with a map, wearing a puzzled look, and someone is bound to offer help, maybe an invitation for coffee. Smile and they'll let you camp in their backyard. Charm them and you'll eat at their table and sleep on their couch with the good comforter.

Japanese rarely invite strangers home. Campgrounds in Japan are few and expensive. I bed down wherever I find myself at dusk: school grounds, golf courses, temples, dikes, construction lots, ruins of castles. Once I slept in a pet cemetery. But I will always love Japan for its endless fascination with miniaturizing nature, its countless sculptured gardens.

At the Seiko Museum, a late busload of Japanese tourists strolls through the garden with a tour guide who is pointing out the leaves' changing colors. They catch me cooking spaghetti on the opposite side of a gurgling brook, my tent staked beside an overgrown bonsai, the bike propped against a carefully assembled mound of rocks. The guide stutters, bewildered at this new exhibition. I wave hello, then bow. They bow. I bow. They bow. I smile, they smile. I bring up my hands, miming them taking photographs. Ahhhh, they agree among themselves, nodding. Cameras come up, flashes going off. Ever the gracious host, I pose for them, stirring the pot, staking the tent, standing with the bike.

They smile and bow their thanks as the guide ushers them toward the main building. I flourish a theatrical obeisance. All quiet again, I eat my spaghetti and sip my green tea, waiting for a security guard to frog-march me out by the cuff of my neck. No one comes. I go to bed, chuckling to myself.

I meander from Narita to the outskirts of Kyoto and back. On my return leg, I am in a hurry to catch a flight. A Japanese friend had urged me to take the train. Having studied abroad at an American university, he was sharp on the differences between American and Japanese cultures. "Take the train," he insisted. "It's safer and the best way to get back to Narita in time for your plane. They probably don't allow bikes on the long-distance trains, but don't worry. Just take your bike on anyway. Japanese people are very polite. They won't say anything."

The November weather is deteriorating so I'm tempted. Already extended beyond my budget, I have no choice but to ride straight into the teeth of it. One day, an English-speaking fisherman tells me a gale warning has even the big freighters heading for ports. All afternoon, a strong wind broadsides me. Around dusk, it quiets. Somewhere south of Shimizu, I find a stretch of clean beach—a rarity in Japan. The thought of a campfire is irresistible. Storm warning forgotten, I cook and eat a meal of hard-boiled eggs and curry with spaghetti next to a crackling driftwood fire, my campsite a good thirty yards from the surf. The wind picks up when I hit the sack. An hour later, it rains. The wind blows harder. My tent, unstaked on the sand, begins to warp, shaking like a lump of Jell-O. I peek out at the surf crashing white in the ambient light. It looks rougher than before. I zip up my sleeping bag, telling myself it will pass. I've sat through plenty of storms. Once I sat in my tent two days waiting for the rain to stop. How bad can it get?

The rain turns pelting. Gusts lift the tent's windward end. I poke my head outside and taste sand and a tang of salt in the air. This is bad. The ocean looks a lot closer, maybe fifteen yards off. The tide is coming in. I am worried. Okay, time to pack up. Holding down the jumping tent, I dress as fast as I can. Although I have a flashlight clipped to my baseball cap, I do everything by feel, instincts gained from months of touring. I can't get out of the tent. Without my weight, it would turn into a kite in this wind. I figure out a way to collapse the tent from inside. The surf rolls in fast. I'm racing the ocean. Frantically, I bundle my gear and drag it up a ten-yard concrete embankment, running, slipping, scrambling back and forth in horizontal rain. It's pitch-dark in the storm and my rain-splattered glasses aren't helping. As I push the bike up to safety, the ocean mats my campsite.

I huddle with my pile of gear on the walkway above the embankment. Trees bow and bushes quiver like slaves before an angry master. The heavens crack, thundering. Lightning scrawls across swollen clouds, tearing up the night and putting the fear of God into me. I mutter thanks to Him, Buddha, and my dead sister Chi. Another minute and things might have turned out very badly. I don't want to think about it. I strap the panniers onto the racks and push the bike to the road. Rain stings my face. I'm drenched, my teeth chattering. A steaming bowl of instant noodles and hot coffee would be really good. I need shelter quickly, but my funds aren't sufficient for a hotel room even if I trip over one. The wind is too strong for riding, so I slog two miles back up the road to a 7-Eleven.

I step inside the heated store. My glasses fog up. I'm smiling gleefully like a maniac. I made it. I beat the storm! I whoop and rip off my helmet, dripping a puddle just inside the door. There's no one besides the clerk, a chubby Japanese guy in his early twenties. He is reading *manga,* a Japanese X-rated comic the size of San Francisco's Yellow Pages.

I'm so happy I want to let him know what a fine place his store is. I pull out my Japanese phrase book and try to strike up a conversation. *"Bad storm, no? Camp on beach. Me. Bad storm! Heh-heh-heh. Hahahahahahaha!"*

He gives me a pained smile and says something I can't understand.

"Me, American. From America."

He lifts a dubious eyebrow.

"San Francisco," I say, and because I am in the mood I start to sing: "I left my heart in San Francisco. High on a hill . . ."

The more I sing and babble the more he looks at me like a bad dream. He flips his *manga,* making a show of reading. I attempt a few more phrases and give up on Manga-man.

Well, bugger him. I settle cross-legged on the floor next to the news rack and slurp my bowl of instant noodles. Heck, I could sit here all night and look at magazine pictures. Who needs to talk anyway? I work my way through two bowls of noodles, two cans of foul Japanese coffee, a carton of custard, and a chocolate bar. The whole time Manga-man doesn't budge from his counter fortress, the phone, and, no doubt, the police–panic button never out of his reach. He doesn't even pick up his comic again. He wipes down the counter a dozen times, waiting for me to do something crazy. After an hour, I feel a twinge of guilt for torturing the poor guy. It's not his fault the storm is bad and my Japanese is worse.

I don my wet gear and go out to face the storm. Manga-man is visibly relieved. I wander in the dark, come upon an all-night gas station, and stand under its awning. The old station attendant looks me up and down from inside his booth. When it is clear I am not a customer, he slides open the window, says something, his words drowned out by the whipping rain. He flicks the back of his hand at me, shooing. I go. All the houses and shops are shut against the storm, making the world look dead. Not a soul stirs. Heavy rain hoods even the streetlamps. Shivers set into me again.

I find it here in Japan where I least expect it: the black-hollow desperation of a runaway.

I luck onto a stone wall, five feet high, enclosing an empty lot. The gate is padlocked. I hoist my gear and bike over the gate. I pitch the tent behind the wall, stake it down good, and crawl inside. The wall shoulders most of the fury. A dozen yards away, the wind howls through a greenhouse, bansheeing on the loose aluminum sheets, jetting through and punching out plastic tarps. I peel off my wet clothes, then do push-ups, sit-ups, and leg lifts until I break a sweat. Things can't get much worse than this. I fall promptly asleep, thinking at last I am ready for Vietnam.

Last-Gamble

On the highway downwind, the Saigon bus driver, at the first whiff of fish, announced, "Phan Thiet, the Fishsauce Capital—two more klics."

I was nine, traveling with Uncle Long back to the town of my birth. The trip initiated my family's second escape attempt from Communist Vietnam. The plan had been hatched half a year before, on the very night my father stumbled home, barefoot and bedraggled, from Minh Luong Prison. For months he paced the attic, fearful of recapture, poring over books and maps, ironing out every detail with my mother's help. This morning, he guided me out the back door saying, "Don't be afraid, son. It'll be fine. You're going home."

The bus rolled into Phan Thiet. It was one of those odd Vietnamese coastal towns steeped in one trade and indecisive about the cloak it wore. In the rainy season, rich red clay swamped the province, pasty on thatched walls, runny on children's faces. In the hot season, blistering shards of wind blasted sand into every crevice so thoroughly that old women complained it gritted their joints. This was the narrow season of transition. It had the air of paradise despite a briny tinge of decomposing fish that haunted the streets and alleys year-round. This town, after all, was famous for its fishsauce.

My step-grandfather Grandpa Le was a fishsauce baron, born into a sea-heritage that dated back before the Japanese and the French occupation. He used to claim that his ancestors invented fishsauce. The whole town was built on this industry. Everyone knew how it was made and at one time most people in town, when they weren't dragging the ocean for fish, were putting fresh fish, unwashed and ungutted, into salt barrels to ferment. While they waited on the decomposition process, all they ever talked about was fishsauce. Which fish produced the best-tasting extract? How to mix various types of fish to make a balanced bouquet. Indeed, there were many varieties of fishsauce, each suitable for a certain style of cooking. The finest batches were flavorful enough to be savored directly from the bottle. In a few weeks, a smelly black ooze seeped out the bottom of the barrel. Fisherfolk diluted and bottled this black gold and sold it all over the country. Blend masters—like Grandpa Le—guarded their secrets zealously and made fortunes. In the old days, the village folk prized bottles of fishsauce concentrate as great gifts, the equivalent of fine wine and cash.

Uncle Long said these days people treated it like an illicit narcotic, hiding their production from the tax collectors, squirreling bottles of it away for bartering. Liberated into Communism or not, Vietnamese needed fishsauce the way we needed air. For us, it was salt and a thousand other spices, the very marrow of the sea to a country of coastal people. It was a good thing Grandpa left us a stockpile of fishsauce when he died.

Grandma Le's house and sundry shop sat five yards from the main road, the national highway. The bus dropped us at the front door. Grandma, Auntie Dung, and all my siblings—Chi, Huy, Tien, and Hien—came out to greet us. Grandma took me into her shop and said I could eat as much candy from her store as I could swallow on account that she hadn't had chance to spoil me as she had my siblings. They had been living with Grandma when we came back from prison. While I was locked up in Saigon, they were running wild with the local kids.

Auntie Dung took all of us out for milkshakes. We walked down the shady avenue, holding hands, singing, our sandals scrunching on sand—this a beach town—to a kiosk that had been in the same spot under a tamarind tree since I could remember. The vendor, whose laughs were as fresh as the sweet fruits she served, hand-shaved ice for us until her arms ached. Huy and Chi had durian milkshakes made with shaved ice and condensed milk. Tien had his favorite, a bread-fruit milkshake. I had soursop.

The feasting started then and lasted until the moment we left. Grandma didn't think she would see us again so she made us our favorite dishes. Grandma and Great-Grandaunt, who was so old and stooped I could touch the top of her head, roasted chickens for Huy and Chi, stewed hams for Tien and Hien, and fried mountains of delicious egg rolls for me. Grandma's little house was full of laughter; the stove in her kitchen, which was separate from the main quarters, never cooled off. They were constantly making treats for us. There was so much to eat, we forgot the rest of the country was beginning to starve.

I could tell people were hungry because I often watched the store for Grandma. It was a mom-and-pop operation, hardly bigger than an average bedroom, carrying a variety of goods: a dozen bolts of cloth, kitchen knives, flour, candles, several shelves of canned foods, spices, dried edibles, and the occasional baked goods from a local baker. Neighbors came in and bought ingredients, one meal at a time: a grab of dried shrimp, a cup of fishsauce, a few spoons of sugar, a scoop of lard. The bin of white rice stayed full. I sold it by the cup to be offered to portraits of dead ancestors. People ate the red rice, a dry, tasteless wild variety that farmers once fed to chickens and pigs.

One afternoon while I was snouting through a jar of candy, the cute girl who lived next door came in. She smiled and gave me a nickel-bill and two chipped teacups.

"My mom needs a tablespoon of cooking oil and half a cup of fishsauce," she said.

"What is she making?" I mumbled, trying to swallow a mouthful of sesame caramel and grinning like a moron. My parents had enrolled me in an expensive boys' prep school. I didn't know any girls except my friend who used to live in the alley behind our house in Saigon.

"Stir-fried spinach and onion omelet."

"Oh." I filled one teacup with cooking oil, the other with fish-sauce. "You want some peppermint candy?" I handed her a fistful.

She shook her head, hesitating.

"It's free!" I said, grinning so wide my face nearly split.

"Really?"

"Yes, it's all mine." I exaggerated, pointing at the row of candy jars.

"Thanks."

"My name is An. What's yours?"

"Hoa."

"What else would you like, Hoa?" I gestured magnanimously at the entire inventory.

Grandma knew I was pilfering her store for a few smiles from Hoa, but she looked the other way, kindly going inside for a nap when Hoa came around. She was letting me grow up the way she had let Chi find her footing.

I could tell Chi was different. She smiled a lot, a lopsided grin brought on by growing up among the coconut palms and basking in Grandma's affection. This place had seeped into her, filled her out, made her a part of it. She was tall and strong. She swam, climbed trees, chopped wood, and practiced martial arts. She bullied the bullies and fasted with Grandma, who was a devout Buddhist. Chi owned the village the way it owned her and she shared it generously with me, something I, the spoiled first son, never expected.

Early every morning, Chi took Huy, Tien, and me down to the bay to teach us to swim. Grandma sent us off with steamed rice cakes filled with peppered pork and sweet beans. We walked down to the beach, our breakfasts warm in our pockets. These were to be saved for after our swim, but we ate them on the road, knowing there was a meal waiting on the beach. In the water, Chi held each of us up by our stomachs and we learned to dog-paddle. We swam, waded, and built sand castles. Entire clans of fisherfolk, from grandfathers to toddlers, gathered on the shore to bring in the morning catch. When they hauled in the nets, we pitched in, digging our feet into the sand, heaving the lines to their rhythm in a tug-of-war with the sea. The net made a great big U in the water, taking a bite of the ocean as we brought it in. Silvery fish came out of the water like coins pouring, bouncing, hopping out of a slot machine. The fisherfolk went mad with laughter, dashing about, scooping up the jackpot into hand-woven baskets, screeching to each other to grab this one or that one before it flopped back into the water. We worked with them, laughing, competing to see who bagged the most. In return, they gave us a couple of fish and lent us a pan and oil. Chi built a driftwood fire on the beach and fried the fish. We pinched the meat from the bones, and ate it off banana leaves with salt and lime, sitting on the sand, watching the sun come up out of the water. It felt as though Chi had never gone to live with Grandma. I never thought we could be so happy again, Chi and me playing as though it had never happened. Like I'd never betrayed her and Leper-boy, three years before.

The village leper didn't have a name. People called him Leper-boy although he was at least a young man. Perhaps that was because he was short, very small-boned—"hardly more than a lame chicken," Grandma used to say. I was in kindergarten then, and he didn't seem all that much bigger than me. He walked on one leg and crutches. His other foot had withered around the ankle like a bad squash. But he was a great traveler, getting around the village more than most two-legged folks. They said he even made it out to the countryside a couple of times a week. It was how he ate.

From house to house, he begged with his one gift, singing in a voice so pure the older folks grieved over his tragedy. That misshapen face, they said, cheated him of a professional career in the opera. But really, it was their way of overlooking his malady. Sad, sad, they hushed, his ancestors must have done something horrible to cause him such misfortune.

An observer of courtesy, Leper-boy made himself scarce in the morning when merchants went to market. Begging from the sellers before they could sell, people believe, brought bad commercial luck. Leper-boy let the vendors returning from market find him in the afternoon sitting by the side of the road, serenading them a cappella. Kind souls gave him bits of what they could not sell. Snack girls, walking with rounds of rice crackers, as big as trays, stacked three feet high on their heads, would stop. They often gave him a little of what they had left. He thanked them and put their gifts into a bag he slung over his shoulder, the bag a gift from some Buddhist monks, who were also, in their fashion, great beggars.

Leper-boy didn't like sesame crackers and shrimp paste as much as he liked tobacco, and he found, in my sister Chi, a suitable trading partner. He exchanged his tidbits with her for cigarette butts she had salvaged from the family's ashtrays. It was a transaction which my father had forbid. Dad said Leper-boy might be contagious and none of us could talk to him or touch anything he touched. But as children, we were not allowed to have money, and sesame rice crackers and shrimp paste were my sister's favorite snack.

Dad came home after work and found Chi snacking. He asked her how she got the food. He knew that without money she couldn't have bought it. Chi said a friend gave it to her. He asked me and I don't know why I said it. Maybe I was angry at Chi. Or, simply, I was just spoiled. Full of a first-son righteousness, I told on her. Dad raged through the house, furious at Chi. *You dare disobey me! I'll teach you how to be respectful in this house!* He laid her out on the living room divan and broke bamboo canes on her, exacting the Vietnamese punishment in a cloud of blind wrath. Neighbors crowded the front door, begging him to stop. Men shook their heads, women beseeched him for mercy. Yet no one crossed the threshold. It was a man's right to beat his child. The police weren't summoned because they wouldn't have intervened. Mom cried, kneeling beside the divan. Dad rose above them, his visage terrible to behold, an angry god, vengeful and unyielding. Thwack! Thwack! Thwack! Chi screamed. Thwack! Thwack! Thwack! Thwack! Thwack! Thwack! Thwack! Thwack! People clamored for mercy. I cried, cowering in the hallway terrified, for I had brought these blows on her. Like striking vipers, the canes blurred through the air, swishing, biting into Chi, one after another. Thwack! Thwack! Thwack! She howled. I cringed, covering my ears, knowing well the taste of bamboo, the way it licks out at flesh, first a jolt like electricity, then sharp like a fang, then hot like a burn. The canes broke over her back. The neighborhood women, wringing their shirttails, muttered that Dad's cruelty was a curse upon our house. The last cane splintered into bits, and Dad stormed away to find another. Mom dragged Chi up and put Chi's hand in mine. Take her to Grandma's, Mom told me. Chi and I fled the house. I returned home that evening, but Chi never wholly came back into our lives again.

Mom came out to Grandma's a week before Dad. When she finally sent word for him that things were ready, he sneaked out of Saigon and arrived in Phan Thiet by hiding on a cargo train. Dad came into Grandma's house like a rat crossing a dark street. We were sitting on straw floor mats in the living room eating dinner. He stepped into the pumpkin warmth of our oil lamp and I, familiar with the carefree beach days, saw him as though I hadn't seen him in months. He was a thin bag of shallow breaths and sweaty skin. Fear had bled away his commanding air. His cheekbones poked out while his eyes sank deeper into his head. His new stoop and rain-sloped shoulders made him small.

In one step, he reunited the whole family for the first time in over a year. And suddenly, I felt Chi withdrawing to the side. She started lurking on the edge of us, constantly on one errand or another when Dad was around. She developed an eerie knack for sensing him around corners, and she had this ability to melt into the furniture when he came into the room. She never looked him in the eye. Fourteen summers old now, she was too young to have fallen permanently from grace with Dad. There was a wedge between them driven, per-haps, deeper by the fact that she lived with Grandma, who was never fond of Dad in the first place.

Our last night in Phan Thiet, Chi and I monkeyed up the star-fruit tree and onto the tin roof of the kitchen shack. We picked star fruits and, dipping the wedges in chili-spiced salt, ate them sitting below a glittering sky. The fruit tasted sun-baked, for in full ripeness it was golden, the color of cloud underbellies tickled by a slanting sun. It had a flowery texture halfway between a melon and an apple, though it was less substantial than either. Its juice was sharp, indecisive between sour and sweet, resulting in a dizzied tanginess that made me think of being out in the sun too long. Chi said it was how sunlight tasted.

I told her a secret game I played when Mom and Dad left me at home alone overnight. I talked to space aliens with my flashlight, flickering photons to the reaches of darkness. Spaceships would come if I ever really needed them, I told her.

"What would you do if a spaceship came?" Chi asked.

"I'd ask them to take us to America. Here, your turn."

Chi beamed her message into the sky.

"What did you say to the spaceships?"

"I sent my wish to the angels."

"Angels? They're up there with space aliens?"

Chi nodded solemnly.

"What did you wish for?"

"I want them to watch over Grandma when we're gone."

Chi wasn't as excited about going to America as I was. She felt at home in Phan Thiet and she loved Grandma. Chi said she'd asked Mom to let her stay with Grandma, but both Mom and Dad wouldn't hear of it. We babbled late into the night, waiting to eavesdrop on the adults discussing the escape inside the kitchen shack. Everyone was there, including the fishermen who would be taking us out onto the ocean. Some of them were angry about Uncle Hung's last-minute decision to stay with Grandma. He said she was too old and needed someone to take care of her. He was convinced that with the continuing food shortages burglars would break into the house and rob her.

"You're a turtle!" Mom mocked her brother. "You never stick your neck out to take a chance. A little noise and—fffthhh—in goes your head, scared of everything." She looked around the room for emphasis and threw up her hands. "There's nothing for you here. We have relatives who will take care of Mother."

Everyone, including Grandma, urged him to go, but nothing could sway him into risking the open sea in a fishing boat. Aunt Dung, his sister, on the other hand, was all for it. She was twenty, and full of fire. A repressed little town with neither opportunity nor food was not for her. Neither were its cowardly men.

"I'll take care of Mother better than any relatives," Uncle Hung said doggedly. "Besides, maybe I'll go back to Saigon and watch your house so that it'll be there if you come back."

At this, joy bled from Mom's face. The house was her greatest treasure, their milestone in life, their monumental accomplishment. Banks didn't make home loans. The house meant security, a departure from their difficult past. They couldn't sell it because that would look suspicious. They had started out with nothing and now they were about to lose everything.

"No." Dad shook his head. "Let it go. The government will confiscate it. I don't want you implicated in our escape. We won't be back. If we return, we are as good as dead." Dad knew if we waited till next spring, he stood a fair chance of being discovered and executed. The cops swept through the neighborhood regularly and dragged people off to labor camps. Properties were "seized" and "redistributed." If they took Dad, they would send us to live in jungle hamlets.

Mom nodded, saying over and over that he was right. She was a smart and resourceful woman who had bribed the prison guards to keep her husband alive, making sure he had the little food and medicine he needed to survive the jungle. Besides rescuing him, she had worked with her brother to find seven fishermen with a boat willing to risk the high seas with us. The crew were young men from Phan Thiet, the oldest twenty-five, the youngest seventeen. Phan Thiet was my mother's hometown so it was the safest place to recruit, but it was also my father's former government station, the place where he was most likely to be recognized. They had been planning for months. The men had been stashing government-rationed diesel by the pint and hoarding spare engine parts. At first, Dad worried it was a trap, for there were many fishermen-turned-pirates who took passengers out to sea to rob and murder. Then he suspected that it was a military sting to capture would-be escapees.

"Tai, the skipper, is Mr. Tang's son," said Uncle Long, introducing his handpicked crew one by one. When he finished, he vouched for them: "I've known every man here since they were kids. All these men are safe. They have as much riding on this escape as you do, Brother Thong. If they're caught, their families can lose their boats and all fishing privileges. They will become beggars."

They began to discuss rations and details of our escape, slated for the next day.

"Oy! An." It was Hoa standing in a tree in her backyard, calling me over the fence.

"Hi, Hoa. You want some star fruit?" I whispered, hoping the adults below couldn't hear me.

"Yes. Meet me out front?"

Chi giggled. My face burned. She said loud enough for Hoa to hear, "Take some chili-salt for your girlfriend."

Too embarrassed to say anything, I stuffed my shirttail into my pants, put some star fruit down my shirt, and ran out. Hoa sat on the front porch with me. Other kids were playing Knock the Can in the street.

"I know what your family is doing," Hoa said, nibbling the point of a star fruit.

I pretended I wasn't listening. Dad had said it was supposed to be a big secret.

"All those men going into the store, then sneaking behind into the house. They don't leave until really late at night. They're fishermen, aren't they? Your family is going to cross the border, aren't you?"

I shook my head, almost feeling my father's cane on my backside. It was my fault she was hanging around the house every day.

"Everybody knows. You can tell me. We're friends, aren't we?" she insisted, calling our friendship into question, which was more than I could bear.

"Yes, we're leaving," I admitted.

We sat quietly. She picked up pebbles with her toes. The kids in the street were laughing, having a good time at their game. I wished I had brought some of my toys from Saigon to give her.

"You'll come back and visit?"

"Sure, I have to visit my grandma, don't I?"

I gave her my flashlight and she let me hold her hand. My palm turned sweaty, but she didn't let go. I liked the feel of her hand. It was soft and it made me dizzy. All my blood was dammed up in my ears.

Early in the morning, Mom ordered us into tattered clothes. The lot of us were going to pass as peasants. She had bought each of us a pair of sandals, known as Viet Cong sandals because they were made out of used tires, the cheapest footwear available. Mom and Aunt Dung hired two rickshaws to take us out of town. Going to visit relatives out in the countryside to have a picnic, Mom explained to the drivers. After they dropped us well beyond the fisherfolk's shanties that ringed the town, we walked for several hours on back roads and trails. The sandals retained their tire curvature and rubbed our feet raw. Huy and Tien began to bawl about the blisters on their toes, but I was too frightened about having told Hoa about our escape to care. If she'd told anyone, we were all going to jail again.

We threw away the sandals and went barefoot. Chi held up bravely, carrying Hien on her back for miles when he was too tired to walk. We were supposed to meet up with Dad sometime late that night, then halfway to dawn our fishermen would come for us. I was frightened that I wouldn't be able to make the swim to the boat. Yet as we walked deeper into the trees, I found myself becoming entranced by the coconut forest. The palms swayed gently in the evening breeze, their naked trunks sweeping into the sky, their splaying leaves, bright green oranging in the sunset, arcing out and down like frozen fireworks. Not a soul traveled the road.

It seemed, then, that we could simply walk out of Vietnam and right into America, beautiful free America, somewhere at the end of this wondrous road. It seemed so easy I didn't think about the thousands of boat people who died trying to escape Vietnam, or about the Vietnamese navy shooting at boats on sight. I almost forgot that this truly was our last gamble.

Mecca-Memory

9 Rain mists the glass pane as the airplane sinks through the clouds and banks into the midnight sky over Ho Chi Minh City. Outside the window a feeble dusting of streetlamps marks the dark sprawl beneath. I search for signs of old Saigon, neon messages, bright boulevards. Nothing familiar in the bombed-out darkness. Gone, too, are the red tracers of bullets ripping the night sky.

I am afraid. This unnameable apprehension isn't something I had anticipated. The hardships of a pilgrimage lend no courage for facing mecca. In the past few months, I have biked 2,357 miles, sleeping in ditches along the road, cooking meager meals of steamed rice and boiled eggs over campfires, and bathing in creeks. I am tired, nearly broke, and scared. Surprise. So I toss back yet another lowball, this one a toast to my twenty-year anniversary since I had forsaken this city. Here's to you, Saigon. I've come for my memories. Give me reconciliation.

The cabin tilts in descent. Passengers, mostly Vietnamese, begin fighting their luggage out of the overhead compartments, spilling packages into the aisles, rallying toward the exit. A Vietnamese couple across the aisle furtively jam uneaten airline cheese and crackers into their handbags, squirreling away the freebies, knowing better but unable to resist old immigrant habits. A middle-aged pair, luggage in hand, rush up from the rear and plop down in the empty seats next to me. Sporting a lavender double-breasted suit and half a pound of gold around his blubbery neck, the man grins at me. At my inquisitive stare, he bobs his head and offers, "Almost there . . . How do you do?"

"How're you doing?" I answer instinctively, the American rhetorical salutation. Then, honoring our common etiquette, I address him in Vietnamese, *"Uncle-friend, are your family-relatives welcoming you at the airport?"*

"Yes, my brothers and sisters," he fumbles, surprised at my Vietnamese, gauging the ethnic shape of my face. *"Brother-friend, you're Vietnamese?"* I nod. *"I was sure you were Japanese or Korean. Sure you're not a half-breed?"*

I shake my head, taking no offense at his bluntness. *"One hundred percent Vietnamese,"* I announce in a tone final enough for anybody.

He laughs, amused at my Americanized idiom. *"Okay! Whole, undiluted-concentrated fishsauce you are!"* Then on a more friendly note: *"Visiting family-relatives?"*

"Yes, perhaps. Distant relatives-neighbors. I don't remember them very well. I'm really just visiting the fatherland." But no Vietnamese American returns unless he has a family to visit. He pauses, eyeing me again, probably thinking I am one of those lost souls he's heard about. America is full of young-old Vietnamese, uncentered, uncertain of their identity. The older generation calls them *mat goch*—lost roots.

"Too bad. What a shame," he mumbles to his moon-faced wife, who concurs with clicks of her tongue. She whispers to him. He scribbles something on the back of a business card. *"Here's the address of my brother's house in Saigon where we're staying. Call us if you get lonely. And don't forget to put ten dollars in your passport for the immigration officials. They'll let you through the gate faster."*

I thank him and wrangle with myself again whether to slip the bureaucrats a little grease. I don't know if my tiny canister of pepper spray or my eight-inch fillet knife is legal. Plenty of Vietnamese Americans who visited Vietnam returned with harrowing tales of the grubby nasties at the airport, and I have been fairly disturbed at the prospect of losing my bike.

He wishes me luck, claps me on the shoulder, then sprints with his wife in tow up to seats closer to the exit. The printed side of his card gives his American profession: a realtor in Santa Ana, a member of Century 21. Another Vietnamese-American immigrant success story coming home all spelled out in jewelry and gaudiness.

Copies of the same fable, some exaggerated, some true, stock the plane, every one of them beside himself with giddiness. Husbands and wives squawk directions at each other, squeezing hands, grinning the victor's grin. Young children caught up in the rush of adrenaline wail. Their triumphant homecoming is at hand.

The Japanese and Koreans, all business travelers, flinch, scorn thinly veiled, drawing back from the Vietnamese. From both ends of the plane, flight attendants, round sensual faces distorted in desperation, scream in Korean-accented English, ordering the horde to put their luggage back into the overheads. On the intercom the captain orders the passengers to return to their seats for the landing. A duffel bag becomes unzipped and rains new toys into the aisle: action figures, fist-sized teddy bears, and Ping-Pong paddles. Somewhere up front, a little boy howls, and on the instant the party shifts into full cry. Mutiny.

A tall European flight attendant spearheads the assault, her smaller Korean counterparts covering her flanks. With small white hands, they wrestle the Vietnamese one by one into seats. They slam closed the overhead compartments. Someone complains about his bruised fingers. Harsh Korean, countered by Vietnamese curses, rattles the cabin. The din alone should send the plane tumbling out of the sky.

Mortified by the Vietnamese's behavior and equally dismayed that I feel an obligatory connection to them, I sink deeper into my seat, resentful, ashamed of their incivility. My grandmother used to say to me when I was unruly: A monkey in a prince's gown is still a monkey.

Eventually the plane touches down and they mob the exit. The flight attendants dive into the fray for another round of taming the animals. Last off the plane, I bang my way out, lugging a helmet, two backpacks, and a rolled sleeping mat. The wet night heat wraps around me. I realize I should have changed during the flight but I was too drunk. Still am. Under my insulated Lycra bicycle tights and fleece, both caked with dirt and sweat, is a full-body thermal. It is winter in Japan, tropical in Vietnam. Early this morning, after forty-five days of touring a thousand miles of Japan, I pumped my bike directly onto the departure ramp at Tokyo's Narita Airport with no time to spare. I tossed my bike and panniers unboxed onto the conveyor belt, fretted through the immigration checkpoint, and ran to the boarding gate, helmet still strapped on my head.

I tail the other passengers across the tarmac toward the docking gate, surprised at Saigon's sleek new facility. I expected something more native, maybe a little burnt-out or run-down, at best a quaint shanty like the Maui airport in Hawaii. Tan Son Nhat International Airport seems fairly modern and in good working condition, comparable in size to an airport of a small Stateside city.

"Visa. Passport," demands a Vietnamese immigration official behind a counter. The sign above him reads: DO NOT PUT MONEY IN YOUR PASSPORT. So I pass over the paperwork minus the grease.

"Pham, Aan-rew," he pronounces, lifting an eyebrow, then rolls the words at me, sneering: *"Viet-kieu."* Foreign Vietnamese.

I ignore the slight, pretending I don't understand Vietnamese, and as I had hoped, his English isn't enough to prolong the questioning regarding my intentions in Vietnam. He makes me pay five dollars to a woman who takes a Polaroid of me *"for extra paperwork."* Fifteen minutes and I collect my papers and pass through immigration.

I edge into the press of people at the baggage claim just in time to see the handler, wearing flip-flops, dragging my bike backward on a moving conveyor belt through a portal. The bike jams in the small door, squeaking loudly against the rubber belt. The idiot was too lazy to lead the bike around the long way. He hollers to someone on the other side to give the bike a good push.

I drop everything, shouting as I blade through the crowd, then leap clear over the moving belts and luggage. I help him work the bike free of the door. One pannier rack is bent. One brake grip on the handlebar is broken off. The rims look irreparable. Something heavy settles on me. This cheap old bike has taken me far, farther than my imagination. Thanks to nitwits in flip-flops, it is practically scrap metal. Oh, God, if this is how I see the Vietnamese, what sorry sights they must be to Western eyes.

"Stupid!" I wrench my bike from him.

Broken bike on one shoulder, one backpack on the other, one backpack on my back, and a set of panniers in hand, I make my way toward the jam of people pressed against the customs gate. People are jostling and elbowing each other to get to the X-ray machines. The officials randomly open boxes and invite their owners into rooms for inspection, doing the routine shakedown dance. White foreigners are off-limits; Viet-kieu are fair game, easy pickings.

Ten minutes in line and I am no closer to the exit. This is a Vietnamese line: shove your way to the front, bumper-car your path through the mess. One Vietnamese-American woman pushes my bags back so she can move her cart forward. It is hot and claustrophobic. Under my thermal, I sweat like a pig next to a roasting pit. Ten more minutes. I snap. I take the offensive, amused at my ability to summon the Vietnamese in me, the grubbing-snatching-edging Vietnamese behavior anathema to the Western me. It doesn't get me far with this crowd, so I spice it up with a dash of American commandeering bullheadedness.

I lift my bike above my head with one arm and bellow: "Out of my way! I'm coming through!"

I swipe two men with the dirt-caked wheels, knock the head of a third with the handlebars. He yipes and falls back, head in his hands. Another man elbows me. I poke him hard in the ribs with a pedal and he too reels back protesting. I throw him a look, angry enough to toss the bike with it. Grandma was right about monkeys.

An uproar. Officials yell in English and Vietnamese. They can't tell whether I am Vietnamese. *You can't go that way.* I barrel through a gap between two X-ray machines, snarling back at them in English: "I'm next! I can't fit this bike through the machine. Can't you see that?"

With the bike over one shoulder, I grab my backpack and panniers coming out of the scanner. I simply turn and walk out the door. The officials are objecting. I become conveniently deaf. Somehow they let me go, giving up on the crazy Asian wearing a bike helmet and filthy clothes.

Outside, the street is wet. The rain has stopped. A crowd of several hundred presses forward, angling for a glimpse inside, each searching for his relatives. There must be a welcoming party of ten for every person coming off the plane. Then there is a brigade of cyclo and taxi drivers hustling for a fare. I search their faces and they search mine.

Twenty years have passed since I've seen Grandaunt Nguyen, my grandmother's cousin-in-law. As a child, I used to play with her sons, whom I must call Uncle despite the fact that we are the same age. I have never written them, nor they me. I half hoped they wouldn't come. I wanted to return, quiet and alone, to fold myself into the city, but my mother learned of my flight number through my brother and told them I was coming.

"An! An!"

Someone calls my Vietnamese name. A man pushes through the crowd. He is smiling and waving at me. I can't place him, so I grin.

"How are you?" he asks in good English.

"Khoe. Chu sau?"—I'm fine. And you, Uncle?

"Noi teing Viet duoc, ha?" He is genuinely surprised I speak the language. *"Remember me? I'm Khuong."*

They emerge from the crowd and surround me, my grandaunt, whom I remember from pictures, and her three sons: Vict, a jovial, dark, portly thirty-five; Khuong, a slim, pockmarked, good-humored thirty-two; and Hung, a fat, pale, mustached playboy of twenty-eight. Two decades stand awkwardly between us, the crowd around us oblivious, pressing in. We exchange pleasantries. How was your trip? I'm so sorry the plane was late and you waited for me. How's your mother? You all waited here two hours in the rain? Did you really bike all this way?

But what I want to do is hug them or shake their hands. No room for either. A hug too familiar. A handshake too disrespectful to an elder. So I grin and bow and sweat profusely in my thermal.

"Is this all you have?" asks my grandaunt in a tone that makes me ashamed.

I nod, coloring, because I have neither money nor gifts for them, only some traveler's checks and camping gear, no room for gifts for fourteen people and not much money to play the good-conquering-son returning home with a cargo of treasure. The Vietnamese I know who came back brought on average three thousand dollars' worth of gifts. Every passenger off the plane has cartloads of goodies: cameras, microwaves, computers, microscopes, tennis rackets, badminton rackets, boom boxes, clothes, soap, shampoo, facial cream, perfumes, cognac, Johnnie Walker by the case, bicycles, electric rice cookers, Walkmans, Discmans, stereo systems, hair dryers, cosmetics, books, music cassettes, CDs, train sets, Japanese geisha dolls in glass display cases, videocassettes, videocams, metal welding kits, car parts, moped parts, tools, and anything else that can be bought and fit into a shipping box.

I didn't have a single gift.

At 2 a.m., we take a taxi-van back to the Nguyens' houses. My three "uncles" ride back on their motorbikes.

Away from the airport, the buildings look dilapidated, water-damaged, their metal doors shut tight. Straying vendors sell food from baskets by the light of oil lamps, feeding the beggars who can't sleep. Thin blankets drawn over their faces to keep the mosquitoes at bay, the homeless sleep on the street, lining the side of the road like casualties of war, scavenged and toe-tagged by the clean-up crew. Around them, an endless crush of buildings, weeping concrete, and clothesline rags hem in narrow streets. At the larger intersections, lighted billboards loom above the dark, odd ornaments at the joints of the city, some sort of somatic dreams hawking Honda motorbikes, Samsung color TVs, IBM computers, Coca-Cola, Pepsi, Suzukis.

There's a cool stink to the city, a scent warped by too many people, too many things, and softened by the wet night. I turn, sniff-swallowing it all snake-like while fielding questions from Grandaunt.

Turning to and fro, desperately trying to penetrate the dark beyond the erratic sweeps of the taxi's headlights, I feel out of phase, a man panning for the memories of a boy. The purr of the van's engine sounds empty in this supposedly live city. The old angst, now unfamiliar, worms back through the years at me. Memories. My man-child fascination. I scan the gutters half expecting discarded uniforms of the deposed South Vietnamese Nationalist Army, like those the boy-me had scavenged off the streets on Saigon's final night. The night of our own downfall.

It was a night of madness and spectacular fires. I was eight and wild with greed for all the loot people had tossed in the street. You could find almost anything that night. The defeated army discarded guns, ammo, helmets, knives, uniforms, boots, water tins, and heaps of things covered with the flat green paint of army-issued equipment. Fugitives, peasants, and city dwellers left belongings where they dropped them: baskets, food, clothes, chairs, sleeping mats, pottery, wads of no-longer-valid currency. The night was choked with those who fled, those who hid, those who scavenged, and those who went mad with fear, or greed, or anger.

The bullies chased me down the alley. I heard them pounding the pavement hard on my heels. They were yelling. BANG! A shot went off. I couldn't tell if they were shooting at me. Maybe they were shooting in another part of the neighborhood. Guns had been going off around the city all day, but I was pretty sure they were shooting at me.

Earlier, I had been down by the empty lot showing off some of my loot to the other kids. Mom and Dad were busy packing suitcases and burning documents, so I was able to sneak out of the house and scavenge the streets. All the kids had something, mostly guns, ammo, and broken telephones. Some had pliers and were using them to take the tips off the bullets to get at the gunpowder. We drew dragons in the dirt with the powder and ignited them. I was firing my name when the older bullies came around. They had pistols and demanded we hand over our loot. The biggest bully wanted my pistol, which wasn't the black metal army kind. It was a shiny, pug-nosed six-shooter.

They started waving their guns at us, just fooling, when a shot went off and hit a boy in the leg. He screamed and blood squirted out of the wound. We scattered. I bolted with my gun and bag of goodies. The bullies yelled for us to stop. I glanced back and a couple of them were after me and my six-shooter.

I fled down a dark alley, running by instinct, feeling my way with the tips of my fingers on the moist walls. Turn right. Run down another alley. Keep the gun. Drop the bag. Too heavy. Turn again. Run through a larger alley. They were closing in on me. I stumbled over trash. Kept going, heading for the clear up ahead.

Then I burst onto the street. Crashed into the flood of refugees swarming in one direction. Refuse covered the ground, stampeded over and over again. The air reeked of smoke, loud with people. Down the road, the fish market was burning unchecked. Gunfire snapped in staccato across the city. Somewhere far away a siren howled. Above, red zipping bullets crossed the night. The sky ruptured with false thunder. Dull flashes of light bruised the city skyline. Growling helicopters skimmed low, their humping air vibrating my ribs, their rope ladders trailing behind like kite tails.

I dove into the tide and was swept along with it. The air swelled with panic, lanced with torchlight. I ran with everyone else, coursing down the avenue. The crowd parted, then closed again around abandoned vehicles like a wild river. In the narrows, people crushed and hammered each other against the brick walls, stampeding, barreling to salvation—the American ships waiting in the harbor.

I had lost the bullies. I ran back to the house and pounded on the metal screen door, suddenly infected with the city's terror. *Let me in! Let me in! I want to come home!*

Strange-Hearth

The Nguyens' building is narrow and long, like a matchbox set on its striking side. Within its alley neighborhood, a two-floor cell block, each residence is sealed with a massive sliding steel door of mesh wire and bars. It is dark and quiet, everyone asleep.

"You should greet Granduncle first," Khuong whispers in my ear as we walk to the house. The alley too narrow, our minivan taxi dropped us off on the main street. *"Don't forget to bow deeply."*

I smile and thank him. He knows it is paramount that I don't give offense in my ignorance. Grandaunt unlocks the sliding gate and beckons her husband gently. Her sons and I wait in the alley. Granduncle comes to the door, smiling. He is a short, wiry man with a round, thinning head of hair.

"Greetings, Granduncle." I bow formally from the waist. *"It is me, your grandnephew, An. Are you well?"*

"Ah! Good! Good! I am well," he bubbles enthusiastically, seizing me by the shoulders. *"Good thing you made it."*

"I'm so sorry the plane was late and customs took so long. I apologize for keeping you up."

"Ah, it is nothing." He waves away my apologies. *"We welcome you inside. Let's go over here."*

Granduncle takes two steps across the alley and opens the steel door to another building. Viet goes into a third home just a door down. In a moment, lights are turned on in all three buildings as the Nguyen clan stirs awake to welcome me. My cousins and aunts step into the alley to touch me on the forearm—a welcoming gesture. They dash from one building to the next to rouse each other out of bed, the alley the communal hallway of their extended residences, all within two big steps of each other. Fourteen adults, children, and servants live here, three generations in three houses.

They give me a quick tour of the main house while a servant girl prepares the welcoming tea on a kerosene stove. Since it is late, the clan gives me a brief welcome around the dinner table with biscuits and tea. When I ask them about road conditions to Hanoi, Grandaunt launches into her litany of why I should abandon my trip.

"The roads are dangerous," she says. *"The country is not safe."*

"People are very poor," Granduncle adds, in agreement. *"This isn't Japan or America. This is worse than Mexico."* He's never been out of the country.

"They'll kill you for a bicycle," says Viet.

"I was stabbed right around the corner by two muggers. They wanted my motorcycle." Hung shows me the scar beneath his shirt.

"One thousand seven hundred kilometers on a bicycle to Hanoi! A bicycle! When your parents find out that you're going to ride a bicycle to Hanoi, they'll be sick with worries. Think about your parents. They didn't bring you into this world so you can waste your life. Be considerate. Don't do it. There's nothing out there but jungle and bandits. You'll die," Grandaunt concludes with absolute certainty.

By the time they bid me good night, I am thoroughly worried. Maybe they are right. After all, they've lived in Vietnam all their lives.

Hung grins at me with his big cherubic face. *"Don't look so glum. Leave it to me. I'll show you a good time in this city. The rest of the country is crap anyway,"* he says with the generosity of a dedicated host.

Hung has cleaned up his corner of the room. He emptied half of his clothes from the closet and drawers to make room for me. Hung offers me half of his queen-sized bed.

Awkward with Eastern sensibilities, I lie—the typical (and acceptable) Vietnamese thing to do. I say, *"Sometimes I get really violent in my sleep. I kick hard—a lot."*

Rubbing his vulnerable teddy-bear belly, Hung quickly acquiesces: *"Let's set you up on the army cot. The bed is a little lumpy anyway."*

Hung has brought his Vespa inside and parked it right next to his bed. Burglars once picked the padlock on the gate and made off with his last motorbike. We unfold an American army cot and wedge it between the Vespa and the dining table. He turns on two oscillating fans, one for each of us. *Mosquitoes,* he explains. I fall onto my cot dead with exhaustion, feeling like a side of meat protected from flies by the whirling fan.

In the morning, Viet, Hung, Khuong, and I go out for breakfast. We walk down the street past scores of diminutive eateries. The neighborhood food scene is the Vietnamese version of the Paris café-bistro life, discounted by a factor of twenty. The streets are twenty times dirtier, and much more crowded and loud. Old women sell food out of baskets. Knuckling their eyes, schoolchildren in white-and-blue uniforms jostle each other, crowding around the women to buy sweet rice, banana rice cakes, fried bread, baked goods, and rice porridge. We take one of the rusted tables lining an alley. A young boy immediately delivers three steaming bowls of beef noodle soup, each starring a six-inch section of ox tail. A rag of a mutt roots around under the tables for bones.

After the hour-long breakfast, we take my bike out to a major "auto shop," a ten-by-fifteen-foot storefront where a dozen mechanics tinker with bicycles and motorbikes. The vehicles are fixed right on the curb by grease-blackened men and boys who work with shoddy hand tools. The cement is runny with oil.

The bike needs a major tune-up after my one thousand miles in Japan, and I'm not up to it. The airport baggage handlers have damaged the rims beyond my ability to true them. The broken brake isn't working properly either, no matter how much I fiddle with it. Then there is the puncture in my "puncture-proof" tire. I carry three types of repair patches and try all of them, but Saigon's humidity foils every one.

The bike guru is a shirtless little Vietnamese, a five-foot-one, silver-haired grandfather. Since he is the shop's revered expert with the most seniority, the other mechanics defer to him the honor of working on my foreign bicycle. He spends a full five minutes marveling at my clunker, going over everything from the quick-release hubs to the grip-shifters to the cleat pedals. When he gets to work, he is amazingly fast. Somehow with a couple of wrenches, pliers, and a hot-patch press, he perfectly trues the wheel, fixes the brake, and gets the bike to purr like a kitten in twenty minutes.

He seems so enamored with the bike that I suggest he give it a test ride. At first he declines, claiming it is too big for him. I insist, and he capitulates with a childlike grin and leaps on it. How he manages to find the little pedals with his rubber flip-flops I don't know, but he speeds off around the city block like a racer, whooping and dodging traffic—wild as a teenager. He returns huffing, wet with sweat, rosy with pleasure. He wants to waive the fees, but I won't let him and settle the bill: $1 U.S.

Around sunset, Viet decides it would be funny to give me a tour of the city at rush hour, when the streets are legally open for trucks and every sort of traffic. Saigon is already so crowded its streets can't handle the large trucks and commercial vehicles during the day. City ordinance requires all vehicles larger than a minivan to park in sprawling dirt lots beyond the city limits and wait until 6 p.m. before assaulting the urbanscape.

Viet laughs when I ask him for a helmet. *"People can't even afford eyeglasses. Prescription glasses! And you're talking about a helmet? A helmet costs sixty American dollars—that's twice as much as a teacher makes a month. Nobody wears them anyway. It's too hot here, and people think you're scared if you wear a helmet."*

With that, he guns the Kawasaki down the alley, narrowly missing the kids playing soccer with a tennis ball. The roads are so people-thick I can reach out and touch four other motorists at any moment. Viet works the horn, the brakes, and the gas constantly. The whole time, all I can say is, *Oh, shit. Oh, God. Look out!* to which his reply is a published fact: head injuries resulting from traffic accidents are the number-one cause of accidental deaths in Saigon. I see no helmets and extremely few eyeglasses.

Nobody gives way to anybody. Everyone just angles, points, dives directly toward his destination, pretending it is an all-or-nothing gamble. People glare at one another and fight for maneuvering space. All parties are equally determined to get the right-of-way—insist on it. They swerve away at the last possible moment, giving scant inches to spare. The victor goes forward, no time for a victory grin, already engaging in another contest of will. Saigon traffic is Vietnamese life, a continuous charade of posturing, bluffing, fast moves, tenacity, and surrenders.

Viet veers, a second from being broadsided by another motorist. I panic, lose balance, and wrap my arms around his torso.

Viet shouts over his shoulder, somewhat embarrassed: *"Hey! Don't worry! It happens all the time. Just stop octopusing me. It's not manly. Only women do that."*

After I reluctantly untangle my arms from around him, he says, *"Now, sit up straight. Don't slouch. And put your hands on your knees. It'll help you keep balanced. If you have to grab something, grab the seat. Just don't grab me."*

"Yeah, right." I don't trust him and prepare to abandon ship at the first sign of an imminent hit. Twice motorbikes graze my legs. Within fifteen minutes, we see three accidents, one of which is serious, involving a cyclo and a motorcycle.

The air becomes toxic, unbreathable as all of Saigon struggles to get home from schools, market, and work, and all the commerce from the rest of the country pours into the crazed streets. In their blue-and-white uniforms, children ant out from their school, eager to go home, to play. High school girls in their impeccable white *ao dai* uniforms, as pretty and perfect as unlit candles, wiggle their bicycles through snarls of minivans, construction rigs, eight-wheeler trucks, cars, and ox-drawn wagons. Construction workers push carts loaded with bricks and sand. Peasants ride motorbikes hitched to produce carts. Pedestrians cross the roads in clusters, holding hands and eyeing the oncoming motorists, mincing through the mad roar slowly, careful to keep their profile to a minimum.

The intersections are the worst, particularly for those who need to make a left. Traffic lights are rare. Where there is one, there is never a turn signal. When Viet wants to make a turn, he simply does it, plunges in ahead of the coming traffic, hoping that his timing is right so they don't run us over. He goes into it, blasting his horn, dodging moving obstacles as aggressively as everyone else.

At the free-for-all junctions, Viet waits until enough traffic going in our direction accumulates—this never takes more than ten or fifteen seconds—and moves forward with the flow when our team inches into the intersection. With such a large contingent, the cross traffic screeches to a halt to prevent collision. But close calls and accidents—if one can call them that—are common, so Viet instinctively worms into the center of the pack to minimize our chances of being hammered on either flank. *Do it the Vietnamese way,* he hollers at me. *Let others take the risk. Travel on their lee and let them take the hits.* It is more difficult than it sounds because everyone else uses the same principles. No one wants to get hit, but there's always a hothead who happily leads the effort.

We park the motorcycle in front of a fancy saloon. Viet hands over his motorcycle to an attendant like a cowboy handing over horse reins. He tosses the boy a dime bill and tells him to wipe down the seat. The boy mumbles, *Yes, sir,* hands Viet a numbered ticket, and walks the vehicle into the sidewalk parking lot, corralled off by ropes.

Inside the bar, Viet introduces me to his friend Binh, a successful tour operator. I flag the waiter for a round of Saigon 333 Beer, a brew waterier than Coors. We start shelling boiled peanuts and exchanging jokes.

Binh is a short, rotund man whose sun-dark face is even merrier than Viet's. *"So, Brother-friend,"* he drawls to me after the third round. *"Brother Viet tells me you're planning to ride your bicycle alone to Hanoi."* He eyes me closely. *"True, no?"*

"First, I'm going to ride out to Vung Tau and sit on the beach. Then I'll ride north to visit Phan Thiet, my hometown. From there, I'll head north on

Highway 1 all the way to Hanoi. What do you think? You're a tour guide, how's the road to Hanoi?"

"Not good. Very dangerous," he replies. "You know that's seventeen hundred kilometers—over one thousand and two hundred of your American miles."

On cue, Viet asks his friend, "Don't you have a group bike tour coming up in a few weeks?"

"Yes, I do. Maybe, you, Brother An, should join my group. I'm organizing a bike tour from Saigon to Hanoi for fifty-two foreigners. Two of them are Viet-kieu like yourself. We'll have two support buses, one in front of the bikers, one behind. We'll be staying in hotels and eating in restaurants all the way up there. It'll be fun and safe. Look, I'll waive my fees. You'll just pay for your own expenses."

"Thanks, Brother-friend, but I've got my mind set on going alone."

Viet and Binh shake their heads. Binh lowers his voice and tells me, "I don't mean to insult you, but I must tell you it is very difficult and very dangerous. I've taken several tour groups to Hanoi. Many people just give up and ride in the bus. I've never biked it myself. I ride in the bus and hand out sodas to people. Listen to me, my friend. Don't do it."

"Why? I've read about one American who did it by himself. I'm sure there must be a few others, maybe Europeans, who have made solo bike tours."

Binh hesitates as though considering whether to let me in on a secret. He draws a deep breath, leans closer, and says with utter conviction, "You won't make it. Trust me, I've been around a long time. Vietnamese just don't have that sort of physical endurance and mental stamina. We are weak. Only Westerners can do it. They are stronger and better than us."

Fallen-Leaves

 11 An was four, playing in cheese-colored dirt, watching his truckload of big brothers feathering the blue horizon with dust. His mother had his nine-year-old sister Chi keep an eye on him lest he decide to eat a rock or something.

The green army truck listed from side to side as it kicked sand into the air. The men were yelling, hollering, whooping. The truck stopped, its cloud dissipating onward. Soldiers vaulted out of its tarpaulin back like grasshoppers. Some ran straight into the big plywood house for beer, others stretched and clapped their hands in great pleasure. Giant white men with hair as gold as the chain around his mother's neck tousled An's black hair. He liked their marble eyes, the colors of sky and shallow water. He liked the way they tried to teach him games. They picked him up, grinning, and said words he did not understand. They smelled strange, different, and they moved about with a booming bigness. They planed him through the air, rocketed him into the sky, and gently parachuted him to the ground every time. His father didn't do that, big government official, big businessman, too busy.

A huge black man came out of the truck. He had a head of curly, crinkly black hair as though someone had singed it with a match. An had never seen a man like that. Chi said the man was an Indian, a black Indian as opposed to the green, purple, and red varieties. She said he was made of chocolate. Try it, Chi told An. He ran up and bit the man's forearm. It was salty.

The man yelped and gave An a stick of spearmint gum to teeth on.

Divergent-Rhythm

Hung is a filmmaker. He wears slacks, a white pin-striped shirt, and a dark thin tie. In sunglasses, he strikes a good image of Jim Belushi. The world moves through his viewfinder as one endless stream of pleasures, ripe for his plucking. He ravishes everything that comes his way. He has a weakness for liquor and women. He has studied art, film, photography, but finds himself making a living at producing wedding videos and studio portraits. He earns a small fortune and enjoys frittering it all away. A prodigious beer drinker who harbors serious aversions to physical labor, he lives his life in spurts, in volcanic bouts of work, frolic, drinking, whoring, and sheer listless idleness where he listens to music lying on his back, staring at the ceiling like one gone permanently vacant.

He has an artist's perspective: *"I'm not fat and I'm not obese. I'm something in between—very beautiful, very lovable—undefinable."*

When his mother scolds him about his lack of savings, he grabs the thick rolls around his belly and gives them a good shake. *"I saved it all right here. This is Cho-Lon, Big Market of concentrated food. I'll never starve."*

His nieces and nephews are afraid of him, as kids often are with someone unstable. Sometimes he gives them exorbitant gifts, other times he slaps and kicks them with such fury one might think him drunk, which usually is the case. It is hard to tell with Hung because, unlike most Vietnamese, he doesn't color when he's drunk. I know he's soaked when he starts talking about himself.

"Shit. I haven't seen my wife and my daughter in four years. If I'm lucky, I'll see them again in four more years. My daughter won't remember me."

His wife had taken their daughter to America. Their immigration was sponsored by her mother, who fled to the States in '75 when Saigon fell. The rules permitted sponsoring immediate family members only, no in-laws. She left during the lean years, when they were suffering like everyone else. Hung thought maybe they would be together in two or three years, but the bureaucrats leeched him of all his savings and now he is no closer to emigrating than he was when she left. He keeps a shoe box full of pictures of her and their daughter by his bed.

He shows me a picture of his wife and daughter in Virginia standing in front of their new Honda Accord parked in the driveway of their house. Eyes lowered, he asks, *"Is . . . is this common in America?"* The material wealth. What he means is, *Can I have this too when I get there? Has my wife passed beyond my means? Does she really need me anymore?*

Much later during one of our drinking binges, he comes out with it: *"Tell me honestly, in your best opinion, can I make a living over there? Is there enough work for a video guy like me? Do I have to learn something else?"*

"No, there aren't many Vietnamese in Virginia. You might be able to make it in Santa Ana, California, or maybe in Houston, Texas, or maybe in the Bay Area, or New York. Video cameras are as common as televisions in America. You might have to start from zero again. Build up your reputation. You'll have to learn to speak English fluently or you'll have to rely on the Vietnamese for all your business. That's tough because plenty of Vietnamese are already doing it."

Then there is Khuong, the good son, the respectable, promising academic. Hardworking, studious, he is the most cosmopolitan of the lot, open to modern attitudes and not so fearful of places outside of Saigon. He is the only one who thinks that a solo bike trip to Hanoi is possible.

"I've met two European women who have done it, but they biked together," he says. *"You could do it, but you should pretend you're Korean or Japanese in case you run into those who don't like Viet-kieu."*

His eldest brother, Viet, holds the opposite view. Viet is sharp and streetwise but he prefers to be the affable bear. I like him immensely. He grills me day and night on English grammar, idiom, and slang.

"How do you say breasts, women's breasts, in English slang?"

"Tits?"

"No, I mean slang. Playing words. Things Americans say on the street."

"Melons, cantaloupes, knockers," I offer. He repeats them carefully. I explain to him the subtleties behind the slang, but I'm not sure of them myself so I make it up as I go.

"Well, melons and cantaloupe, that should be self-explanatory. The shape and the perfume, I guess. Knockers *are these things people mount on their door. They've got handles that you grab and bang to let the people know that you're at the front door. Like a doorbell."*

"Ha, ha, ha. I get it! Grabbing women's breasts so they'll let you in. Give me another one."

"Hmm. Headlights."

"Headlights? Like on motorbikes?"

"Well, everyone has a car in America. A car has a pair of headlights. Big, round, very bright."

"Ha, ha, ha!" He doubles over, clutching his belly, slapping his thighs. *"That's great! Lowbeam. Highbeam. You're blinded! Ooooo-hooo!"* He sighs with satisfaction. *"That's great! What do Americans call a butt licker?"*

"A brownnoser," I tell him. *"That's like a sycophant. A brownnoser kisses his boss's butt and his nose is brown with his boss's shit."* This one is his favorite. He pens it on the front page of the pocket notebook he carries with his wallet. Viet is trying to solicit Western business partners and worries they might use similar terms on him.

Viet holds a master's degree in chemistry. This is no small feat in a school system with a seventy-percent attrition rate. He has worked in various factories, making anything from soap to pesticide. He struck gold four years ago when he perfected a soda flavor that could compete with Tribeco, the dominant soft-drink producer at the time. His one-man company rocketed into a thirty-employee operation that manufactured and distributed soft drinks throughout southern Vietnam. His backslide began two years ago, when Pepsi appeared on the scene. By the time Coca-Cola returned to Vietnam's market, his operation had dwindled to seven employees. He says the American giants are selling their drinks below cost to steal his market share.

"Look, I'm selling soda that's mixed and bottled by hand. Labor cost is almost nil for me. I don't build big plants. No executives and no managers. No bribes. You know how I handle the bad cops? Sodas! I give them sodas! All foreign companies pay tax-bribes. You tell me, how can they sell a better-tasting soft drink cheaper!"

Now he's deep in debt, teetering on the verge of bankruptcy, but he keeps a grin on his broad, dark face and tastes all the imitation cola flavors Japanese and Korean vendors hawk to him. Within a few months, he will lose his business and his home. Pepsi and Coca-Cola will win.

I suspect I will remember my days in Saigon through an alcoholic haze. We drank when I arrived, then we drink just about every other day thereafter. One at a time, they take turns dragging me to street-corner saloons, Vietnamese equivalents of the Spanish *tapas* bars that serve little food dishes to accompany alcohol. We squeeze ourselves into child-sized plastic chairs and drink beer from plastic one-liter jugs and nibble on barbecued beef, steamed intestines, pan-fried frogs, and boiled peanuts. We eat goat stew and drink goat liquor, two parts rice wine mixed with one part fresh goat's blood. Halfway through the meal, my bowels heave and I sprint to the toilet.

During the second week, Viet, Khuong, Hung, and I motorbike out to Snake Village, a good jaunt from Saigon. Their restaurant-bar of choice has thatched walls and a low ceiling made of corrugated aluminum. In the back, a fine mesh of chicken wire fences in two trees and a snake pit. A young woman is standing in one of the trees pulling poisonous snakes out of the branches by their tails.

We take a coffee table with wooden stools. The waiter serves us a platter of appetizers, an array of pickled fish, fresh herbs, sliced cucumber, and vegetables.

Khuong seems irritated. *"Why don't you eat the vegetables? They're washed."*

"Viet-kieu's fickleness causes a lot of problems. Refusing to eat the same food as your hosts makes them think that you think you're too good for them.

Their food is filthy, unfit for you," Hung carols to me, joking, but I get his drift.

"Well, I've eaten everything you've handed me and I've got the runs twice in two weeks," I reply in mock reproach. *"I can't go anywhere without looking for the toilet, thanks to you guys. Isn't that enough?"*

They laugh, mollified. The waiter arrives with warm beer, pours it into plastic mugs, and drops chunks of ice into them. I snatch one without ice.

"Ice. Why are you afraid of ice? All the bacteria are dead, frozen," Viet complains.

I look at him, incredulous. *"And you have a master's in chemistry? Guess that didn't include a biology class, did it?"*

The bartender, a shriveled man with the pinched face of someone bitten a hundred times, lugs a basket of live, two-foot-long cobras to the table. He reaches inside casually—a magician going for a rabbit— and pulls out a cobra. He whacks its head sharply with a mallet. The snake goes limp in his hand. With a deft glide of his short knife, he opens a slit in the scales, a perfect surgical incision. Blood drips onto his hand. Puffing a cigarette held at the corner of his mouth, he plucks open the skin and shows the beating heart, the size of a chocolate chip, to everyone at the table. Working with the boredom of a shrimper, he severs the arteries and transplants the heart into a shot glass half filled with rice wine. The heart pulses swirling red streamers of blood into the clear liquor.

Viet seizes the glass and shoots it down his throat. The idea is to swallow the concoction before the heart stops beating. Viet smacks his lips, grunts, and grins blissfully. The snake master tosses the carcass to the waiter, who flays it and has the meat grilling over coals before it is Hung's turn to drink. After Khuong, it is my turn.

"No, I can't do it," I object flatly.

"You've got to."

"It's good for your libido."

"I'm not worried about my libido."

The bartender, sensing some fun to be had, becomes animated. *"Young man,"* he says, gesturing grandly with the bleeding cobra in hand. *"I've drunk heart-liquor once every week for forty-three years. Keeps me healthy. Eleven children, six grandchildren,"* he announces, tapping his chest with the handle of the knife. *"It's good for you. Gives you strength. Look at me, I'm not dead."*

"Don't be such a wimp, drink up!" They pound the table.

I look at the bartender's poisoned body with misgivings. By now the entire place, some two dozen drinkers, has taken an interest in my cowardice. A few enthusiastically cheer me on, spieling a list of beneficial properties and incredible cures.

"Drink up," orders Hung, serious now. It is his show, his idea to blow a week's earnings on this excursion, and he has counted on me to reciprocate his friendship with my follow-through. *"You said you want to be Vietnamese. You want to try everything we do. It doesn't get more Vietnamese than this."*

I nod.

The heart drops into the glass. I toss it back, my throat locks. I feel the squishy live organ, tapioca-like, on my tongue. I double over and retch it onto the floor, alcohol up my nose, burning. Hung pounds my back. The audience hoots with laughter.

That is how Vietnamese men bond. We only talk when we drink. Two nights a week, the three brothers and I drink at home on the floor, a bottle of Johnnie Walker in the center of our circle like a campfire. Viet sends his nephew Nghia down the alley to bang on the door of a neighbor who sells dried fish and squid. Nghia's mother roasts the fish over coals and serves it to us with plates of pickles and chili paste.

The women and children always keep clear of the men when we drink. Viet is fond of declaring loud enough for everyone to hear, *"We are dealing in men's business. Let us be."*

Viet, the oldest male present, ceremoniously starts us off. He pours himself a shot, tosses it back, harrumphs, grins, pours another shot into the same glass, and passes it clockwise. While the next comrade regards his shot of whiskey, Viet gnaws on bits of smoked fish. The four of us do the rounds, drink the shot, pour another, pass it on, eat a piece of fish, over and over until Johnnie is gone. As long as the booze flows, we are free to talk about anything we want. Free to confide our hopes and fears. We chase it all down with a couple of beers, then disband, each to his own bed to sleep it off. The women clean up our mess as we pass out.

A night like this runs about twenty-five dollars. Many Vietnamese men drink up half of what they make, treating each other to round after round of beer, liquor, whatever is at hand. Their women make do with the money left over, splurging on things for themselves, like material for a new dress, bowls of noodle soup at the market, maybe a cyclo ride.

The Nguyen women are mysteries to me. Thuy is the dutiful daughter. Viet's wife, Mo, is the respectful and obedient daughter-in-law. Together Thuy and Mo devote half of their days to cooking, cleaning, and caring for the entire clan, sharing labor and responsibilities. Mo dotes on her two children. Thuy has a passion for Western clothing. Her husband is a tailor. She likes to sew new clothes fashioned after styles she sees in Western magazines.

The oldest daughter, Hanh, teaches English for a living. Her husband was a Vietnamese Nationalist soldier who was exposed to Agent Orange during his tour of duty. He died eleven years ago when Han, their only child, was four. Han suffers from mental disorders, retardation, and epileptic seizures. Her spine is deformed and she has a clawed hand, which the family covers with a knitted mitt tied so securely she cannot tear it off.

Hanh is an aging orchid, a gentle beauty who cannot understand why her womb birthed such pain in her only child. She is poor, and without her family there would be no way she could care for Han. At thirty-six, her prospects for a second marriage are dim. Vietnamese men, even much older ones, prefer to marry young women, certainly not an older woman with a handicapped child.

Moving in the rhythm of their lives, I grow fond of them all. I hear their quiet arguments. Through their amiable ways, I learn about myself and what would have been. But it is Hung who unwittingly shows me his Saigon, a Saigon that I could never forget. Hung and I are the same age, both artists after a fashion. Rebels even, by our own reckoning. He takes me into the depths of the city, parades me on the back of his beat-up '68 Vespa through every hole and dive. He introduces me to Son.

I believe there are only a handful of men like Son in the world. Likable men who embrace vices in such measure and style that it is difficult to hate them. Son is a womanizer, a photographer, a pimp, a Taoist, a poet, a Buddhist, a drunk, a Catholic, a polygamist, a philosopher—a dreamer. One of the two living Vietnamese Green Berets and a survivor of four plane crashes, he believes he is blessed, living a roguish life at top volume like a child, almost innocent by amorality. Together, Hung and Son show me every vice, depravity. They seek generously to share their world with me, never realizing that their diverting marvels are my wounding horrors.

Dying-Angels

The stars gleamed around an emptied moon. A cool breeze rolled off the ocean over the surf, across a road that paralleled the beach, and into the coconut field, combing up the foothills where we hid among the sounding crickets. We hunkered down in the brush, twenty yards of coconut palms separating us and the road. Tien huddled with Huy on my right, whispering so softly I could not make out his words. Bundled in a blanket at my feet, Hien, the four-year-old, wheezed through his snot, eased from crying into slumber by Mom's sleeping pills. She crouched nearby, keeping one eye on us, the other on the road, where Auntie Dung and Chi waited to flag down Dad. We had been hiding since dusk, nearly six hours in one spot. I was crumbling with fear that my friend Hoa had told someone who might have gone to the police. Mom thought I had eaten something bad. She kept urging me to go up the hill and empty my bowels. I wanted to confess. I was sure Dad had been caught. It was 11 p.m. He was two hours late.

Sounds of shuffling. Chi came hunched over, then Auntie Dung and Dad. He checked on us and reassured us, patting each in turn. We lay on the sand and waited. Midnight came and went without sign of the boat. Dad said that they had agreed to wait an hour beyond midnight for the fishermen. We waited, but I could tell Mom and Dad were very worried, their panic rising with every minute.

I prayed with all my heart that we wouldn't get caught, that my big mouth hadn't brought the police on the entire family. The wind shook loose a star and it flashed down the sky. Chi, lying beside me, said each star was an angel, and a falling star was a dying angel. She said angels died to balance the world's good and evil. I counted three disappearing and, feeling very sick, I kept the omen to myself.

Standing ahead of us and wearing dark clothes almost indistinguishable from the trunks of the palms, Chi and Auntie scanned the ocean for signs of the boat. Huy, Tien, and Hien dozed side by side. Mom and Dad crouched a few feet from me, arguing about why the boat was over an hour late. Dad said to Mom that they should stick with the plan and abandon the beach. Mom shook her head, saying she had a strong hunch that the boat was on its way. He gave in as he usually did when she had a strong feeling about something. Another hour ticked by. Dad became jittery, constantly fumbling with the flashlight intended for signaling the boat if it ever came.

"We've got to go back now," he whispered to Mom. "We wait anymore and sunrise will catch us out on the road." The plan was for everyone but Dad to return to Grandma's house. He would hide out somewhere else until Mom sent word that everything was all right.

"They're coming. Just bear it out a little longer," Mom said calmly. She had entered her strange state of total conviction based on her gut feeling. Nothing could sway her.

Chi and Auntie came back, pointing at a blotch of darkness edging into the bay. It was very faint, its outline blending with the rippling water. Wringing the flashlight, Dad groaned that it might be a patrol boat or worse—one in disguise. Mom urged him to flash them. At last, Dad held out the flashlight covered with a cardboard cone he fashioned to focus the beam. One short flick of the button. The torch stabbed out at the darkness, giving us a sudden jolt of exposure.

No reply. Chi woke Huy and Tien. We had to run soon, either to the beach or into the hills, but we were moving for sure. Wait. Dad aimed the flashlight again and gave it another flick. Nothing. Mom was mumbling now, not so sure anymore. Dad wrung the flashlight in his hands. Mom and Dad eyed each other. The third flash was to be last, that was the plan. No reply meant the mission was aborted. The boat hadn't moved for five minutes. Dad raised the flashlight and sent the last beam out to the ocean.

A light winked back from the boat, twice. Dad flicked out the code: short–long–short. Back came long–short–short: everything fine. Dad gave the word and we dashed to the beach. Dad carried Hien. Everyone except Huy and Tien had a bag to carry. I ran after them, bringing up the rear.

A fallen branch tangled my feet and I pitched face first into the sand with a yelp. Disoriented, I fumbled for my bag, digging the sand out of my eye. Terrified of being left behind, I wanted to call out but I didn't dare. I was flailing when a hand lifted me by the elbow.

It was Chi. "I've got your bag," she whispered. "Hold onto my hand."

I clung to it fiercely with one hand and knuckled sand out of my eyes with the other. We crossed the road and stumbled to the beach. Men ran out of the waves toward us. They came out of the night ocean, swimming, running like fish growing legs, becoming men. The water exploded moonlight around them. I was terrified, unsure of who they were until they were upon us. Our young fishermen were as frightened as we were. Silently, they grabbed our luggage and tugged us into the waves. Three men swept up Huy, Tien, and Hien, piggybacking them into the water. Mom, Dad, Auntie, and Chi ran into the surf and began to swim for the boat. I splashed in after them. It wasn't as cold as I'd anticipated. Maybe I was so scared I couldn't feel the sting. Although the boat was only fifty yards from shore, it seemed a mile off. I kicked and windmilled my arms as hard as I could, but the waves kept nudging me back to shore. I fell behind. Panic set in as my limbs began to tire. No. I don't want to be left behind. I shouted for them to wait, but saltwater filled my mouth. The only sound was me sputtering.

A dark form turned back toward me. It was Tai, the captain. With me clinging to his neck, he plowed over the swell like a fish. He heaved me into the boat and climbed in, the last one aboard. There was barely any room to sit. The boat wasn't much bigger than the ones Chi and I found abandoned on the beach. It was ten meters,

roughly thirty feet, about the length of five big beds placed end to
end. Dad was talking furiously with Tai and Hanh, the first mate.
Mom hissed for them to get going.

Someone started the engine. It rattled, coughed. Nothing. He tried
it again and again. Same result. Mom was clutching the jade Buddha
pendant around her neck. A sick silence engulfed us. Dad looked afraid,
his face so very gaunt in the moonlight. We crouched helplessly, watching the man inside the tiny engine house mid-deck. On the fourth try,
the engine heaved to life, and the pilot pointed us out to the dark.

Huddling on the smooth wooden deck, I steadied myself against
the gunwale as the boat rose and dipped with the waves. I flattened my
palms against the smooth planks and felt the engine vibrating, clacking
like a big baby rattle. Hien was snoring, drugged to the whole experience. Huy and Tien changed into dry clothes and, already bored,
curled up to sleep. I was cold, tired, but I was too scared and excited to
sleep. I had never been in a boat before.

The fishing boat had four sections. The foredeck was used to store
sailing gear. It was also the head, the toilet a gallon tin can. We
crowded just aft, on the holding deck where the fish usually go. There
wasn't enough room for everyone to lie down so we took turns. I sat
against the shallow gunwale, hugging my knees to save space, worried
that one good lurch of the boat could pitch me overboard. Behind
me was the engine house. It provided access to our stash of food,
water, and diesel below deck. One man always stayed inside to keep
an eye on the engine and the seawater sloshing in the bilge. Most of
the crew congregated in the stern cockpit. It was slightly larger than
the mid-deck, but, with the pilot and the big tiller, two men had to
sit on the roof of the engine house.

Dad was arguing with Tai at the stern, furious about the two extra
young men whom he had never met. They weren't part of the plan.
He didn't trust them. Seventeen people were too much for a tiny
boat. How could we clear land before sunrise? Tai shrugged, they
were his cousins. He pointed at the beach, saying that he had forgotten about the tide change. The grounded boat wouldn't budge until
the tide returned. Dad was angry that the new deckhands were too
inexperienced. They were both seventeen. Tai was twenty-five and

his first mate, Hanh, was twenty-two. The crew milled about, re-arranging bags of provisions and jugs of water, looking uncomfortable.

A faint seam of violet was opening on the horizon when every-thing happened at once. Without enough room to sit on deck, the men started to throw their fishing net overboard, pretending to be laying out their net in case someone was watching from ashore. As the net was paid out to port, the boat was turned slightly in the same direction to keep the net from fouling the propeller. Within minutes, the engine died. The man in the engine house was frantic, shouting that it sounded as though something inside the engine broke. The boat slowed, then stopped, bobbing in the swells like a cork. The men scrambled, trying to figure out what happened.

"The net is caught in the propeller!" a crewman cried. Our inex-perienced pilot had not kept the boat on a steady port curve. When a large swell had gone under the keel, he overcorrected to starboard, swinging the stern directly into the net-curtain. The propeller sucked up the lines until it choked.

Someone pointed to a pinpoint light—a patrol boat—rounding the peninsula behind us to port. "Down, down! Everybody down," ordered Tai. "Keep working the net like you're fishing."

We lay down. I peeped over the side at the white dot in the dis-tance. It seemed to just hover on the water. Not coming closer, not going away. Waiting. One of the men slipped over the side with a knife to cut the propeller loose. Another followed with a flashlight. We bobbed in the waves, helpless. A man surfaced, sputtering that the other man was tangled in the net. Three more went over the side with knives. An eternity sloshed by. They all came up. The rescued man was pulled onboard, coughing seawater, his leg bleeding from a superficial cut. Someone muttered that blood attracted sharks.

Two men went back down to hack the net from the propeller. They couldn't get it off. The strands were too strong, wound too tightly around the shaft. There wasn't a knife sharp enough among them, though they all had knives to fight Thai pirates. Six men, all capable divers, took their turns against the net. Tai, the best swimmer and strongest man aboard, was under hacking madly until they pulled him aboard like a dead fish. Mom burrowed into her bags and produced a cooking knife she had impulsively seized from the family altar the day before during prayer. Hanh slid into the water with it. Mom was in the throes of her "feeling" again, whispering to everyone that her "prayer-sent knife" was equal to the job. The outline of the patrol boat came toward us slowly from port. Standing on the foredeck, a pair of crewmen made a show of pulling in the net.

Tai surfaced on the starboard side, hidden from the patrol boat. The knife was sharp, he gasped. It was cutting through the net. Tai relayed the blade to Tieu, who slipped overboard to take his turn underwater. The patrol boat was only a few hundred yards off. A pair of crewmen stood, fussing with the net. The rest of us lay flat on deck, out of sight. The patrol boat slowed, then veered slightly from us, heading to shore. The sun's crown was nudging out of the water, its aurora blossoming a nub of orange. Figures of men were visible on the other boat. They must have thought we were fishermen since our net was out and we weren't making for the open sea.

A quiet cheer went up when Tieu surfaced and announced that the propeller was freed. They waited until the patrol boat was well out of sight and started up the engine. Again we headed out, this time toward the sunrise. There was no doubt among the crew that, had our boat been running, the patrol would have given chase. Our misfortune saved us.

Afternoon of our first day on the ocean, we sighted a small freighter. Although the fishermen claimed it was a good sailing day, sunny, moderate wind, average seven-foot waves, we were seasick. Except for Dad, who seemed to be holding up, Mom, Chi, Auntie, and us boys vomited, making the deck slippery. I felt horrible. My stomach fisted. Sour mush gushed out of my mouth. I broke out in a cold sweat, curling up in my own fish-smelling fluid. The sun yo-yoed across the sky. It was hot, white, and round—like the pearls Mom had sewn into the crotch of my pants for safekeeping. My skin hurt, burning. I couldn't keep food down. None of the women and children could. The men, on the other hand, were in high spirits, joking and singing as though we were all on a holiday.

It was a long time after they sighted the ship that I could distinguish it from the sea behind us. No one could tell what type of ship it was.

With neither radio nor binoculars, there was no way to tell from which country the ship hailed. The men agreed that it must be a Vietnamese or a Russian ship because we hadn't gone far since dawn. At full speed, our fishing boat made eight, maybe nine knots—a little under ten miles per hour. We couldn't have been more than fifty miles offshore. Tai took the tiller and swung us away from the direction of the ship, but, a few minutes later, it seemed as though the ship had changed course. It was coming closer, and now we could make out its bow, pointing straight at us. Dad told Mom to make a Japanese flag. One of the men dove below and brought up her satchel. Mom started working furiously, digging out her red dress and a white sheet she brought in case we needed it for bandages. She couldn't thread a needle in the lurching boat, so she used safety pins. In minutes, we had a Japanese flag, a red dot on a white sheet. They hoisted it high at the stern. Tai kept us steady on course. Then all we could do was sit and wait.

The younger crewmen started to panic. There was talk of getting rammed or captured. Manh, who couldn't swim, was terrified. I didn't know enough to be scared until I saw Dad's face. The last time he looked like that, we were imprisoned and he nearly got executed. Mom shut her eyes tightly, head bowed, and prayed and prayed so hard I was sure we were as good as caught. I thought what a shame it was since I was just beginning to feel less seasick. And it was such a nice day to be out on the ocean—water, sky, and sunshine all the way around as far as my eyes could see.

Alley-World

14   I sit at the table with my bicycle, sweating. The mid-morning breeze curling in from the alley singes. Granduncle Nguyen brings me a hot cup of espresso sweetened with condensed milk. He has made me one every morning since I came back to Saigon. It is a considerate courtesy which he can ill afford and which I cannot drink because it is too sweet. Telling him would be an unbearable breach of manners. So I bow saying, *Thank you, Granduncle. You shouldn't have. Mmmm, it's delicious.* And dump it down the toilet.

I take a cup of tea up a creaky ladder to the sun-drenched roof. In tropical Vietnam, the roof serves the same function as the American basement: a junk depot. I spider across the ramshackle storage shed, rainwater cisterns, and garden, entangling myself in a maze of laundry lines. Toward the front of the building, right up against the barbed wire that discourages burglars from prowling the rooftop, I duck under the wet laundry and settle down on a large old U.S. Army ammunition box, rusted in jungle-green paint, the rectangular kind that makes a good field stool. I rearrange the wet clothes into a shelter to soften the sun's sting. Under cotton underwear and fake Levi's, between a potted pepper plant and a tomato plant, I sip my tea and watch life unfolding in the alley. Nostalgia descends on me like a sweet sickness. I have done this often, long ago in my tower above the alley of my childhood.

My room overlooked the lane behind our house. Back then, the city streets forbidden to me, I spent the bulk of my childhood in a nook, scarcely larger than a closet, but hardly big enough to be called a room. I had fancied it a nest or a sort of treehouse, for it was built into the landing of the stairwell between the first and second floors, almost a secret space, above the kitchen and below the bathroom. It was six by eight feet with a single bare light bulb screwed into a socket on a low ceiling I could touch standing on a footstool. In the far corner, two small windows were set together at a right angle like a contracted bay window so that they jutted out the back of the building, giving a prime view of all the happenings up and down the alley.

Two bookcases lined the opposing walls. The shelves sagged with books, some mine, most my father's. A portable AM radio sat next to the pen and inkwell on a board nailed into the wall nearest the windows to serve as a writing ledge. I used the varnished flat top of a wooden trunk set against the fourth wall as a napping spot. In the sunny season, the wooden planks were cool to the touch, but my sweat would make the varnish sticky. In the rainy season, the planks were cold and I would cover them with a straw mat.

From the windowsill, my favorite reading spot, I watched, smelled, and listened to the alley-world outside. A stone's throw down the path, the alley dead-ended at the side of a sooty building with a big dark door. That was where my uncle Hung, who stayed with us months at a time, sent me bodily out of the house, with a smack behind the head and a boot on the rear, to fetch his favorite snacks—beer, cigarettes, and ginger-roasted dog meat.

They dragged five or six dogs in there each day. The dogs barked, howled often through the night. In the morning, they hung the dogs just inside the door by their hind legs and used a cleaver to cut their throats. Sometimes the wind skirled in the alley and brought the reek of guts and blood mingled with smoke to my window.

But there were many other odors of the market that came up

from the alley. A dumpling bar crowded a corner three doors down from ours. A fat woman sat in the center surrounded by four big pans on which she poured, steamed, and rolled pork dumplings like crepes. Two low bars fenced in the woman and her daughter, who helped from behind. One the other side, customers crouched on footstools and ate her fresh dumplings with garlic-chili fishsauce. Across from the alley, the Chinese medicine shop, a narrow one-door one-window establishment, smelled of pungent herbs and faintly sweet medicines.

Then there were those who brought their business to the alley in baskets to sell as they sat on wood blocks, backs to the walls. Up and down the crowded alley shoppers, pressing past each other, bargained with vegetable vendors, tofu women, noodle sellers, sausage makers, fortune-tellers, and trinket merchants. The aromas of food battered the stink of the alley. Above the din of the market were the shouts of playing children.

As a child, I spent all my time in this room, especially when my parents locked me in the house for days while they went out of town on business trips. It wasn't too bad because I had a friend. She was my age and she lived on the first floor of the building behind ours. It had a folding metal rail door that her parents always kept locked. At night, when the shops closed and the alley merchants had gone home, she came to the front. Hands on the bars and face looking out between them, she talked with me.

"What happened at school today?" she hollered up across the alley.

"Not much. The teacher hit my hand with the ruler."

"Again? I thought you studied."

"I did. I always get so nervous in front of class I can't recite my lesson. What about you?"

She grinned. "I got good marks for my lessons. They don't hit us so much at my school."

"I wish I could go to your school. I don't belong in mine."

She went to a public school and so did all my brothers and older sister. I was the first son, so my parents put aside a small fortune to enroll me in the best school in the country, a private French institution for boys. All the other kids were rich and smart. I was neither. My clothes were always older than theirs and they all had private tutors.

I turned on my radio, the volume way up, and we sang along and danced. Then she shifted her television so I could watch cartoons with my father's pocket binoculars. She was my best friend, although we never met beyond her bars and my window.

Things changed after the country fell. Mom and I came back to the house after our imprisonment. Chi, Huy, and Hien boarded with Grandma Le. Tien went back to live with Grandma and Grandpa Pham. I stayed with Mom. She busied herself with getting Dad out of prison. We always went out to Minh Luong Prison and Labor Camp together, but I stayed home alone when she went to various cities to petition for Dad's release. As part of her preparation, she cooked me her "magic pot" of catfish. She'd take half of the fish to eat on her journey and leave me the clay pot with the other half, giving me the choicest meat, the part just behind the head.

She locked me inside our three-story building and said, "By the time you finish this pot, I'll be home."

So I ate it fast. It was all gone in two days. There was nothing left in the clay pot except sauce, bones, and the big catfish head. I had saved every scrap of fish, bones and all, like Mom told me, and put them back into the pot after every meal. Then I would give it a squirt of fishsauce and bring the pot to a boil. For the next meal, I would add a little water, maybe a dash of pepper, and boil it again. When there was no more meat, the pot magically kept on yielding plenty of pep-pery, fishy, sweet, salty, buttery sauce, tasty enough to be poured on plain white rice for a meal. And sure enough, Mom came home before the clay-pot catfish ran out of magic.

After tea, I bike out to Ly Thai To Boulevard where we used to live. The street has become one of Saigon's major arteries. Nothing looks familiar. The buildings have been renumbered, but some have the new numbers, some the old numbers, some none at all. The block is mangy with signs and billboards, and the whole place looks, smells, and feels grimy with oil and soot. On the third pass, I find our house. It has been converted into a community health clinic, a big Red Cross sign out front.

My heart dips at the sight of it. The front of the building has been demolished and rebuilt farther back to make room for motorbike parking. I peek inside. There have been some major structural modifications. The head nurse greets me at the door. When I tell her that my family once lived here, she expresses concern that I might be one of those Viet-kieu returning to reclaim properties the government or squatters seized. I assure her I am only here for my childhood memories. Sighing relief, she tours me through the clinic. The building seems new, small, strange. There is nothing left of my youth. After fifteen minutes, she returns to work, leaving me milling about the house trying to—as she puts it—*"visit the humble life that came before."*

The staff and the patients begin to stare, which makes me feel misplaced. What was I thinking? Did I really believe that coming here would bring back dead memories? I guess I was hoping something miraculous would happen. Something spontaneous that would make everything all right and justify all the hardships I have gone through. I had been banking on a stupid Hollywood ending, too embarrassed to admit as much to myself.

Too many things changed. Too much time passed. I'm different now, a man with a pocketful of unconnected but terribly vivid memories. I was looking to dredge up what I'd long forgotten. Most of all, I am wishing for something to fasten all these gems, maybe something to hold them in a continuity that I can comprehend.

I thank the nurse and step outside. On the sidewalk, it feels infinitely odd that I am standing in the same place where I had played as a boy, twenty years ago. Here, I had waited for my school bus. Locked inside the house most of the day, I yearned to play on this hot pavement, my domain. Of the people who crossed my kingdom, I remember one peasant woman most poignantly.

It was the day before the fall of Saigon. She had paused in front of my house. Her plastic sandal had slipped off her foot. She lowered to the ground the two baskets that hung from the ends of the bamboo staff she shouldered. In one basket, a baby wailed. Quieting her child with a sliver of sugarcane, she tipped back the rim of her conical hat fashioned of palm leaves and dragged a soiled white sleeve across her brow. Fear flickered over her face as she looked behind.

Hundreds of people were fleeing the column of smoke rising to the gray sky. Some came on bicycles laden with belongings. Most scrambled on foot, peasants with possessions in their baskets. Fathers pushed carts. Little children rode piggyback on their older siblings. Mothers lugged bundles with young ones in tow.

A few cars, horns blaring, plowed a path through the mass that spilled into the street. When the cars ran out of gas, drivers abandoned their vehicles and fled with their families on foot. Children screamed. Gunshots crackled sporadically somewhere in the neighborhood. People shouted, urging each other to hurry. Some pushed against the tide, calling the names of those they'd lost in flight, craning their heads above the crowd. Clothing, baggage, carts, baskets, and bicycles littered the street, left where their owners had dropped them.

The scene frightened me. I ventured onto the sidewalk and asked the woman with her baby where she was going.

"To the harbor," she said. "There are American ships there. It's over. The Viet Cong are coming!" Her answer panicked her. The baby bawled.

She was thirsty. I fetched her a glass of water. She asked me why my family wasn't leaving. Was it because we owned land and this house?

I told her I didn't know. I only knew my mother cried this morning when my uncle told her the country fell. Maybe we were leaving, too. Where, I didn't know, but we were going somewhere. My mother had been packing all day and my father had been gone since this morning to bring all my brothers back home from grandparents' house and uncle's house where they boarded. Even without the madness outside, I knew it was a big occasion because I couldn't remember the last time that we were all under one roof.

I would have gone on, but she wasn't listening. As suddenly as she had stopped, the woman shouldered her load and her baby and hurried away, her sandals slapping on the concrete.

———

A fat, dark woman comes out of the building next to the clinic and asks me, *"Uncle, what are you looking for?"*

She uses the honorific "uncle" although she is older than me, so I bow in return. *"Older Sister, I used to live here with my parents before the Liberation. I've returned to see the old neighborhood."*

"Really! Are you Uncle Pham's son?"

I nod, amazed that anyone remembered my father. It had been two decades and we hadn't lived here more than two years.

My return excites her. She touches my arm. *"How are your parents? Is your mother, Aunt Anh, doing well? Are all of you in America or Europe?"*

"Yes, they are doing very well. Healthy and prosperous in America."

"I knew it! Your father was wise to leave when he did. A week after he left, the police came to your house."

I don't need to press her on the details. Any business that brought the police out to one's home at night was very bad. I realize now how narrow our escape was, how it was common for neighbors to turn informers.

"Forgive me, Older Sister, I was so young, I don't recall your name."

"Oh, Lord, you don't remember me? I'm Fourth Sister. Ask your parents about me. They remember. Are you An or Huy?"

"An."

"It's so fortunate to see you again. Anything about our neighborhood look familiar?"

"No, Fourth Sister. I was hoping you could walk me around the neighborhood. I don't remember the alleys too well. A lot must have happened since the Liberation."

Fourth Sister laughs and tells me to lock my bike inside her house. She takes me into the alleys and introduces me to the people living there, but no one remembers me nor I them. Old houses have been felled, newer ones, dingier ones, have taken their place, and my old playground, the nooks, the corridors, the hidden alcoves have long been paved over. Yet the place isn't as dirty as I'd expected. In fact, it seethes a headiness of incense, frying garlic, and the sweat of too many people.

"Where is the dog-meat restaurant?" I ask Fourth Sister.

"Gone. After Saigon opened up a few years ago, things got better, so people don't eat dogs much anymore. It's sinful."

"Where is the Chinese apothecary? The dumpling bar, the tofu women?"

"All gone."

"No, no." I couldn't have come all this way for naught. *"What about the house behind mine—the one in the alley? I just want to see that alley house behind mine."*

"They smashed all the alley homes a long time ago. New homes are built right against the back of all the street-front houses. No more alley."

"But what about the people who used to live there? The Vo family."

"Gone. All gone. Who do you remember?"

"The daughter. I don't remember her name."

"Come. Meet the new people and some of the old ones who are still here."

I want to leave. This place is empty. But she draws me by my elbow deeper into the concrete shade of the back byways gauzy with crisscrossing laundry lines and green with cheap paint. She steers me, nudging me sideways through the crowd of short men, invalid seniors, black-toothed matrons, and naked children who squat in the alley eating stinky, pungent noodles sold out of home kitchens. She walks me past the meat sellers whose wares are single sides of pork displayed on banana leaves on the ground, introduces me to the women who scrub their laundry at the front steps, tells the cigarette-suckling men where I am from. She shoves me into strangers' homes, shouting jubilantly: *A Viet-kieu, our own neighborhood Viet-kieu comes back to see his roots. Let him in to see your house. Let him see how humbly we live.*

They rush questions at me. *Do you live in the Country of Oranges* [Orange County] *in the sate of Cali* [California]? *I hear all Viet-kieu live there. What do you do for a living? How much do you make? Are you married? Would you like me to be your matchmaker? I'll find you a good wife. Meet my sister. You bring us gifts? How about a hundred dollars? Here's my uncle's address in New York; find him and ask him why he stopped writing and sending us money. Here's my photo, find me an American husband.*

They laugh with me, at me. I desperately want to be away from this foreign place. *So sorry, but I must go now. I'm late for an appointment.* I leave, bowing, nodding, smiling, running. Fourth Sister trails me all the way back to her house. As I fumble with my bike lock, she pours a cup of tea, stale-cold, and presses the blistered porcelain into my hand.

She speaks with an urgency that makes me pause. *"We are so poor. Life is so tough here. People who have Viet-kieu in their family live better. They buy motorbikes, open big business, make good living. I'm poor. My family is poor. Can you help us? Will you be our benefactor?"*

I try to explain something to her about life in America. And that I don't know her. I try not to let my disappointment show. I come searching for truths, hoping for redeeming grace, a touch of gentility. But, no. The abrasiveness of Saigon has stripped away my protective layers. I am raw and bare and I ask myself, Who are these strangers? These Vietnamese, these wanting-wanting-wanting people. The bitter bile of finding a world I don't remember colors my disconsolate reconciliation between my Saigon of Old and their muddy-grubby Saigon of Now. Saigon gnaws at me . . . its noise . . . its uncompromising want . . . its constant . . . Memememememememememe . . .

Beggar-Grace

15 The Saigon I see isn't visceral. I'd be deceiving you if I took your hand to walk you through it. It isn't just something you see. It's what you feel, an echo in the blood that courses through you. It is a collage, a vanishing flavor, a poison, a metallic tinge, a barbarous joy, strange impressions indefinable in the usual ways.

It is easy for me to say because I am cowering in a bar, exclusive, situated high above the muck. Easy, for today I was wounded, my armor finally pierced. Now, through this tinted window, I see a Saigon evening like the dozens of others before. I see the setting sun grinding down on the ancient treetops and the prickly antennas atop the shouldering buildings. It glowers, a fist of coal in a sea of smog thick as dishwater. In the glimmering heat, the narrow roads swarm with headlights of motorbikes, bright beams wildly fingering the asphalt arteries, companions of the horns, the screeching, badgering, warring horns, persistent always. The air throbs, salty, wet with exhaust, dank with perspiration. The people, the skinny dark people suffocate, enduring.

Kiosks hedge the street, no sidewalks, catching the drift of humanity churned up by the traffic. The sandwich makers, old ladies with oily hands, dusty skin like yesterday's bread, lather pork fat onto tiny loaves. On the curbs, the shirtless men of sun-jerked sinew in boxer shorts and rubber sandals, squatting on their hams, grill meat over coals in metal pans. A dog, patchy fur over ribs, sniffs the droppings of another. In an alley, a mother and daughter fry dough cakes, selling them wrapped in dirty newspapers. Next to them, laborers hunch on plastic footstools slurping noodle soup from chipped bowls. TVs squawk, flickering foreign images to a score of spectators each. They're watching an American travelogue dubbed in Vietnamese. Tonight, we tour Yosemite and luxuriate in the hospitality of the Ahwahnee Hotel.

People shout, curse, barter, laugh, whine, edging words into the traffic, hustling for money. The buildings press narrow, ten feet wide, and stretch thrice as long, every other one a storefront, open for business, selling, selling, selling anything, everything. Food, paper, spare parts, clothes, candies, color TVs, fake watches, cheap Chinese fabric, screwdrivers, wrenches, rice dishes, Coca-Cola, cigarettes, gasoline in soda bottles, penny-lottery tickets, imported tins of biscuits, and everything has a buyer, everyone is for sale.

Across the city on a darker avenue in a place they call Hang Bong—the Row of Flowers—life drifts in on the evening breeze. First come the snack vendors, two-basket merchants of sweet jelly drinks and tapioca desserts, each armed with a bead flame winking from an oil lamp. They cater to the buyers and sellers of perfumed nights. Next, the police make their entrance in ill-fitting olive uniforms, black knee-boots, and white vinyl belts, nightsticks and Russian pistols riding awkwardly on their hips, here for their cut of the night's transactions.

Then, the flowers blossom from nowhere onto the nightscape: women who look like girls, and girls who look like women, and hags who hug the darkest shadows, cosmetics of another sort. They stroll out from the maw of dark alleys. They walk in from afar by twos and threes, hand in hand like sisters going to the market. They ride in on motorbikes, ferried to the Row of Flowers by friends, family, lovers, others.

Last come the buyers. The upwardly mobile and the raving destitute. Locals who squander weeks of wages for a moment of release. And down by the well-lit sections of the avenue not far from the big hotels and the sewer that is the Saigon River, foreigners pluck the choice bouquets that blossom here. They flourish on this street, women of sheikhs. Everything for sale. Up front.

There is a place called the Turtle Fountain not far from my old elementary school, the French Catholic institution I had dreaded. I had spent many a joyful afternoon dallying at this spot as a boy. It was a place in the city where I went to be alone, although no one is really alone in this city of nine million. The smog and heat are more bearable out on these old boulevards under the tall trees planted long ago by French civic designers. This fountain is one of the few remnants built by the deposed Nationalists that the Communist regime has allowed to stand. Now the hoboes and the homeless families cling to it, camping under its elaborate awnings and washing in the fountain.

Six streets pour traffic into this intersection. The honks and purrs spin counterclockwise around the fountain with its fringe lawn-garden, footpaths, and benches. A bustling trade of sidewalk concessions rings the traffic. Cafés and food stands mark their territory by the foot. In addition to these is a steady stream of vendors passing through with their pushcarts, their baskets of food, bells clanging, calling out their wares. The acrid bite of exhaust is blunted by the smell of food: sweet meat grilling on coal, soy-sauce-soaked liver sizzling, roasting ears of corn dripping with pork fat and scallions, pork buns warming in tiers of great bamboo steamers, pork chops sautéing in fishsauce and garlic, sesame dough balls browning in woks of oil. From the tattered folding lawn chairs, all facing the traffic—amphitheater seats—Vietnamese congregate to drink and nibble on bits of food. Most just watch the traffic go by.

Earlier this afternoon, Viet, Nghia, and I came out to the Turtle Fountain for a round of iced coconuts at my usual table. The proprietor reluctantly pulled herself from a card game, nabbed three coconuts from a Styrofoam cooler, cleaved the tops off, plunked them down, and rejoined her game. The beggars began to make their way toward us. I had grown inured to the daily pleas of beggars and no longer felt the instinctive urge to reach for my wallet, especially in front of Viet, who got into a fit whenever he saw me giving money.

Saigon was thick with almsfolk, every market, every street corner maggoty with misshapen men and women hawking their open sores and pus–yellow faces for pennies. The air near them stank with the pepperiness of red boils, rotting flesh. Crippled boys lay on crude skateboards and crabbed along with sandal-covered hands, a begging cup clamped between their brown teeth. Old women with hungry, vacant eyes sat in the gutter, cradling one-eyed babies with heads the size of watermelons. Then there were begging bards: duets of one-legged guitarists and quadriplegic singers who sang supine on a wheeled board.

Last week, I visited Grandaunt at her stall in the Ben Thanh Market. It had taken her four years of selling in the street to save enough money to buy the leasing contract of this five-by-five-foot stall. While we were chatting, a child and her blind mother begged me for two pennies. I reached for my wallet, but Grandaunt, who had caught me giving money to beggars before, placed a restraining hand on my arm. I wanted to give the child my paltry change, but it would mean disobeying Grandaunt, and thereby causing her to lose face. Seeing my discomfort, Grandaunt said gently to the little girl, *"He's family, little one."*

The child bowed and moved on to the next stall, leading her milky-eyed mother by the hand. This tiny girl whom I could lift with one arm respected the custom: beggars forgo shopkeepers. This child had shown more grace than I in our empty transaction. I stood in her wake, moved by something I couldn't name.

By the time we were through with our coconuts, we had turned away six or seven beggars. We were about to leave when she came. She was six, maybe seven, maybe ten. It was difficult to tell because street children were generally so malnourished that their growth lagged by several years. She carried a baby in a shoulder sling on her chest. They were both ragged and thin.

I looked in her face and the breath went out of me. She looked back, an exact image—a younger image of Trieu, a former lover I had thought someday would be my wife. I must be crazy, but the likeness was there. The war had orphaned Trieu and the only token of her childhood was a yellowed photo that I had committed to memory. This beggar-child had the same braided ponytail and huge gleaming eyes set in a persimmon face. The resemblance resonated a hundred what-ifs and I heard them as though I were trapped in a time portal.

I wanted to give this child something. A wild thought needled my mind: I could be her godfather. Send her a monthly stipend for schooling and food. I wanted to hug her. But I sat helpless and wordless, as though saying she would have no mercy, not a single penny from me.

Viet shook his head at me, a warning against giving handouts. Annoyed, he dismissed the child with a flick of his hand.

Knowing her work had reached its end, she pointed at our empty coconuts. Scabs tattooed the length of her arm. She whispered, *"Uncle, if you are finished with these, may I have them?"*

I could not move, watching with the impotence of a specter. Viet grunted his assent, motioning her to move on.

"Thank you, Uncle," she said, and gathered two shells, one in each small hand. She wanted to take the third as well, but couldn't with the baby hanging on her chest. She sat down not ten steps from us and tilted each shell above her mouth. A few drops. I was mesmerized by her fingers. Dirty little fingers scraping bits of white coconut. Licking fingers. Sweet juice. Sharing slivers with the baby.

I was her. She, me. She was Trieu. Could be my sister Chi. Could be my own daughter. Random. My world—her world. But for my parents' money, I could be any one of the thousands of cyclo drivers, vacant-eyed men wilting in cafés, hollow-cheeked merchants angling for a sale. Everything could shift, and nothing would change. No difference. The shoes to be filled were the same.

She left our coconut shells on the ground and skipped away across the busy street, the baby jostling awkwardly on her hip.

Something awoke in me. Silent minutes passed and at last I stood up.

"Where are you going?" Viet asked.

"Nowhere."

He looked slighted, but it no longer mattered to me, his feelings, his culture. Vietnamese. Honor. Obligations. Respect. I hated it all.

I climbed on my bike and rode after the beggar-child, going in the opposite direction of the circling traffic. Frantically, I searched for her braided ponytail bobbing among the tables. From café to café I went, stopping on the curb and peering into the dark. She appeared just coming out of the kitchen diner, sucking on an orange wedge, the baby riding her hip.

I waved her to me. She came warily.

"Here, Little Niece, take this and buy something to eat for yourself and the baby." I gave her all the money in my pocket. Not much.

She looked at it, shocked, eyeing me with such gratitude that I was ashamed. She bowed. Voice trembling, she mumbled, *"Thank-you-very-much-Uncle, thank-you-very-much. Little-Niece-thanks-Uncle-very-much."*

And she seemed to want to say something else but didn't. And I wanted to say something, but couldn't. In that moment, she seemed so awfully old. I felt terribly young. She jammed the bills into a pocket on her shirt where she held the baby. She hurried away, a lightness in her step. From across the street, she turned, waved bye, and smiled.

Abruptly, the easing of tension I had felt as I gave her the money vanished. It was only my selfish conscience. I stood there sickened for her, gasping at her tragedy and my part in it. Oh, child. What have they done to you? What have I done? Her parents will send her back here again and again on the off chance of a windfall like today's. Oh, God. Why is she here? This beautiful child. What is her birth-fortune?

But on this afternoon in this city of webbed intentions on this hot sidewalk, I stood rotten with doubts, more lost than I had ever been in my life. Why do I care for this persimmon-faced child? Is it simply because she bears a likeness to someone I once knew? Is that what it takes to remind me that I am Vietnamese? That I am human, capable of feeling the misery of another? If so, I am a worse bigot than those I despise, those who have hounded me in America.

A grayness swept through me, but I wanted to feel the pain. Deserve it. All my life I have held pain in check, kept grief at a distance. I got on my bike and pedaled into the traffic, spooling into the six-way intersection. I could not stop. I felt a spark ignite something flammable in me, and my insides combusting. I couldn't stop and I didn't trust—didn't know—the wetness welling up behind my eyes. So my legs pumped me headlong with the traffic, round and round the park I flew. Blue exhaust teared my eyes, seared my nostrils. In the circling, my mood spiraled downward, inward, powerless. There was nothing I could tear down. Nothing to smash my fists into. Roaring. A monster eating my heart.

I raced around the intersection. A madman. I went faster than cars and motorcycles. Reckless young men gave chase, but I left them behind. I rode, hands on the bars, not fingering the brake. A dark Herculean strength burst forth from the pit of me. Faster and faster I raced and I knew I was heading toward an accident, but the realization was remote, misty behind my red anger. Drivers honked, swerved. I went faster still. Sweat slanted down my forehead and salted my eyes. My chest burned.

My Saigon was a whore, a saint, an infanticidal maniac. She sold her body to any taker, dreams of a better future, visions turned inward, eyes to the sky of the skyscrapers foreign to the land, away from the festering sores at her feet. The bastards in her belly—tainted by war, pardoned by need, obscured by time—clamored for food. They laughed, for it is all they know. She hoped for a better tomorrow, hoped for goodness.

Then there was nothing. The wildfire swept past. Ashen, I pulled over. Without a word, Viet, his nephew, and I went home. At the house, I parked my bike just inside the gate. The tears came without warning and I had to turn away from my uncles and aunts and nephews and nieces. I cried into the wall, the sobs racking my shoulders. There was nowhere to go, nowhere to hide in this little house, in this crowded neighborhood. I wept uncontrollably, as I did when I heard my sister Chi had committed suicide—my father cutting her free from a yellow nylon rope. I had known then, as I knew now, that I was weeping for her and I was weeping for myself because I was not there in the months before her death. Although we had lived in the same city, I had avoided her, too engrossed in my own life, my own problems.

This time my tears made my relatives ashamed for me. Yet, in this alley-world of theirs where there was no space, no privacy, they gave me both. My aunt said to her son, *"He got dust in his eyes. It's painful. Nghia, go upstairs and fetch him the bottle of eyedrops."*

When the eyedropper was in my hand, they dispersed. They never mentioned my shame, my unmanliness. Never asked me why. And in all my time here, they never once mentioned my sister's suicide.

Never once spoke of her unspeakable act. The only thing they said, they said it thrice: *Poor Chi. Poor Chi. Poor Chi.* These wonderful, generous people, they gave me face when I deserved none.

I wept for my sister Chi. I wept for myself. I wept for the disparity between my world and the world of these people. And I wept for my sorry soul. When the tears eased, I bathed. In the breezeway behind the bathroom, a servant girl, washing dishes, sang to herself. A wall and two feet between us, I cried and she sang of monsoon rain in the countryside. I emptied the cistern of cold water over my head, one tin at a time.

Baptized, I went alone to a bar—an expensive, exclusive, air-conditioned oasis, carpeted and lavishly upholstered, with a guard at the door to keep the beggars out. And I drank myself into a stupor, watching crusty people through leaded glass.

Now, in the grip of the tequila—this toast to Tyle, my shipwrecked Viking—I sense a terrible doubt. I wasn't there when my sister needed me. I did not turn my life into a crusade for runaways. Did not volunteer to help the homeless or to counsel troubled people. For these starving children of Saigon, I have no intention of sacrificing my life to change theirs. Then, perhaps, my grief is but a compensatory facade.

I am drunk and I am tired. Whether my journey is a pilgrimage or a farce, I am ready and anxious to see this last leg through. Tomorrow I will head north to Hanoi.

Fallen-Leaves

 Tonight, Anh was with her old friend Bich in downtown Saigon having tea and strawberry ice cream, a middle-class luxury she had come to adore.

Bich, I brought you some green mangoes. Ahhhh, Older Sister Anh, look at me craving green mangoes and fishsauce-syrup just like a peasant girl. They chortled madly. Remember how we could tell which one of your girls was in trouble when she started eating green mangoes like bread? They sang the chorus in unison: Quick—Brew the root-tea—Call the midwife—Catch the Jeep before they take him back to the front lines. They were laughing, but they were holding hands, comforting each other, their weathered peasant fingers interlacing like roots, wrists bound by matching circlets of blood jade. Bich, you aren't going to Paris with Claude, are you? Yes, I am and I'll have him reserve plane seats for your family. No, Bich, we can't. We have too much here. Our family, our home. Listen, Older Sister Anh, we're leaving, all your girls are leaving. Uyen is leaving with Jack. He says Saigon will fall any day now. Ly and Paul are going to America with her family. We've come a long way. We can't lose everything again. You must come with us. Anh shook her head sadly.

They were women of the same harvest, strong women who did what they had to for the survival of their families. They knew pain and they knew joy and all the selflessness that was required to take a person from that one place to the other.

Anh scanned the park lawn, wondering where her boy went. He wanted to go to the movies, but she didn't want to take him, not with all the recent bombings. He was a strange one, that An. Always burrowing into one fix after another, off in his own world, constantly getting into trouble.

An was angry when the crowd jostled him and his scoop of chocolate ice cream tumbled out of its sugar cone. He was reaching down when a woman stepped on it then cursed him for the mess on her sandal. An ran. He squirmed between adults' legs and popped out in front of the crowd. The heat of the fire on his face made him forget the taste of chocolate on his tongue.

He thought there ought to be a bittersweet odor of burnt meat, but there wasn't. Just gasoline fumes. People gathered to watch robes of flame dance brightly against a whitewashed backdrop of a wall. Black smoke billowed to the night sky. A blackened form silhouetted amid unfurling orange. A Buddhist monk aflame. His last sacrifice.

Hope-Adrift

The engine was running, but the sea had us in its palm. Our poor fishing vessel bobbed directionless, putting no distance between us and the mysterious ship in pursuit. The crew looked defeated. Mom muttered that it was terrible luck. First the net fouling the propeller, now this. She said to Dad, How could this be? The calendar showed today to be auspicious. All the celestial signs were good—clear sky, good wind. She shook her head, looking at her Japanese flag, a patch of red on a white sheet, flapping noisily. Our hopes were pinned on that fraudulent banner.

We waited. Time sagged. I counted the waves surging beneath our keel. There was nothing to do. The men's lips were moving, mumbling prayers. Eyes closed, Mom had her jade Buddha in her palms. Miracle. Miracle. Our boat seemed to plead with the ocean. Please send a miracle.

It happened. The men stirred, but no one uttered a word. They looked hopeful, fearing that saying something might jinx whatever was happening. Another minute, I could tell that the ship was veering away from us. They cheered. Tai instructed us to stay hidden, knowing that the ship had us in its binoculars. Mom was shaking with relief. Eventually, the ship went over the horizon and the men celebrated with a meal.

The ocean grew more restless by evening. We were exhausted, dehydrated, and hungry, but couldn't eat because food made us vomit. This was fine with the men who ate and drank our portions. The night was chilly. We put on our sweaters. Dad pointed out the constellations to the men. As soon as I fell asleep, a spray of water would wake me up. My face was crusty with salt. I wanted to get up and stretch my legs, but Dad forbade it. No standing. He didn't want to lose us overboard.

Clouds puffed into the sky the morning of our second day. A ten-foot sea rose up from nowhere. Stress was beginning to show among the crew. They were sullen and irritable with each other. Some of the men washed their faces with our dwindling supply of fresh water. They were also in the habit of rinsing their cups with fresh water before drinking. Dad protested. They cussed him. Tai, the leader, looked on without comment. Dad shrugged, resigned to the young men's foolishness. We couldn't afford a quarrel.

The sea continued to build through the afternoon. Occasionally, a rogue wave broke over us. We were drenched and cold. A shark nosed by our boat, the fishermen panicked. Some started lashing themselves to the boat, others had their knives in hand.

Tai asked his first mate, "Did you make an offering at the Shark Temple?"

"Yes, I did. I lit two batches of incense, just in case."

"Are you sure?"

"Yes!"

"You didn't drink the money, did you?"

"Fuck, no! I swear to heaven I made the offering!"

This mollified the crew, but they were still nervous. The weather worsened and the shark went away. The wind picked up. Shivering, we changed into our last set of dry clothing. As the sun slipped toward the water, flying fish took wing, shooting out of the waves like silver bullets. Long fins out tricking the wind, they skimmed the sea in straight lines, in curves, in banking dives like tiny, shiny jets on a raid. When golden rays caught them broadside, they shimmered like splinters of the sun-gilded ocean shaken loose by a breaking wave. A pair kamikazed into our boat. They flopped about stunned. I asked Mom if she would cook them for dinner. She rolled her eyes at me and threw the fish back into the water, saying it was bad luck to let flying fish die in the boat, much less eat them.

Then dolphins came, arcing beside us. We waved at the visitors. Cheering, the fishermen took it as a very good omen and devoured the rest of our food, which was supposed to have lasted us a week. None of them had brought food. Apparently, they had drunk the money Mom had given them to buy their own supplies. Dad tried to stop them from eating everything. A nasty argument broke out and they nearly came to blows. Tai and Anh simply watched their rabble of a crew snarling at each other over bits of food. It dawned on us all then that unless we chanced on a boat with a kind captain, we were going to die at sea. There wasn't enough fuel to turn around and we were nearly out of food and water.

Just when the ocean was about to nibble the foot of the sun, we sighted a tall white ship, aft to starboard. Tai turned the boat around and pointed us at the ship. It was a French vessel, a beautiful white ship slicing across the ocean. Some sort of freighter-cruiser. We cheered. We screamed. We laughed, giddy. The men embraced each other, arguments forgotten. Salvation had never looked more beautiful than a tall white ship shouldering through waves in the sunset. Mom gathered her bags. Dad readied his flashlight, mentally reviewing his Morse code. Unwrapping a set of signal flags Mom had fashioned, Dad started signaling S-O-S. My brothers and I were hollering, yelling, waving as though it were the biggest parade boat we'd ever seen.

"We are very fortunate," Dad told everyone. "It's a French ship—a friendly ship." His face was lit up with what must have been memories of himself, the young son of an aristocrat who had thrived under French colonialism. Dad adored everything French, from their bad-smelling cheese to their classical poets.

The fishermen were excited, too. They knew Dad was fluent in French and that France had given refuge to many Vietnamese since the fall of Saigon. As the ship drew closer, we screamed ourselves hoarse. I thought the ship had vaults full of chocolate and cookies and roast chicken. I told my brothers as much, then we howled happily. We cheered so long and loud that we didn't notice the adults' hooray had tapered off. When we did, an ill-fitting quiet netted the boat. The men exchanged uncertain glances. Our tiny fishing boat chugged faithfully toward the ship. Someone muttered a curse. The others shook their heads in disbelief. Tai's broad face grew grim, a hint of anger. Dad was clearly worried, frowning in a state of shock. The ship did not change direction. It didn't slow. Was it speeding up? We were so close, they couldn't possibly not see us. The ship was going so fast, it would pass us within minutes. Go directly at them, Dad ordered Tai, make them stop. It looked as though we were going to ram the white ship's flank. Dad signaled them in French, then in English. No reply, not even a warning horn. We drew closer, dead set on a right-angle collision course.

At the last moment, Tai idled the engine and we coasted, inert, impotent, unable to reach out to beg for help. The ship sailed by, its white side rearing up in front of us like a great wall. It was so close, we wished we could just swim over and grab on, but the ship was going too fast. The current would have dragged us under. We shouted, waving. Dad worked his flashlight, spelling out our desperate plight with dots and dashes. Dad had us all stand up on the listing deck to show them we had women and children aboard. I could see people aboard the white ship looking at us through portholes. They did not wave back. The ship slipped past us, an untouchable dream. The fishermen looked on in silence. Nothing to say. I saw an officer standing on the upper deck at the stern of the ship, hands bracing on the rail, regarding us. He was white, perhaps French, and he wore a beautiful white uniform. Mom was moaning, Oh my God, oh my God. They are going to let us die. Chi had her arms around Mom. Auntie Dung was shouting, not giving up. The fishermen made drinking motions to the ship's officers, tilting imaginary cups and pointing into their mouths. We begged them to help us, they looked on without interest, our boat and our pathetic lives but flotsam in their wake. I was so angry I thought I could hit the officer on deck if I had my slingshot.

The ship hummed by, its stern receding from us. Suddenly, the ocean leaped up. A wall of water—the ship's wake—maybe two stories high, bore down on us. EVERYBODY DOWN! Tai shouted, throwing the throttle into full forward. Hang on! The diesel stuttered under the urgent load. The boat nosed into the barrier of water, head-on like a car trying to scale a building it was supposed to hit. Up we went. Mom screamed. We screamed. Up, up. Up until we were sliding back on the deck. Up until I thought the boat would pitch-pole backward. Then, in a breath, we teetered on the crest of the wave, looking down to the white trough. Down we plunged. Water foamed white, swirling energy. The bottom looked hard, asphalt-like. My stomach lurched up as we fell over the back of the wave. The boat slid sideways. Tai wrestled the tiller, fighting the ocean from rolling his boat. The cords in his neck stood out. Screams. The boat was lifting to port, about to pour us over starboard. I jammed my feet against the toe rail, grabbing on to Tien and Huy. Then the boat dropped into the trough, the sea blasting over the bow and abeam. The hull groaned. The wooden planks strained against the sea, creaking sick-like. A moment. The boat popped up like a plastic ball.

As we caught our breath, the boat climbed again. This time Tai was ready. He guided us over the series of waves, each smaller as the ship's wake diminished. When we looked up at the French ship again, it looked like an iceberg moving ponderously along its course, imperturbable, oblivious to us, to everything. An empty-stomach feeling wrapped itself around our small vessel. The white ship dwindled. Dusk folded around it until its mighty bulk was no more than a speck on the water, indistinguishable from the breaking waves.

Things grew desperate the third day. My brothers and I shared a can of water laced with sweetened condensed milk among the four of us. There were a couple of packets of instant ramen left for seventeen people. Without a stove to boil water, we crushed the dried noodles and ate them like crackers. Two gallons of water remained. The younger fishermen realized their mistake and accepted Dad's rationing, one sip for everyone. The weather fattened the dark clouds and fouled the waves up another few feet. The sea god was bouncing us mercilessly on his belly. Our inexperienced crew fretted. There was talk of turning around. Some suggested heading toward Thailand, though, of course, with no bearings and only a compass, we had one chance in ten of pick-ing the right direction.

When the argument grew heated among the crew, Mom got up unsteadily on her feet. "This is my boat," she said, looking each man in the eyes. "I paid for it. I paid all of you to come with us. We agreed on Malaysia: we *go* to Malaysia! We are not going to Thailand unless I say so."

"Big Sister," Truong protested, "you shouldn't worry about Thai pirates. They wouldn't be out sailing in this bad weather. Our chances are better heading to Thailand."

A murmur of assent from the others.

"No. We are not changing course," she said, scanning their faces. "If you change course, I will not pay the second half of your fee."

She had them where it counted. The gold was secure with Grandma in Vietnam, and without Mom's word, none of it would be transferred to the fishermen's families. The crew cast their eyes away from her, their resolve faltering before hers. So onward we plowed, dangerously low on fuel.

Our boat sat low in the water, sinking gradually. One day in a con-fused sea was enough to crack open wooden seams. The boat sipped enough water to wallow like a tub. The pump couldn't keep up with the leaks. By the time the crew noticed, the bilge was calf-deep in seawater. A panic bailing ensued and didn't stop while we were aboard. There was only enough room below for two persons, so the crew set up a frantic bucket relay to keep the boat afloat. The combi-nation of rough seas, diesel exhaust, and cold water began to make even the tougher fishermen sick. Chi took her turn in the hold, bail-ing as hard as the men. We threw overboard all the excess weight— baggage, net, anchors, lines. Incense sticks were lit and the praying began in earnest because our skipper admitted that there was a fair chance our boat might fall apart within twenty-four hours.

Toward evening, the men were muttering that the boat might not make it through the night. Turning around wasn't an option now. It was too late, without water and food. Our leaky boat was perilously low on fuel. We were so sick and exhausted, no one protested the talk of doom. It seemed we all came to a fatigued acceptance of the inevitable. Our end was written all over a sky as impenetrable as stone. All day we hadn't seen a single shaft of sunlight. It was a day without shadow.

"SHIP! SHIP!" someone shouted. At once everyone picked up the call though no one else saw the ship. Then our arms oriented in one direction like compass needles. "Ship! Ship! Ship!" we sang, flushed with relief, thrilled. Mom prayed her thanks aloud as she lit joss sticks.

Tai took the helm and swung the boat back around, pointing it northwest toward the ship. It was just a dot, vanishing and reappearing on the crinkling gray ocean. One moment we saw it, the next we didn't. Tai ordered his first mate to open the engine's throttle completely. An all-or-nothing push. Big ships moved so fast that they could travel out of view within twenty minutes. Our tiny fishing vessel could easily slip under a ship's radar. When the ship grew to the size of a button at arm's length, Dad used his flashlight. Tai ordered the women and children to stand up and wave so that the ship's officers could see we posed no danger to them. We followed his instructions, but there was no cheering. The memory of the French ship was still fresh in our minds. Friend or foe, this ship must be our savior.

It was a huge freighter with a black hull and red trim, coming into hailing distance just as the last of the light bled from the day. It slowed and we cheered. The ship was an Indonesian freighter. It allowed us to come alongside and Dad used his flashlight to communicate with the dark-skinned sailors on its deck. Flashes of light reached out, back and forth between the vessels.

Dad's voice was shaky, choking with joy. "They're offering us refuge!"

We cheered. Mom sobbed.

Tai brought our boat alongside the black hull. The ocean was too rough for them to lower the gangplank. The waves were heaving our boat over fifteen vertical feet. A rope ladder tumbled over the rail of the ship. Tai brought us closer and the waves slammed our tiny boat against the freighter. The few spare tires on the side of the boat saved our wooden hull from breaking. Tai veered us away before the next blow. The men moved all the spare tires onto the same side and Tai made another pass at the ladder. A wave threw our boat against the black metal hull, the tires flattened like sponge. The men were using poles and oars to soften the collision, trying to hold us off the metal hull. Oars snapped, bamboo poles splintered. The boat itself was coming apart and taking on water as though the pump was running in reverse. Tai yelled for everyone to hurry, women and children first.

The boat jumped all over the waves like an ice cube on a hot griddle, and only the men could grab hold of the ladder. Tai, Hanh, and Tieu, our strongest men, took turns carrying the women and children aboard. With a hand from one of the crew, Chi grabbed the ladder and climbed up on her own. Tai came back down and piggybacked me. He waited until the boat crested the next wave and lunged for the ladder. Waves splashed against the ship. I tasted saltwater. I was wet and blue with cold. The boat dropped, and suddenly we were dangling fifteen feet above the deck. Tai scrambled, fearing the next wave might bring the boat back up and squash us against the hull. Up and up we went, shimmying up the rope ladder.

It was his second trip so Tai was tired and slow climbing up. I was exhausted and weak. I couldn't hold on much longer. Somehow, I knew I wouldn't make it onto the ship. I felt my arms surrendering, my legs going limp around his waist. I couldn't keep myself from looking down. He was going up and I was slipping off his back. I tried hard to hang on, but my arms slipped from his wet neck. I looked down to see where I might fall. Maybe on the boat forty feet below. Maybe in the water between the boat and the ship, where I would be crushed. I was falling. Tai screamed over the howling wind, reaching back to grab me. The rope ladder twisted. I fell. A shoulder-wrenching jerk. I was hanging by one arm.

A sailor gripped my wrist. He was leaning way over the rail; someone else was holding him back from falling in with me. He held my eyes for what seemed an awfully long time as I dangled in the air. Then another arm reached down and they pulled me aboard. I sprawled on the deck of the giant ship shaking, very aware of how bad things might have turned out for me.

In minutes, we abandoned our fishing boat. The Indonesian sailors urged us inside but no one moved. We lingered at the rail to watch our life raft bobbing in the sea. Even from the deck, we could see it sat very low in the water. In minutes there was only the top of the engine house showing, and the ocean swallowed it in the next wave. The weather deteriorated fast and even the big freighter was swaying. We prayed, thanking God, Buddha, and our dead ancestors for our deliverance.

The captain told Dad that our boat was almost out of the shipping lane. The weather had pushed us a hundred miles off course. Pointing at the dark horizon, the captain said that another half day and we would have been shipwrecked on the eastern reefs beyond the shipping lane.

Gift-Marriage

"Baaaannh Teeeeeett, ooooi! Baaaannh Teeeeeett, daaay!"

The banana-rice-cake vendor whinnies her wares as she waddles on her first morning round through the neighborhood. Night still shades the sky, and her calls echo down the alley like a lonely mother beckoning a willful son home.

I crawl out of my sleeping bag. My head feels thick, my stomach hurts. Too much liquor paired with chili peppers and fried anchovies at the bar last night. I feel dry, scooped out. My rush of emotional madness left powdery residue. I am glad to be leaving today.

I wait for the rice-cake woman on the stoop. Normally, I mimic her cry from any part of the house, and no matter how noisy the neighborhood is, she hears and waits for me in the alley. I buy a mug of tea and two rice cakes—Vietnamese Twinkies wrapped in banana leaves. The gooey grains of glutinous rice, green and fragrant with the banana leaves, taste fat and fruit-sweet, like candied caviar. Embedded at the center, the ladyfinger banana has changed to a lavender hue haloing an ivory core. Hot tea in hand, I savor them, standing in the alley, back against the wall, watching the strip of sky navying over.

One by one the breakfast women weave through the alleys. The parade of food baskets ribbons the morning air with the varied aromas from every region of Vietnam: *banh canh* (udon in chicken broth), *bun bo hue* (spicy beef and anchovy-paste noodle soup), *hu tieu* (Chinese-style noodle soup), *banh beo* (rice dumpling with shrimp powder and fishsauce), *tau hu* (soft tofu with ginger syrup), *banh cuon* (rice crepes with Vietnamese sausage and fishsauce), *soi* (sweet rice with mung beans and coconut shavings), *banh mi thit* (ham-and-pickled-daikon sandwiches), and a host of other morning food. Vietnam is a country of food, a country of skinny people obsessed with eating.

As I prepare for the ride, methodically stowing gear in the panniers to balance the load, I realize how out of shape I am. I haven't been on the road for a month now. My days in Vietnam have been a series of food binges, libation excesses, and bouts of diarrhea. It has been nearly two months since I cranked out two eighty-mile days in a row. Saigon to Vung Tau, today's destination, is about seventy miles.

I sent a postcard to Huy and his boyfriend, Sean, from Japan, telling them I was heading to Vietnam. Sean mentioned this to his mother, who owned a modest beach house in Vung Tau. She lives in San Francisco and comes back two months out of the year. She graciously offered me the use of her house, though she regretted not being able to offer me her entire estate because the Communists had seized everything. She was only able to buy back a fraction of what she once owned.

I tell Grandaunt and Granduncle that I am going out to the beach house to recuperate. Saigon's smog and heat have given me a persistent hack. I cough up black phlegm and have recurring stomachaches, which medications stem but cannot dispel. The latter problem concerns me most because on the road I will be eating whatever is convenient, and diarrhea is a fiendish curse when you're in the saddle—as I discovered in Mexico.

The entire clan sends me off at dawn. Grandaunt and Granduncle, still in their pajamas, shuffle up and down the alley, boasting to the neighbors who come out to watch that their grandnephew is riding out to Vung Tau on a bicycle. One hundred twenty kilometers! What do you think of that? He comes from a long line of sportsmen. Anyone want to ride with him? Hahahahahaha. Next door, Mr. Tinh asks, why doesn't he simply ride a motorcycle, it's a lot less tiring. Granduncle exclaims, *Sport!* as though it is the clever answer to a riddle. The neighbors ooh and ahh, all fairly impressed with my ride because physical exertion, manual activities, are not a part of their culture. Sports are seen on television, something they might have dabbled in as schoolchildren. In fact, as one grows older, it is more prestigious to engage in fewer manual activities, sports included. Who ever heard of a grown man "doing" a sport? A solo sport and no prize! Bafflement plainly on their faces.

While Granduncle embarrasses me, Grandaunt wags a finger in my face: *"Don't even think about sneaking off to bike to Hanoi. Don't you dare. Go and recuperate. Get better. We'll all take a vacation and come out there to visit you soon."*

"Yes, Grandaunt," I lie, bowing, nodding as I have been taught to do all my life. Never disagree with your elders to their faces. Don't make them lose face. Whatever you must do, do it behind their backs. If you're caught, take the punishment eagerly, earnestly, like a true repentant. If not, stow the deed among the others.

Viet and Khuong are decked out in their riding gear, jeans, windbreakers, and Los Angeles Lakers caps, raring to go. Grandaunt has decided her sons will take the day off to escort me out to Vung Tau because, she says, the road is dangerous and full of bandits. Cousin Nghia tags along for fun. The three of them pile on one 100cc motorcycle, Nghia sandwiched tightly between his uncle Viet and his uncle Khuong. Viet, the driver, takes both of my panniers. He sets the larger pair over the gas tank, balancing it against his belly. The smaller pair he bungees to the tiny book rack on the back of the motorbike. The little Honda sags dangerously under 450 pounds.

By the time we leave, the sun peeks orange through the screen of trees lining the road. Already, the roads are congested. Within two miles, I sweat with nervous exhaustion in the toxic air, negotiating the dangerous traffic. A group of students gather around me. Soon, I lead a motorcade of fifteen motorbikes. They bump one another, jockeying for a position closer to me. I smile at them. They beam back. Emboldened, they shout questions over the din of traffic.

"Halloo! Where rrrre you phrrom?"

"Good morningsss. Where do you go?"

"My name is Trung. May I talk wip you?"

"Welcome to Viet Nam. You come drink *café* with me? I . . . in . . . invite."

I tell them I'm Vietnamese American. They shriek, *"Viet-kieu!"* It sounds like a disease. The news travels down the procession and the excitement subsides. Half of the group peels away, losing interest since I am not a real foreigner. The others continue to tag along to talk, quite impressed with my trip, which I relay as they ride several miles out of their way to escort me to the city limit. I feel safe inside a buffer zone two riders deep.

On Highway 1, a concrete divider keeps the chaos going in one direction from colliding head-on with the chaos going in the other direction. Though the road is wide enough for three lanes in each direction, there are no lane markings, no shoulders, not even oil tracks, just one big long river of asphalt boiling with Brownian motion. If there are laws concerning what types of vehicle or creature are allowed on the national highway, the traffic cops aren't enforcing them, too busy extorting bribes—unofficial fines, they call them—from truck and bus drivers who prove more lucrative prey than single travelers. Besides the pedestrians who walk along the edge of the road and occasionally attempt mad sprints across the highway, the road teems with cattle-drawn carts, horse-drawn wagons, load ponies, wheelbarrows, herders with cattle, cyclos, bicyclists, and everything motorized. Dust cloaks everything. The air, a metallic blue fog, makes the road murky, twilight-like. With the tropical humidity, it doesn't so much settle as it condenses on the skin like a poisonous mist. The engines roar, the animals bleat, the horns, the curses, and the screams boil into a fantastic cacophony. Set back from the road under the shade of a few scraggly trees, the spectator cafés dot the length of the highway on both sides, their sooty lawn chairs all facing the traffic.

I draft behind Viet's motorcycle, struggling to keep up, but I am out of shape. We turn off the highway onto a smaller road going out toward the coast. The shanties continue to bank the road. There is no break in the land or the crowd. Remnants of a tropical forest, trees rise above the lumpy plain, scattered like stubble on a drunkard's face. At a shed with a concrete slab floor, we slurp down vile bowls of beef noodle soup. I eat with one hand and swat flies with the other. Viet, the scientist, comes up with a bright idea and beckons our waiter, a shirtless ten-year-old boy, to bring us the electric fan. Sure enough, it banishes the flies, but blows the road dust right into our faces and soup. No one else seems to mind, so I buckle up and slurp my noodles, determined not to be "Viet-kieu crybaby." Maybe when grit and grime infuse every cell of my body, I will truly be Vietnamese again.

The terrain is flat all the way out to the coast. Rice paddies and fruit groves stretch away to the hills on either side of the road. Saigoners, mostly laughing young couples and students, buzz past us, also heading out to the beach for the weekend. People wave at me, shouting greetings exuberantly, beckoning me to come and eat at their cafés.

Five hours later, we arrive in Vung Tau, a sleepy tourist town geared for the foreign oil workers and executives. Viet leads us down to the tourist beach for a quick swim. We rent sun chaises. A mob of vendors descend on us, plucking at our sleeves and thrusting bowls of clams and snails in our hands. Teenage girls shove baskets of fruit, warm cans of sodas, and Evian bottles at us. Sellers outnumber prospective buyers five to one.

Clusters of Russians scatter along the two miles of sandy beach. They started vacationing in Vietnam soon after the country's reunification. Many are part of the Russian oil interest headquartered in this resort town. They sprawl on the sand with their entire clans, children and grandparents. They are big, obese, in fact, great with food, and either pale-skinned (recent arrivals) or baked as red as steamed lobsters, buttery with suntan oil. Gangs of vendors squat around them, looking like scrawny mutts waiting for table scraps.

"You help me. You buy crab? Fresh. Very good."

"No. No. No buy. You go. We no buy."

"Coca-Cola? Evian? Chocolate?"

"No. We want sit alone. No buy!"

"Banana? Oranges?"

The two groups despise each other, one taking the other hostage. A two-yard neutral zone separates the warring factions. There are so many vendors that the Russians have difficulty getting to the luscious warm water. The unwilling foreign buyers resent the intrusive, persistent native sellers, shooing them away like strays to no avail. The merchants, having nowhere else to go, nothing better to do, no one else to whom they could sell food and drink at five or ten times the going price, wait patiently, socializing among themselves. They only have to wait. The aromas of their garlic mussels broiling over coal eventually overcome even the most trenchant babushka.

Clink, clink, clink. The entire cliff face sounds like a giant wall of a clock-repair shop, boasting a thousand broken timepieces knocking out of tune, out of time. A thousand clinks a minute, metal on stone. Clink, clink, clink, beckons the cliff. As the road to the back side of the peninsula dips out of the sun, into the cool shade of the cliff, I come to a stop, my eyes fumbling with the change of light. "Oy! Oy!" Someone calling hello. The stonecutters stand up high on the raw face of the cliff, their plastic-sandaled feet finding purchase on shingles and shards of irregular, brittle rocks. These waifs are serrating the very bone of the earth, clawing, eating their way ragged into the gray, red, ivory rock. They are everywhere, like termites. Little men in shorts and baseball caps, women in dusty pajamas and conical straw hats cling to the cliff, their holds invisible from where I stand. They look disposable, little spiders ready to be plucked by a breeze. They are scaling the vertical jags, agile and fearless with neither safety harnesses nor guidelines. Their passage releases drizzles of dust and pebbles. They fracture the stone face of the hill in coffin-sized slabs, sending them down to explode at the bottom. An army of cart pushers and basket carriers scrambles over the rubble to bring the crumbs to safety for measuring and shaping. Then they load the processed bits of the mountain onto waiting Russian trucks. All this to make room for a tourist seaside boulevard.

On the other side of the peninsula is a strip of settlements, mostly fisherfolk homes and two dilapidated motels. There are no street numbers so I ask around until I find the house. Viet and his musketeers bid me goodbye and roar back to Saigon. Mr. Ba, the housekeeper, and his wife greet me at the door and, after many bows, show me to the master studio accessed through the servant quarters where they live. The one-room studio sits apart from the front building, on a lip of land, its balcony jutting out over the water. Waves lap the rock embankment three feet below. The roof is flat and tiled with terra-cotta. A thatched awning turns the roof into a veranda. Two coconut palms shade the side of the house. Mr. Ba scats up the ladder as easily as a boy and cuts me a fresh coconut for my welcoming drink. *I've been saving it for you,* he says as he hacks open the coconut with a machete in that casual, loose-limbed, flailing manner Vietnamese wield a machete. Mrs. Ba cooks a dinner with clams and fish we bought from the boy next door, who casts his net every day from the breakwater behind his house.

I sit up late on the balcony exchanging stories with Mr. and Mrs. Ba. The couple describe the terrible, hungry years following the fall of Saigon. Shaking with decades-old emotions, Mr. Ba tells me of how he had to serve the French, then the Japanese, then the Americans, a lifetime of servitude without rewards.

Woodpeckers wake me to a pale morning, the sun hardly up. I bow the drapes to the walls, throw wide the balcony glass doors, and step into light, a robe about me against the cool. There are no woodpeckers. The tide has fled out twenty yards during the night, and women crab over exposed rocks, plastic sandals holding them on sharp shoals. They chip loose clams with miniature sickle-like picks. Their wide, conical hats shadow their white peasant shirts, dark pants. My mouth recalls the clams and oysters, the shellfish sweetness of yesterday's dinner.

At once, perhaps feeling my eyes, they turn, looking up at my whitewashed balcony, at me—the prodigal scion—resplendent in a white terry-cloth robe, hands on rail, peering down from towering heights at their toils. Their seashell-shaped hats tilt back, revealing their human faces, their luminous eyes. Unnerved, I retreat inside, and with deliberate casualness free the drapes from their wall ribbons. Through a slit in the curtain, I spy the clam women pecking at the rocks.

In the afternoon, unable to take a siesta the way the Vietnamese do, I hike downtown to look for a gym. The cliff workers, napping in the shade, beckon me to join them. *Come and rest. Where are you going in this noon sun? It'll boil your brain. Crazy Viet-kieu!* A mile farther along the paved main drag, cyclo drivers pack the shade of a street-corner tree, each expiring in his own cab like a barber on a slow day.

Catching wind of me a hundred yards off, they perk up like coyotes. I see them drawing lots among themselves. The winner eases out of the cab, mounts the saddle of his cyclo, and lazily swoops toward me, in no hurry at all. I groan inwardly. He pulls along calm and friendly for the kill, pretending to be interested in practicing English and making a friend. "How are you? Where you from? You like Vietnam? What's you name?" After a minute of chatting and pedaling next to me, he invites me to ride his cyclo. I tell him in Vietnamese, *"No, thanks, Brother. I really want to walk."* His eyes flip to the back of his head. *"Fuck!"* he exclaims, then laughs as he abandons the chase, shouting over his shoulder at me. *"Shit. I thought you were Japanese."* He banks the pedicab back to the pack, tosses up his arms, and shouts to his buddies, *"He's a Viet-kieu!"* They hoot, laughing at his misfortune.

The weight gym is the size of a three-car garage with prison-barred windows. A movie poster of Arnold Schwarzenegger is plastered over the main wall, where images of Uncle Ho should have been. Arnold preens his beef in six more images predating his meteoric rise in Hollywood. Hoang, the seriously muscle-bound owner of the gym, enrolls me as a member for two dollars a month even though I tell him I'll only be in town for a day or two. He seems pleased that I chose his gym over the big hotel Nautilus and spas geared for foreigners. The muscle boys of Vung Tau stomp around the hot, smelly room in various states of nudity, dripping pools of sweat. Some are in jeans, others are in boxer shorts. Half are wearing rubber flip-flops, the other half are barefoot. One old guy with sprung ribs and chopstick arms is benching in his white cotton briefs.

I slap a big fat grin on my face, a very un-Vietnamese thing to do, but there is plenty of testosterone sloshing around in the cramped space and I don't want to step on anyone's toes. One by one, the muscle boys approach me tentatively with preambles like *I have an uncle in America; Someday I'll go to America; My sister is sponsoring me. My family tried to escape in '75, but we got caught; I'm going to America next year; My fiancée is sponsoring me to immigrate there, but I love this town and my family so much I don't think I can go.*

Tam, a musician my age, introduces himself. Solely on his salutation, I know we will be friends. This is easy because the Vietnamese form of address allows two people to assess each other and extend overtures of friendship. It has several tiers, each indicating the nature of acquaintance (informal, formal, business, friends, intimate) as well as the hierarchy. Just by pronouns used, one can discern the type of relationship between two people. For instance, if Tam refers to himself as *toi* (I) and calls me *anh* (big brother, or, in this context, you), then the relationship is formal and equal, with neither having the upper hand despite age; however, if Tam is in fact younger than me, then unless there is something else—social, economic status—to normalize the age difference, Tam is being disrespectful by not referring to himself as *em* (little brother). And if I were, say, fifteen years older than he, Tam should use *chu* (uncle) and *chau* (nephew). There are many forms, including regional variations.

Tam calls me *ban:* friend.

I like him instantly. He reminds me of an old childhood friend from my days at the French Catholic school in Saigon, who used his own name, in the third person, instead of "I" and called me "friend" rather than "you." Tam invites me to one of his regular gigs at a hotel disco.

After dinner with Mr. and Mrs. Ba, I walk to the Grand Hotel. It sits not all that grandly on a side street near the beachfront boulevard, one of the two top dogs in this sleepy tourist town. It lodges bureaucrats, foreign oil moguls, and high-caliber journalists. It is the only place with live music every night.

The red-coated bellhop directs me past the faux-marble fountain and up the spiraling staircase to the nightclub on the second floor next to the expensive restaurant. I tread carefully through the chambers replete with Oriental rugs, linen tables, and mirrors. The place is empty save menial servants—and fourteen stunning women sitting around a table. In unison, they turn to look at me. I feel a jolt—a finger-in-light-bulb-socket charge. A hitch in my stride. This must be a meeting for the most beautiful women in the city. I am keenly aware of my faded black jeans, grimy cycling shoes, and sun-bleached mock turtleneck, my only good shirt. I grin like an idiot and hurry down the hall into the nightclub.

Tam greets me the moment I step inside, shaking my hand and maneuvering me through the dark room. "I'm so glad you came," he shouts in careful English, over Mick Jagger howling from the stereo.

He is wearing the requisite white shirt, dark slacks, and a garish polka-dot tie as broad as a meat cleaver. "I am very happy," he says, smiling. "We can talk now. I play with my band soon, but we talk."

We sink down into black leather sofas. Tam tries to say something in English but his vocabulary fails and so he switches to Vietnamese. *"Friend, Tam is very pleased friend has come to see Tam at Tam's workplace. It means much to Tam to have friend here as Tam's guest. It is an honor."*

I return his formal words: *"It is an honor to be with you, friend. Thanks for the invitation."*

Tam grins, his Boy Scout face as bright as a good deed. "Now we practice English, okay?"

"Okay."

"You are very on time. You are very American."

"Why is being on time so American?"

"Because American people value time. My teacher say time is money for American people. American people work very, very much. More than Vietnamese. So America is better, stronger than us."

"But Vietnamese work six days every week. Americans only work five days. Americans have many holidays. Vietnamese have only the New Year."

He reconsiders the point. The waitress comes, and Tam asks me what I want to drink. Beer, wine, cognac? Etiquette requires him to offer me the best in the house. I insist on having whatever he is drinking, which happens to be a diluted orange juice sweetened with sugar. The drink of the day for everyone. A beer in this place would cost him a day's wage.

An older woman herds the roundtable beauties into the room—stunning girls of all shapes and sizes, the youngest probably in her teens, the oldest not over thirty, each clad in satin slips of creative cuts. They spool automatically on the deserted dance floor and begin to move. They cavort in pairs to the throbbing rhythm, turning, swaying fronds in waves. The black lights make their smiles glow. The disco ball runs hands of light across their taut bodies. My desires, the red light strobing on their faces.

Tam chuckles good-naturedly. *"Little sisters think they have a guest: You-friend."*

"Me?"

He chuckles. *"Does friend see anyone else here besides the band and the bartender? It doesn't matter that friend doesn't dress well. Friend is a foreigner—a Viet-kieu. Friend can have any girl friend wants. They all think friend has money. No one can be a tourist in another country without being very rich."*

"I'd disappoint them."

"Don't worry. Friend is here as my guest. Besides, we are like family, the cua ve and the band. The same hand feeds us. We eat from the same dish," says Tam.

Cua ve are taxi dancers / hospitality girls. The price of a dance with them is a drink. A man goes to the bar and buys two drinks, one for himself and one for the woman of his choice. The bartender brings the woman the drink, usually a diluted orange juice or colored water, and directs her to the man who bought the drink. A man who doesn't want to dance can take the woman back to his table for a chat and, usually, light fondling.

A party of six Chinese businessmen marches into the club. The instant they drop their hefty bottoms into the vacuum suction of the leather sofas—even before the waiter has a chance to take their drink orders—the savvy suits sense there are greater predators than themselves in the room. They struggle to sit upright in the quicksand couches, their fatty necks sprung taut, nervous. The *cua ve* spread out, blanketing the empty room, closing in on succulent prey. The suits whisper-negotiate fiercely among themselves—probably debating who ought to be sacrificed. As one unit, they heave and pop themselves out of the couch and buck through the door. I hear the collective sigh of the *cua ve* over the thumping music.

Not another soul comes through the door. No money to be made tonight. Madame rolls her eyes in disgust and clicks her stilettos into the kitchen. A retired string of marionettes, the *cua ve* drape their limbs over the chairs along the wall, collapsing against each other, yawning. Two girls curl up together and doze off like Siamese twins; the spunkier ones joke among themselves. A card game starts at one table. A pair of girls rumba slowly around the room, enjoying themselves completely at ease in the absence of patrons. They are very good. I like watching them.

When the song ends, Tam waves them over. They cross the room toward us, each holding a glass of diluted orange juice in front of her like a truce flag—a polite and thoughtful declaration that they don't expect us to buy them drinks. They are smiling.

"*Hello, Brother Tam,*" says the taller girl, with straight black hair spilling down to her waist. She bows, showing proper respect to Tam, who is a few years her senior. To me she also bows and says, "*Hello, Brother.*"

The other young woman, with short hair and a tight red body dress, echoes her friend's greeting. Tam makes the introductions and invites them to join us.

We take turns talking, shouting in that awkward mode of communicating in a disco. They are a lively pair, polite and full of curiosity. We chat and dance until the club shuts down early due to zero business. Kim and I make a date for lunch the next day.

I simply forget I have to leave for Hanoi. First, it is lunch. Then lunch and dinner. Then breakfast, lunch, dinner, breakfast, lunch, dinner. Kim and I wrap our days around each other. It seems so natural, as though this is part of my itinerary, a scheduled stop on my journey. She takes me to all her favorite haunts. When we dine out, she insists on taking turns paying. "*I want to pay,*" she says. "*I want to do like Western women do. We're friends, aren't we?*" I nod. "*Then let's do it like Westerners do. Let's take turns. I don't want to be a Vietnamese girl who always waits for her male friend to pay.*" I protest that she makes so little during this off-season. She hushes me, looking upset.

She has a mane of black hair, straight and long, as fine as silk, as supple as thoughts on a breeze. It is a veil that threads across her face, her musings unknowable to me. It curtains her off and lifts only when she is ready. But she is always ready, I forget things lurk backstage. When she chooses, she is up-front, honest. There is no false churchy demureness about her. We are eating in a restaurant and I tell her I notice people treat her differently, look at her in a way I do not like.

"*It doesn't matter,*" she says, shrugging. "*I am an untouchable in this town. People know where I work and what I do. I am like trash. So it doesn't matter that we're seen together in public. It's not like I'm a nice girl or any-thing. No nice girl can ever be seen talking to a Viet-kieu. If they are, people will call them used material. It doesn't matter with me. I like you, and maybe part of the reason why I like you is because you're a Viet-kieu. You might like me, but it doesn't matter, I'm only a taxi dancer."* She turns and smiles at me with dark eyes. *"Let's go swimming down at the beach."*

And we are off, just like that. Somber moments forgotten like shadows of errant clouds on a sunny day. I pass in and out of her flickering sadness so quickly I take it for granted. How can I think of dusky places when she vibrates beside me, laughing mischievously as she wreaks minor pranks: feeding me a hot chili pepper craftily stuffed inside a green bean; leaving me alone in a temple with praying Buddhist monks; pulling wild stunts with her motorbike, me scream-ing for mercy on the seat behind her.

When the end comes, it all seems to have lasted so much longer—yet not long enough, the hours we shared. We are sitting on my bal-cony watching the day's fiery death. It is high tide and the sea laps close beneath us. The sun is going down over the water. The sky is aflame, the clouds baking, heavenly beds of hot coals. Her face is flushed with the light, her hair not so dark now.

Kim inspects me with her inscrutable eyes half-curtained behind the cascade of her hair. She asks me, *"Am I beautiful to you?"*

"Very."

"I think I love you . . . If what I am feeling is not love, it will grow to be love. Do you love me?"

"I don't think I've ever truly loved anyone."

"Why?"

"I've left everyone I loved. I've failed people I loved."

"You can leave me, too. I don't mind. Things always work out."

"Do they? That's what I want to believe."

"I don't want to stay here in Vietnam. Take me to America."

"I can't."

"Why? Viet-kieu do it all the time. Four of my friends have been married to Viet-kieu, two married Australians."

"I can't."

"We don't have to stay married. We can get a divorce after I get a green

card. You don't even have to support me. I have five thousand dollars saved. My family will give me more. I speak English. I can get a job. I have a degree in French literature. I can go back to school."

"I can't."

"Please, don't leave me in this life. Look at me. Look. Look at my face. I am not young anymore. I'm twenty-five. My friends have children already. There are so many young and beautiful girls at the hotel now. I won't last there much longer."

"You are incredibly beautiful. You are very intelligent."

"Please, take me. You can save me. I can save my family. And they and all my children and their children and their grandchildren will be indebted to you."

"Don't put it that way."

"But it's true. Think about it. When you have children, they will be Americans. They will have food, clothing, and education. They will grow up and have jobs and have their own children. And their children and their grandchildren will all benefit from your coming to America."

"I had nothing to do with my coming to America. My parents brought me."

"Do the same for me. How can you deny me this when it costs you so little? You have the power to give me, my family, a better life."

"It's not right."

"Why? You like me. You might even grow to love me. Can't we try?"

"I can't."

And for the life of me, I don't know why I can't.

It is very cool the instant the clouds stop burning.

I feel her slipping from me. An unenthusiastic reply. A canceled lunch here. A missed dinner there. One evening, I see Kim strolling down the beachfront boulevard in the company of a tall white tourist, her tiny hand looping the crook of his arm. She catches my eyes, and when her companion isn't looking, she smiles brightly at me: Friends.

Kim has never looked more beautiful. It is too late, but I wish I could tell her of the warmth and respect I harbor for her—for her tenacity, for her unblinking honesty, her selfless devotion to her family. She is very Vietnamese and very un-Vietnamese all at once. Fate is an obligation I don't understand—the reasons that random beast passed over her deserving soul in favor of mine.

Jade-Giant

19 A great hue-and-cry rang throughout the refugee compound, wails and curses the likes of which were never heard again. A mob howled that their water supply had been poisoned.

We heard it from the railroad track where we were playing among the warehouses and freight yards. Within a few months of being stranded at the facility, Huy, Tien, and I, unable to enroll at the local Indonesian elementary school, had turned into dock rats. We scooted through a gap under the wall and brought up the tail of the mob. They were chasing someone along the edge of the compound, which wasn't really a refugee facility—Jakarta didn't officially have one. It was a low-security prison for petty foreign criminals and illegal aliens awaiting deportation, a sort of holding pen for live cargo in transition.

Apart from the crooks, there were four groups at the compound: refugees like our family; dock clerks and government officials; guards who kept an eye on everything; and the compound staff, which included servants, caretakers, and kitchen hands. It was the staff who were up in arms, screaming that the culprit had disgraced them, soiled them. They shouted horrible things. A terrible humiliation on their heads.

The chase turned the corner and rumbled through the front garden, right across the dignitary parking lot. The horde funneled back and forth through the warren of single-story structures that sprawled out into four wings, within which was a ramshackle of minor annexes, lean-tos, and two central courtyards. Shaking their fists, angry Indonesians in sarongs—poor running outfits—flip-flopped after their antagonist through offices and storage rooms, disrupting over a hundred inmates and clerks. We didn't see the culprit until he raced down the other side of the compound, a little black head blitzing along a fence sprouting barbed-wire foliage. It was Hien.

I cornered one of the cooks, a massive old woman curtained in swaths of fabric. She babbled furiously about her drinking water. Each wing of the complex drew drinking, cooking, and bathing water from the central water tower into private cisterns via garden hoses. Breathing like a great dying beast, she swore to give five-year-old Hien a good whipping. She croaked that she had caught him with his pants down, his penis inserted into the garden hose feeding directly into the staff's water supply. Peeing! Peeing!

No one knew, but once Hien discovered that his penis and the garden hose were a perfect fit, he had been using the same personal urinal for months. Hien escaped the lynching mob that day but didn't leave our quarters for a week. Whenever he crossed the path of a staff member, he got a smack on the back of the head for the disgrace he had dealt. From then on, hoses were coiled and put away in a safe place.

For the length of our stay in Indonesia, eighteen months, we were quartered in a single fourteen-by-twenty-five-foot room. Our fishermen shared one of the two dormitories with other inmates. The food was bad. There was no privacy. People bickered. Quarrels often came to blows. The men lasted ten months and jumped on the first opportunity to leave. They wanted to go to America, but the paperwork took too long and was an uncertainty at best because none of them had relatives living Stateside. To a man, they elected to go to France. It was the last we ever saw of them.

During the first three months we shared a room with a Chinese couple from Hong Kong. They were nice and solicitous, giving us candies and toys they bought in town. Mom liked them immensely because they had daily town-passes and they grocery-shopped for her. They were particularly nice to Chi and Auntie Dung.

One night, with my parents' permission, they took Chi and Dung into town for dinner and a movie. The evening's real destination, their little surprise, followed the sanctioned part of the outing. They pedicabbed the girls to a massage parlor on the far, and seamier, side of town. It was a place I later visited with a big-brother-friend, an Indonesian soldier stationed at the dock compound; on his payday spree I drank sodas while he did his thing. Local patrons called this corner of the city the Perfumed Quarters. It was a rubble-tossed jungle of plywood huts running along a river of reeking sewage. Pavement and streetlamps hadn't found purchase among the mountains of sundered concrete.

They ushered Chi and Dung into one of those lice hooches and gave them cold sodas. A couple of girls who worked there joined them for a chat. Neither Chi nor Dung spoke much Indonesian. Mr. Ho, the husband, commanded a smattering of Vietnamese and translated for the girls. While they were there, men came in and paired off with Indonesian girls who led their newfound boyfriends to the rooms in the back. The operation dawned on both Chi and Dung.

Mr. Ho whipped out a thick roll of bills. "You like money? You want to make lots of money?"

Chi and Dung nodded and shook their heads simultaneously. Food was barely sufficient at the compound, and no one had any money to buy as much as a new shirt or a pair of plastic slippers. Mom sold her earrings to the cooks to buy rice, eggs, and vegetables for the family, but besides these extra staples to line our stomachs, there was not a nickel to be had by anyone.

Smiling goodwill, Mrs. Ho, a slim, attractive woman in her mid-thirties, took the girls' hands and urged them toward a rickety corridor of rooms with unevenly boarded walls leaking raucous laughter and moans. Mrs. Ho let them peek into the rooms to make certain there was no mistaking the terms of her proposition. She led them back to the waiting room, where Mr. Ho was talking with some Chinese-Indonesian men. Pulling a stack of bills out of her purse, she nudged it at them, then gestured at the men.

Grabbing Chi's hand, Dung cried, "No! We want to go home!"

Dung and Chi fled outside and caught a pedicab home with the money Mom had given them. At the compound, they spilled the story to Mom and us boys—Huy, Tien, and me. I was thinking there was going to be a fist fight, but Mom didn't seem all that angry about the whole thing. In fact, she didn't want us to tell Dad. She just said we couldn't trust the Hos anymore and reminded us that Mr. Ho out-weighed Dad by forty pounds. It seemed odd to me that Mom didn't want to have it out with the Hos. I vowed to Chi and Dung that us boys would exact vengeance and redeem the family's honor. The Hos returned early in the morning and retreated to their corner of the room, sectioned off by bedsheets, and pretended nothing unusual had happened.

The next afternoon when the lunch bell rang, the Hos were going away at it, passionate and noisy behind their fabric walls. The whole family had always turned a deaf ear to their frequent husband-and-wife business. Since seven-year-old Tien was the most innocent look-ing, we had him spearhead the operation. We waited until the men of our group came by, as they usually did, to go with the family down to the kitchen for lunch.

Tien, trailed by Huy and me, marched into the room and pulled open the Hos' curtains. Tien announced in his peeping voice, "Mr. and Mrs. Ho, it's lunchtime! Do you want to come with us?"

Mrs. Ho was naked on her back atop the bed, her red panties shackling her knees. And Mr. Ho, equally bare, looked up from where he was busying himself, his head between her legs. Our fisher-men got a good view. Tien dropped the curtain and the men yanked us out of the room by our ears.

We followed this stunt by slipping a batch of live cockroaches under their blankets and trapping them inside the mosquito netting. Next were cat litter beneath their bed and food scraps in their clothes drawers to attract fire ants. They screamed and threatened, but they never caught us in the act, so we went unpunished. Our series of pranks lasted three days, until the Hos, with a little official bribing, finagled quarters in another wing.

Life in the compound was intolerably boring. Breakfast was a lump of bread and a cup of instant coffee, or milk-tea for the children. Lunch was rice and vegetables boiled with oily onion water. Dinner was a fillet of fried fish, rice, and more boiled vegetables. Little variation. The morning was cool, the afternoon muggy, the evening alive with mosquitoes. Huy, Tien, and I picked up a hobby—burning anthills—until we inadvertently torched an ancient tree.

Besides the maintenance staff, most of the compound denizens liked us because our pranks gave them something to talk about. We picked up foster brothers. Tien's favorite friend was Jatook, a guard who lived in town and often brought him candies. Huy's big brother was a tall Indonesian lieutenant, an avid golfer who accidentally whacked Huy in the head with a driver. Wong, the Chinese giant, was my friend.

He was the gentlest lifer, a loner in his late forties. He towered a head and a half over everyone at the compound, but no one feared him. He was well-liked because he was soft-spoken, kind, and kept to himself. Wong had a broad, plain face, a wide nose, round cheeks, and a stone set mouth, hard and silent. He was a jade cutter. Eight to ten hours every day, seven days a week, he labored on the steps under the roof overhang just out of the sun and rain. Perching on a comically low stool, an animated gargoyle, he hunched his great shoulders over a grindstone mounted on a block of wood, shaping a shard of jade clamped between his vise fingers.

Shk-shk-shk-shk. The sound of him grinding in the courtyard outside our quarters became as natural to us as cricket song. Once, to end my pestering, he lent me a shaping stone and a drop of red jade and had me try. I lasted an hour. Wong spoke fluent Cantonese, Mandarin, Vietnamese, and Indonesian. He often told me Chinese fables, which I committed to memory and retold to my brothers. My mother was fond of him because he gave estimates on the value of her jade bracelets. She hoped they might help us if we ever found ourselves in a tight spot in America.

"The nature of the stone is its will to remain stone. The stone's will is strong. To shape it, your will must be stronger than the stone's. To do this you must be the stone of stones."

"A diamond?" I asked, and Wong tweaked my ear.

Wong was a permanent prison fixture, and white-bearded Mr. Ling, the longest resident and oldest lifer, said that all lifers cracked sooner or later. Wong had been there twelve years and every year he sent an appeal to whatever country he thought he belonged to. Every year he was rejected. So he polished jade for jewelers in town. The compound's officials allowed him to work and took a cut of his earnings.

The day Wong cracked, he started drinking from morning until late afternoon. Wong went over his limit around sunset. Maybe another one of his appeals got rejected. Maybe someone in his family died. Maybe his big old heart just broke after all those years. Maybe the sunset pushed him over the edge. The orange hours were the toughest behind the walls because it was always hot and clammy and the latrine stank and there was nowhere to walk off that jittery energy in cooped-up legs. Inmates paced like overwound clocks. Wong's alarm finally went off.

It was hard to tell why he cracked because no one but I, a snot-nosed kid, really talked to him. Wong dwelt in a dark corner of the cavernous but windowless west hall, with its single row of rectangular air holes at the top, not large enough for an adult's head. His cubby-hole of a decade was nine by six feet, curtained off with old bedsheets hanging on bailing wire and a modest folding screen.

All day, every day, the compound cronies, inmates and staff, convened for bingo. By the time the sun slipped horizontally through the air vents, the gamblers had puffed their cheap tobacco into a wheaty haze. The humid hotness was dense. Except for the caller croaking out numbers, the chips rattling in plastic jars, and the halfhearted curses of the players, the place was rather quiet. I was hanging around, hoping for a soda errand. They usually wanted cigarettes or sodas while they played.

Wong broke the hour with a wordless sound, a blast from the bull-horn of his throat. It was a groan, a scream, a cry, a screech, but it was the depth and the power of his rage that made it a howl. It was throaty and it was brittle. Something was breaking in him. I had never heard anything like it. A chill flushed through me. The hall reverberated, the echoes chasing each other back and forth and away. The cronies jumped, then froze, bingo chips pebbling the floor, as Wong came alive behind his cell of cotton sheets.

He tore up his corner, shredding his mattress, and with one sweep of his arm the shelves he had fashioned of salvaged bamboo exploded and all the fine stones he had polished and all the figurines he had cut shrapneled across the room. His fingers balled and formed a wild pair of hammers levered on his shoulders. Down went the hammer, the table shattered. Down went the hammer, the folding screen splintered. Down went the hammer, the chair collapsed. Wong tornadoed through his small world, letting loose the demon inside him. And the demon became Wong as the sham of his existence was reduced to rubble.

All the people to whom he was too shy to talk were there to witness his destruction, his shame, his hurt bare in the wreckage, fine stones ground to bits and howls that gave odd time to his fevered dance. They watched him exorcise their demon, the frustrated boil of confinement, the bleeding of hope. Wong's wet red eyes mopped across me without recognition. I was afraid for him when the guards came. They beat and jumped on him, piling four deep, tearing off his shirt. Wong roared. He threw them aside like clothes. Out from the front building came officials and bureaucrats, brandishing sticks, beating Wong. The matadors converged on the bull, teased him, herded him into a tower, and locked him inside. His throat venting inhuman cries, Wong sledged himself against the door, but it did not give. On the strength of his fingertips, he clawed his way thirty feet up the brick wall of the hollow tower, right into the rafters. He punched through the roof and burst into the orange sunset. Half-naked in the curving light, he hurled tiles into the empty courtyard. The guards didn't want to shoot Wong. Shaking their heads in pity, they stood in the breezeway out of the spray of tile fragments and murmured that this would all have to come out of Wong's jade-earnings. The day was failing him. He had scalped the roof, nothing left to throw. He jumped. I wished we could go to America.

Fullcircle-Halflives

20 5 a.m. The night couldn't have passed quickly enough. I want to be away from here. Away from Kim. I want to go north. I want to go to Hanoi and forget, but I need to pay homage to one more place in South Vietnam. I need to find Minh Luong Prison, perhaps even more than touring the rest of the country. Somehow, I have long thought of it as the end of my journey—as if by finding Minh Luong and returning to the exact spot where I had watched my father working the minefield, I will have come full circle. I spent the night mulling over my choices and nursing beers on the balcony. An hour before daybreak, I strap on my backpack and strike out for a brisk four-mile hike to the market, where a fleet of minivans shuttles people into Saigon hourly, sunrise to sunset. Hanoi must wait.

A wolf-faced man and his partner collect my two dollars and pack me into a minivan along with thirteen other people, including the driver. Two torturous hours later, they drop us at Ben Thanh Market in downtown Saigon. I take a motorbike taxi out to the main bus depot at the southern fringe of the city. It accommodates all the traffic to and from the Mekong Delta.

I trudge up and down the dusty, diesel-slicked lot the size of four football fields, inquiring for the next bus out to Rach Gia. The place is a hive of activity, sellers hawking food, last-minute gifts, and what-nots, porters moving cargo, travelers hurrying to their buses, motor-bike-taxi drivers pestering for fares, and mechanics banging away, repairing buses. A constant stream of noisy, fuming vehicles moves through the gate in both directions. Most of the raw materials that sustain Saigon are channeled through three major bus depots. Farmers bring in produce and livestock from the countryside. Young men and women come to the City looking for work even as Saigon sends its manufactured and imported goods out to the provinces. The frenzy seethes with ant-like industry.

Busing in Vietnam is a freewheeling enterprise, somewhat akin to the stagecoaches of the old American West. Privately owned buses, driven by the owners and their relatives, go bumping from town to town hailing freight, livestock, and produce and picking up riders standing on the side of the road like hitchhikers. A stripped-down traveling show, they roar along, working every minute, shooting from village to village, laughing and cajoling a livelihood from the highway boredom. They haul on a skeleton crew of four—any more and there are too many mouths to feed, any less and they're liable to be cheated by their customers. The driver is always and only the driver, keeping his eyes on the road and muttering prayers to the Buddha mounted on the dashboard. There couldn't be a more serious lot of drivers in the world. These guys deal in life and death daily, their whole family riding on their performance, the bus their vehicle, the whole family's savings and possibly their coffin on wheels. In my brief travels here, I've seen several dead buses, smashed, rolled belly-up, and disembow-eled by salvagers.

I board the next bus out of town, trusting myself to its plastic deity. It is going to Chau Doc, then Rach Gia. Like most others, it is a Russian-made death trap, halfway into its own graveyard. I negotiate my way to the back of the bus, climbing over luggage, crates, and tin tanks of fishsauce. The bus has been gutted and crudely regaffed to double its passenger capacity, the thinly upholstered benches crammed so tight that even small Vietnamese have trouble sitting without knock-ing their knees. The floor is decked with wooden planks sporting gaps big enough to swallow a boot.

Combing the aisle checking passenger tickets, the bus driver arches an eyebrow at my accent: Viet-kieu, eh? Yes, I tell him. He tows me back to the front of the bus. Sit right here, then, the best seat in the house. No, not there, here right behind me. He steers me into the seat and whispers in my ear. You don't want to sit back there. Too noisy. Sit here, good view for sightseeing and you can stretch your legs. He shows me where to put my legs, right beside his seat, inches from the stick shift. You're the first Viet-kieu on our bus, he tells me excitedly, grinning around his cigarette, his teeth chewed up and stained like spent spark plugs. Why don't you rent a car instead? Too expensive, I tell him, this is more fun anyway. He looks at me incredulously then starts mining me for information about the bus business in America.

The owner is a woman in her fifties with a round, generous face, white and soft like a steamed pork bun. Swathed in yards of expensive red satin of a peasant cut, she waves a prospective fare aboard, saying in a quacking voice (a tone my mother often condescendingly refers to as that of a fishmonger): No, no we go straight through. This is the fastest bus there is. You can't get to Chau Doc any faster if you fly like a bird. We're safe, of course, we're safe. This here is my brother (pointing at Driver). He has been driving since he was old enough to get a license. His mother delivered him on a bus. It's natural for him.

I stifle a laugh. Driver plays his poker face. I have heard this line so often I figure the only people driving buses are the ones born on them.

They are a smooth crew, the four of them: the driver, the owner, the mechanic, and the bagman. The owner collects the cash and handles all financial matters, from buying petrol to bribing cops. The mechanic doubles as a relief driver and a baggage handler. The bagman, their barker, leans out the open door when the bus is under way and shouts fares-destinations to prospective passengers standing on the side of the road. Most crew are family members or relatives. Fares are standard. Buses equipped with air-conditioning, televisions, or karaoke machines charge about twenty percent more.

Passengers arrive sporadically, carrying anything from luggage to live chickens. The bus eventually leaves ninety minutes after its scheduled time, filled to seating capacity. Just as we pull out of the gate, two men bang on the door and swing aboard. The bus owner, whom I call Madame, casts a distasteful glance but doesn't ask them for fares. They stand next to the driver. As the bus lists out onto the street, the crew becomes nervous, craning their necks on the lookout for cops. Even the passengers seem agitated. Along the side of the busy road, a string of seven buses have their engines in idle as traffic cops scan passengers and prod luggage.

Faster, Madame urges Driver. He thumps the accelerator and the crew heaves a big sigh as the bus grunts past the busy traffic cops. Around the next turn a cop steps out from a soda kiosk and points at Driver, who obediently edges the bus to the side of the road. Bagman jumps off and lopes toward the cop, wearing a big friendly grin. He pumps a couple of bills into the cop's waiting palm with everyone watching. The cop nods Bagman back on the bus, thumbs up to Driver. Again, the bus shudders and farts into motion. Half a mile later, the incident is repeated and this time Madame is pissed, yelling to her passenger witnesses: *Oh, my God, what's going on. The cops got all their relatives out here collecting or what? They can't peel and gut us twice like this. How are we supposed to eat?*

Cops usually collect anywhere from five to thirty percent of the bus's net income.

No sooner than we clear the city, the duo who boarded the bus at the gate open their satchels. One man pulls a bullhorn on the passengers, the other brandishes long ticker tapes of pills in cellophane. The pitch begins. *May I have your attention, ladies and gentlemen. Please quiet down. Quiet, please. QUIET! Thank you, everyone. Hey, sister, you there, make your kid shut up. Thank you. Ladies and gentlemen, have you ever had a headache that just won't go away? One of those that feels like a spike driven from the base of your skull through the top of your head?*

I groan, feeling the very pains he is describing. The smooth-skinned, sharp-eyed man fires off his singsong pitch in a nasally tenor, the battery-amplified words shot out like bullets from a Gatling gun. My head is three feet away. *The drug is positively a miracle of science,* he claims. I try turning my head away from the horn. *Everything you'll ever need to cure everything.* My eardrums are about to implode. *Let me tell you about Doctor Nguyen Le Van Truc, the esteemed doctor of Saigon who invented this miracle drug. Look, look here is a photo of him.* I try to politely cover my ears. *You. You, uncle in the green shirt. What ails you? Backache, you say? Well, this drug will cure your backache. Make you feel like a kid again.*

The dealer's compatriot works the aisle, shaking people awake, dangling his string of pills in their faces. There are a few takers. After all, a string of ten pills costs less than a bowl of noodles, about as cheap as medicine gets. The tirade of medicinal benefits keeps getting longer. Then I hear the real breakthrough: It cures cancer, all cancers. More buyers. A fair quarter of the passengers have coughed up cash for the miracle medicine, but not enough to please the pair. They go on the aggressive, publicly interrogating passengers individually to see why each failed to jump on this spectacular one-time offer. Thirty minutes into the intimidation program, they have extricated money from three-quarters of the passengers. The peasant woman next to me explains in my ear that the pair are part of large gangs that prey on buses throughout southern Vietnam. If the bus owners don't let them aboard, they'll slash the bus tires. Buses have been known to be put to the torch by gangsters. She has seen them slash a girl's face.

Madame acts as though the snake-oil salesmen aren't raping her passengers. Driver concentrates on the road. Bagman and Mechanic sit dejectedly on crates, putting up with the salesmen without a word.

"What about you?" Snake turns to me. *"You're a Viet-kieu, aren't you?"*

I nod.

"Buy some of this medicine and take it home with you."

It is an order. I shake my head. *"No, thank you, Brother. I don't need any medicine."*

"DON'T you shake your head at me!" Snake roars. *"If you don't want my medicine, don't buy it, but don't you dare shake your head at me!"*

Oh, shit. I scramble to my feet, thinking: It's going down. They're going to make an example of me. Snake's partner is moving slowly up from the back of the bus. There is no time to look for the pepper spray I'd tossed into my backpack. I brace myself against the seat, trying to keep an eye on both of them.

"You Viet-kieu think you're better than everyone else, don't you!"

"Sorry, Brother. I don't want any trouble."

"You don't have to shake your head at me, you son of a bitch!" Snake is working himself up to a frenzy.

I know his type too well. I've dealt with this kind since I was a kid fresh to America. When you cross paths with anyone who doesn't take kindly to your kind of gook, Chink, nip, you must come at him swinging. It doesn't matter if he beats the crap out of you, you've got to fight back or it will only get worse. The only thing that will save you is the bottomless rage that burns in your deepest pit.

"FUCKING ASSHOLES! You-wanna-fight? Come-on-you-mother-fuckers! COME-ON!" I bring up my fist, churning, ready to swing. Burning with fury, I have no idea I am cussing them in English.

They pause. People ogle me as though I am an alien that has just inadvertently dropped its mask.

Before Snake recovers, Madame wedges herself between us. I can't see her face but I hear the edge in her.

"Brother," she says, eerily calm, *"this is my cousin. I will buy a pill string for myself."* She holds out a fifty-cent bill. Bagman and Mechanic are on their feet, poised to back up their mistress.

A moment of silence inflates the bus. All eyes on our showdown. Snake stares at Madame, murder plain in his eyes. I can see him weighing the odds, calculating.

"Very smart decision, Big Sister," Snake declares, and takes her money with a flourish. *"Smarter than your cousin."* Snake smirks at me.

Snake orders Driver to stop. The pair jump off. As we pull away, they cross the street to hail another bus, heading back into Saigon. Madame pats me on the shoulder and takes her seat, clearly as shaken as I am.

Four hours out, Bagman licks his chops and bellows, *"Bridge stop,"* which in Vietnamese means rest-room break. Our asthmatic vehicle wheezes into a dirt lot in front of a roadside diner built specifically for bus traffic. Barely large enough to host one busload of diners at a time, it is a corrugated tin roof on wooden poles with picnic tables on packed dirt. *"Everybody out!"* Bagman bellows. *"We're locking up the bus for your protection. Come in the shade and have lunch."* I accept Madame's invitation and join the crew at their table as an honorary guest. *"Eat up,"* Driver encourages me with a wink. *"It's on the house."* On cue, the proprietor marches food to the table and we dig into it with gusto.

Most of the passengers refuse to dine and squat on their hams in the parking lot, glaring at the crew. Impatient, Bagman gets up and waves them inside. *"Come on, have lunch. Get out of the sun everybody. Rice here is good and cheap."* No one budges. Bagman throws up his hands in disgust. *"Go ahead, sit in the sun if you like, but we're not leaving for another hour and a half."*

He goes back to his bowl and starts scarfing down everything in sight, zigzagging across the table and popping morsels into his big mouth. He chopsticks a morsel into my bowl in a gesture of friendship. Madame gives me a stewed egg. Driver picks me a choice piece of fish. Mechanic spoons me some vegetables. We eat a hearty meal. The crew heaps on me the standard questions every Vietnamese asks about the West, and I answer them between mouthfuls, my bowl never empty.

Half an hour later, Driver groans to his feet, rubs his belly, and drags his bones over to a hammock hung from mango trees off to the side of the diner. At the sight of Driver slouching into the hammock like a dead man and draping an arm over his eyes, the crowd, suffering in the noon sun, clearly swindled, moans. By twos and threes, they stagger like captives into the shade of the diner and order peasant lunches of steamed rice with pork chops sautéed in fishsauce and scallions. Even tight-pursed elders eke out a dime-bill for iced tea.

I swing onto a hammock next to Driver, who peeks at me from beneath his arm, apparently feigning a nap. *"What's it like in Japan?"* he whispers without shifting his reposed position, keeping up the charade for the benefit of his passengers.

I feel funny telling a traveling man about traveling, and, in fact, telling a second party about the culture of a third party, a little like snitching, gossiping. But I oblige anyway, giving him a look at Japan, the jewel of the East, through Western eyes. Perhaps Western eyes have rose-colored lenses particularly suitable for adventurers because my tales of mountains after mountains of skyscrapers and glass and concrete and asphalt and smog, overrun with a bewildering sea of people, excite him.

"Sometimes, I wish I could go," he says, eyes looking off to someplace devised by his wanderlust. *"I just want to rip out the seats on the bus, put in a table and a bed. And ten fifty-gallon drums of diesel. And drive. Drive all the way to Hanoi, then right into China, then up and up and up through Russia until I see snow—you know, I've never seen snow—and then just go West. Aim for the sun and drive at it . . . Drive until I hit Poland and France and right into the end of the world, right into England."* He pauses, perplexed. *"You think there's a road like that, a road over all that land, over all those countries?"* I tell him there probably is and if there isn't, a couple of side trips wouldn't be bad either. Adventure is but a collection of detours. He asks me how I got the courage to go. I say I'd realized that the surest way forward was to burn all the bridges behind. I am really good at that. He rambles on about all his *"crazy notions,"* yakking passionately about exploration and adventure. He does all this without moving, so that, to everyone else, he is still napping.

"Fuck, I must sound pretty crazy wanting to take off like this."

"Don't worry about it."

I tell him about Frank, an eighty-five-year-old retired farmer I met while riding through Napa, California. I had stopped on his porch to ask for some water from his garden hose. "Damn. Damn," Frank said over and over. "I wish I was a young fella again. Bicycle. I used to do that when I was a boy. I'd make me a peanut-butter-and-jelly sandwich and I'd ride my bike on down the road and over the bridge outside of town to the edge of the woods. I'd always wished I could keep going. Wondering what I'd see round the next bend." And he is still wondering, although he is too sick and poor to go far beyond his porch and his oxygen tanks. "What do you like to drink?" he asked me. Water is fine, I said—Frank was proud of his water, a well he'd drilled himself some forty years earlier. "A real drink, I mean. Beer, wine, whiskey?" It was summer so I said I'd fancy a slushy margarita. Frank dug into his high-draped white trousers, pulled out a fiver, then stabbed me with it saying, "Drink one on your trip for me." I accepted his money, drank a margarita to Frank twenty miles down the road, then fell flat on my ass because in my dehydration, the tequila lambadaed straight to my head.

Driver laughs himself off the hammock. By the time we leave, practically all the passengers have spent money in the diner. I see the proprietor discreetly pressing a rolled bill into Madame's hand as she comes out of the rest room.

With the passengers barely in their seats, Driver guns the bus down the road and is back humping the horn, never laying off more than a minute. Soon after we take off, a little boy pisses all over himself and the bus reeks. Madame, finger jabbing over the heads of the crowd, vows to charge the mother extra if her kid whizzes again. The whole miserable bus, packed tighter than eels in a bucket, grumbles in agreement. Still, Bagman and Mechanic hang out the doors and scoop up more passengers. They make a game of bagging people on the fly. One little guy, shouldering a heavy bag, flip-flops frantically after the bus like a three-legged dog. Bagman and Mechanic reach down and monkey-yank the man aboard without losing their cigarettes. The poor guy is huffing open-mouthed with either terror or exhaustion, but then he suddenly grins. This and his narrow face and popping jawbreaker eyes make him look like a Chihuahua. Madame sits Chihuahua next to me and tells both of us to lift our legs for Bagman to slide Chihuahua's luggage, a huge block of wood, into our foot space. Now we are both crouching in our seats. I tell myself it could be worse. We could be sitting on the five-gallon drums of stinking fishsauce sloshing in the aisle like the two new passengers. Chihuahua-man says he used to be a deer and boar hunter, but he hasn't seen much game in the last five years so he's turned to cutting rare hardwood and selling it to artisans and carpenters in town, one cord at a time. *"Fuck!"* he exclaims with his everlasting fat grin. *"It's better than churning mud or busting rocks for two bucks a day."* I present him with a new baseball cap Kim gave me. He puts it on over his moppy jungle of black hair. A couple of sizes too big, it slips down and catches on his ears. He grins, happy. He is such a jovial, nature-happy guy, I feel like giving him a hug and calling him my lost brother, but don't want to startle him. So I show my teeth and dip my head in a bow of sorts. He returns the courtesy and we perch together, looking out of our rattling cage at naked kids playing in the Mekong tributaries, the color of Dijon mustard. Since Saigon, the land has been a hundred

and fifty miles of rustic farms and thatched huts. Brown mud and clay-
ish red earth peek through like stitching in the mat of intense, lush
green, almost violent, a hundred shades of green. In the distant rice
paddies, plodding water buffalo are moving rocks; white ducks drift
like patches of snow. But it is hot and humid and the smell of the land is
thick in the air. From certain angles, it is a testament to coffee-table
books. I count my weeks in Vietnam: broken roads; children playing
hopscotch on the asphalt; peasants drying their pickling vegetables and
fans of joss sticks on the side of the road; unbroken strings of shanties
fencing both sides of the highway for hundreds of miles. And I see it all
equaling a land of abject poverty, the smiles of its people its only hope.

In the late afternoon, the bus groans into Chau Doc. Driver complains that the engine isn't running well. Mechanic will be tinkering
with it all night, so they'll leave for Rach Gia first thing tomorrow
morning. Sleep on the bus, Driver urges me, there's plenty of room.
The combination of diesel fumes, fishsauce, urine, and chicken feath-
ers is making me nauseous. I beg off to look for a room. To get into
town, I decide to try a mini-rickshaw hinged to the seat post of a regular bicycle. In the rural south, bicycle rickshaws are more practical.
Unlike big-city cyclos designed for short distances, say, under five
miles at a snail's pace, the country bicycle rickshaw easily belts out ten
miles a haul over unimproved roads.

The sun slashes down mercilessly; my skin browns like carameliz-
ing onions. The dead river air smells bloated. Without much debate, I
commit the mistake of hopping on a bicycle rickshaw without settling on a definite price. How far to the closest inn? Pretty far in this
heat, sir, the skinny man replies around his cigarette. How much?
Whatever you think is appropriate, sir. I nod.

He hauls us onto a sandy road that reminds me of some dusty
Mexican mining towns. I mention that it is very hot. *"White people
smell,"* he says without preamble, *"especially when they sweat. Most of
them use cologne and perfume and that chalky stuff they rub in their armpits.
But, oh, God, they can really stink."* I laugh and offer that maybe it has a
lot to do with their diet. Maybe Vietnamese stink pretty bad as well
because we eat so much fishsauce. But we can't smell each other
because we all eat the same thing. He snorts and delivers me to an inn

a hundred yards from the station. I feel about as brilliant as a jackass, handing him a fifty-cent bill—several times the going rate. His chummy face sours as though I have wedged him a slice of lemon. *"Oh, come on, Big Brother, can't you be more generous than that?"* I explain that I could have just walked the distance. He raises his voice demanding more. People crane their necks in our direction and I feel the flush of embarrassment rising on my cheek. To stem off his tirade, I sheepishly surrender another fifty-cent bill. He pockets it quickly and bawls, *"Come on, how about two dollars. Give me two U.S. dollars. You're a Viet-kieu, be generous to your Vietnamese brother."*

I shake my head and zip into the inn, leaving him cursing me outside. Beat and dizzy with a full day of diesel exhaust, I take a room and order a meal. After a boy delivers the food, the owner invites himself into my room, strolling in with southern informality. I ask him if he would like to join me for an early supper.

"No, no. Thank you. It's very kind of you. My wife expects me for dinner. If I don't have a big appetite, she'll think I have a mistress!" He pops with mirth, laughing at his own joke.

"It depends on how you eat. A cook always appreciates a diner with a whetted appetite," I reply lamely, using a well-worn line. The double entendre hits him a second late. He claps his hands gleefully like a boy, and laughter rolls up from his round belly. I expect his laughter to taper off, but it grows. Soon, he is hammering the wall, hooting, spewing spittle. I try to cover my rice bowl, worrying that my host is a few bricks shy of a load. Nothing contagious, I hope.

Finally, he wipes the tears from his eyes. *"Brother, are you a tourist? Visiting relatives?"*

"Neither. My bus broke down. I'm just here for the night."

"Ah, too bad," he bubbles with genuine sympathy. *"This province is beautiful. I grew up here. A village up-River."*

"Up the Mekong River?"

"Uh, yes." He looks puzzled as though there exists no other river in the world. Like everyone I meet who lives or makes a living on the Mekong River, he refers to it the way peasants refer to Saigon as the City. *"I was born up-River, but I traveled the length of the River many times."* He pauses significantly, very proud of this accomplishment. *"I*

ferried bananas down the Mekong for thirty-five years and saved enough to buy this place. Believe me, there is a lot of beautiful scenery here."

"Like what? The River?"

"No, no. The River is the River. There is a wonderful forest up near the mountain. There is a big temple there with a huge statue of Buddha. There is a garden, a pond, a trail for strolling, and a little waterfall."

I keep eating and nod encouragingly for him to continue, though have no intention of sticking my head into another tourist trap. He announces that he has been noticing a steady stream of foreign tourists trickling into town, mostly through one of the two major hotels up the street. Word has been going around that the hotels are operating day tours up the mountain and around the River, and charging thirty dollars a Western head. He pops his eyes at me: Thirty American dollars a head! That is more than what his little inn makes on an average day. He wants to get in on the action, so he is going to offer me an irresistible deal: fifteen dollars for a full day's tour provided I advise him on every aspect of hosting tours for Westerners. How to attract Westerners to his tours? What do they like to eat, drink, and see? Do they like roughing it or do they prefer air-conditioned minivans? How much will they pay? My corpulent host dreams of one day owning a minor monopoly on the tourist trade. He'll pick them up in Saigon, transport them to Chau Doc, lodge them at his inn, serve them food from his kitchen, motor them around the province, and deliver them back to Saigon—naturally, collecting every dollar they spend while in his charge from beginning to end.

I have heard this all before. Everyone has a plan for getting rich off foreigners. And as one who is privy to both worlds, I am perceived as a gold mine of free advice. I am used to entrepreneurs of every creed ribbing me: What the heck, Brother, they say, spill the beans. Let us in on the secret so we can roll in the dough. I have been propositioned many times, there is no graceful way to back down.

He is smiling the conspirator's grin. I wince and grab my stomach, doubling over, grunting.

He jumps to his feet. *"What's wrong? Stomachache? Is it the food?"*

"Maybe. Maybe it's something I ate on the bus," I moan, lying.

"Yes. Yes, it must be the food you ate on the road. You should never buy food on the side of the road. Very risky."

"Excuse me. I have to go to the bathroom."

"Yes, yes. But what about the tour?"

"I'm too sick to think about touring," I cry, pushing him out and locking the door. I plop down on the bed, pitying the Vietnamese who believe with all their hearts that Vietnam, indeed, is the most gorgeous place on earth.

They have no idea that they have gnawed away their nature. There is not much left and they don't even know it. They tell me: All the foreigners go to see this. All the foreigners go to see that. You should go, too. Go and behold big trees on big mountain. Go see this monument and that temple. They say it with such conviction that I don't have the heart to tell them, you are lemonade-stand children gouging five bucks for a paper cup of Kool-Aid. Their only fault is the fact that they don't know anything better exists beyond their borders. So they always ask me why foreigners are disgruntled after paying five U.S. dollars to look at a forty-foot waterfall or a pile of bricks.

No, my friends, I wish I could tell them, they are here to gawk at you. You small, dark people who in all your craziness defeated them. You smiling simple people who haunt their dreams, torture their fine sons now old with wrecked lives.

For me, there is only one man-made wonder in Vietnam worth the price of admission. In the month and a half I have been in Vietnam, I've dutifully trekked to nearly every museum, park, and point of interest listed in a pamphlet supplied by my cousin Viet. Most of the time, Viet accompanied me, using the occasion to practice his English. Of all the places we visited, there is only one that embodies the national psyche like nothing else I've seen since.

It was not far from one of the most palatial war memorials in Vietnam—a temple-like structure, sculpted and painted in gold, its monolithic walls etched with tens of thousands of names of war heroes killed in combat, a conceptual copy of the U.S. Vietnam War Memorial. We wandered about and came to a restaurant where a group of construction workers was building a resort for foreigners. There was a sad little black bear in a ten-by-ten-foot cage. With the exception of the dense forest of flagpole trees, cottonwood-like, covering the Cu Chi Tunnel, the local region had been transformed into farmland uninterrupted for scores of miles. We rode our motorbike along a scenic river, touring the countryside, and came to a gate at the edge of a forest. A large hand-painted billboard marked the entrance to the Cu Chi Tunnel.

An old soldier, nothing but a coatrack in uniform, handed us our tickets at the gate. Seeing that it was our first time, he took on an air of importance and rasped, *"In Asia, there are two man-made wonders: one you can see from outer space, one you can't see even when you're standing on it."*

He was liberally equating the Great Wall of China with the Viet Cong's Cu Chi Tunnel, both products of wars. The greatest war tunnel in the history of man, Cu Chi was over 260 kilometers of tunnels, traps, barracks, ammunition dumps, and military headquarters, all designed for the final assault on Saigon.

Now it is a major tourist attraction and a venue for government propaganda. Tourists, two-thirds foreigners, one-third Vietnamese, come by the busloads. The staff are soldiers and civilians, some dressed in black pajamas and handwoven scarves, uniforms of Viet Cong guerrillas. We were grouped with other Vietnamese visitors seated in a large gazebo to watch a war video about American atrocities spiced with a hefty dose of commentary on the evil of Western capitalism. A young soldier led us into a maze of trails twisting back and forth through the jungle. Great bomb-gouged pits, now weeded with vegetation, gaped like giant satellite dishes, testimonies of unsuccessful U.S. attempts to destroy the tunnels. He showed us invisible trapdoors, tiger pits for men, and grenade-rigged manholes.

We shimmied down ladders into caverns, hand-dug in secrecy one scoop of earth at a time. These once served as the headquarters of the Cu Chi operation. Although some areas had been enlarged to accommodate foreign tourists, the chambers were anything but spacious. Most were barely five feet ten inches in height, the tunnels three feet tall. The air was hot and wet, full of the mustiness of packed earth. It was difficult to take a lungful. It had to be breathed in sips. In some sections, the subterranean structure had three tiers, brilliantly designed to withstand prolonged bombing and surface siege. The network of corridors was riddled with booby traps. There were all sorts of amenities, from sleeping quarters to kitchens to training centers. It was a cross between the warren of Peter Pan and his band of lost children and the Stone Mountain Kingdom of Tolkien's dwarfs. Only it was real and crazy and deadly.

After half an hour tunneling on our hands and knees, we escaped to the surface, gasping. Another group headed down. A well-fed British woman in her fifties was desperately wriggling into the opening. Her male companion and a Vietnamese tour guide struggled to help her into the passage. One tried to keep the woman from getting stuck, the other tried to prevent her from falling through. Standing next to us, two Vietnamese soldiers watched with amazement plain on their faces. They were both about five feet tall and a hundred pounds—roughly the size of the Vietnamese Rat People who built the Cu Chi Tunnels.

"How do Westerners get so fat?" one soldier asked another.

After due reflection, the man replied, *"Eggs and butter."* His companion nodded in deep agreement, both of them mentally calculating—the wealth—how many dozen eggs and pounds of butter it took to amass a three-hundred-pound body.

I wake early and return to the Chau Doc bus depot at 4 a.m. The whole crew is already up and prepping the vehicle. The engine's idling. It sounds no better to me than it did yesterday. Madame is haggling with a woman at the back of the bus. Driver greets me with a slug to the shoulder and offers me the same prize seat behind him. I decline. *"No way. You drivers scare me. I get heart attacks watching you play chicken."* Driver and Mechanic roar as if it is a joke. I shrug and go to the rear of the bus. They pull out of the lot at 4:30 a.m. with only half the seats filled. A mile down the road, they pick up what must have been the ten fattest Vietnamese I've ever seen. Madame argues privately with one of the new passengers. A thin-faced man sits down gingerly next to me and I see his obesity is all in padding of odd rectangular shapes straining against his trousers and jacket. No one else seems to take any notice so I do the same. Our bus hiccups onward.

A bus traveling in the opposite direction flicks its headlights madly. As it blows by, the drivers exchange hand signals. Our vehicle slows down. Madame gives an order. The fat people hop to their feet and begin to strip, pulling out from under jackets and trousers cartons of bootlegged cigarettes, not the expensive American brands but ordinary tobacco grown and rolled locally. They distribute the contraband to other passengers, begging people to "hold" the cigarettes for them until the bus crosses into the next province. Some refuse, most accept the legal limit of one carton. Madame drops four on my lap, saying *"Help me out, Brother. Don't worry. It's fine."* Seeing my hesitation, she shoves them down the front of my windbreaker. *"Try not to smash them. I'll come back for them later."*

Sure enough we roll into a checkpoint a few minutes later. Two other buses languish by the side of the road being inspected by a handful of cops. I have an urge to kick myself in the head. I look under my seat for a place to stash the cigarettes. No luck. Around me is a riot of produce and luggage. If I put them on the floor, they have a good chance of falling through the cracks and right onto the road. A cop climbs aboard, commands Driver to kill the engine. Madame tries chatting him up, but he marches brusquely down the aisle and sweeps passengers with his flashlight. My hands are clammy. Sinking lower in my seat, I take off my spectacles and pull my baseball cap down over my eyes. The cop opens luggage randomly and inspects the contents, Madame at his elbow babbling in her friendliest voice. I have a flashback of the Viet Cong nabbing my family outside Rach Gia. The cigarette cartons feel dangerous, like the stacks of American dollars my mother had made me carry the day we all went to prison.

"What is this?" the cop asks a woman, shoving a bag at her.

"Don't know. That's not mine," the woman bubbles, shaking her head vigorously.

The cop holds up the duffel bag, which is filled with maybe a dozen cigarette cartons. *"Who owns these?"* he shouts at the rest of the passengers.

No one answers. He simply walks off the bus with the booty. Madame follows the cop out. When she comes back, Driver starts the engine and rolls us back on the road. I ask Madame why the cop didn't search the rest of the bus. He must have known we are hiding ten times what he found. She smiles at my naïveté. *"No,"* she explains, *"they don't do that, Brother. If they get too efficient at search and seizure, no one will be smuggling anymore. And where would they be? No more free cigarettes. Understand?"*

We arrive at the Rach Gia bus depot around noon. I bid the crew a sad farewell and thank them for their hospitality. We trade addresses, but being folks of the road, they know as well as I do that it is unlikely that we will ever cross paths again. So I teach them the truest farewell I know, the one I received from Tom and Patty when I left Portland, Oregon: "So long, I'll see you when I see you."

I take a Tuk-tuk—the cheapest transportation available—into Rach Gia some seven miles away. The vehicle looks like an army truck shrunk to clown size. It has the footprint of a Volkswagen Beetle and a tiny two-stroke engine hardly larger than that of a lawn mower. I cram into the toy vehicle with fourteen other people, including the driver and his sidekick, and one duck. Knees up around his ears, the young driver, a lanky Vietnamese with the build of a second-string basketball player, handles the three-wheeled vehicle like a madman, jerking it this way and that, punishing it like a go-cart, scaring the fleas off me but delivering me intact nonetheless to downtown Rach Gia.

I wander through the waterfront district, which is like any other waterfront district in the Third World, festooned with the rags and shards of the poor. I look out of place with my jeans and backpack, and women start catcalling me from doorways and the dirty men with their sandals slopping in the mud urge me to take up the ladies' offers. I try to talk to them but soon grow bored with their single-minded pursuit of earning a living. Around dinner, I splurge on the most expensive room available at a cold-water hostel in the fisherfolk's quarter: $2.50 a night for a windowless partitioned room with a padlock. All night cat-sized rats scurry in the rafters and on the floor under my bed.

Morning, I go down to the market and follow the smell of Vietnamese doughnuts to a pushcart where a young husband and wife are frying sweet dough. They wrap me four pieces in newspaper, the oil waxing through the newsprint. The fried dough is doughnut-sized except without the hole and nowhere as sweet. I munch on them, walking up and down the crazy waterfront, trying to find a trust-worthy motorbike driver to take me out to Minh Luong Prison. I have no idea where it is, and I don't even know if anyone knows what I'm looking for. I pick a middle-aged man on a hunch and offer him five bucks for driving me around all day. He introduces himself as Truong and accepts my offer. I hand him one of my doughnuts to start our day properly.

Narrating local history, he loops us through Rach Gia, while I sit on the back of his ancient 50cc Honda cub. When he seems comfort-able talking to me, I ask him if he knows anything about Minh Luong Prison.

"Of course, I almost died there," he shouts matter-of-factly over the wind. *"You know, it used to be a garrison?"* Yes, yes, I say, go on. *"I was in the South Vietnamese army,"* he says. *"Stationed there. Can you believe it: I got to go on leave the day the Viet Cong attacked the garrison. I went home to see my family in the afternoon and that night, THAT night, the Viet Cong came in and wiped out everybody. No survivors. No prisoners. I came back the next day and everybody was dead."*

"Why did you join the army? Did you hate Communism?"

"Ha!" he snorts. *"Drafted. I was a kid. Nineteen. Never even seen a Viet Cong in my life. I didn't know what they looked like. They might as well have had horns for all I knew."*

Truong was incarcerated and sent to reeducation camp for two years. On his release, he couldn't get a job because he was a former Nationalist soldier. His application to open a shop was repeatedly denied. So his wife sold produce in the fish market and he worked as a motorbike-taxi driver. He is bitter, but hopeful that things will change.

He rambles freely as he coaxes the motorbike down the gnarly asphalt, dodging trucks and bicyclists. Bam. Rattle. The chain has snapped out of the gears and lodges between the cogs and the frame. We bang it loose, reset it, and continue. A mile later, we roll onto a red dirt road and the tire pops. We walk it to a shop and wait while an old man burns on a patch. Hours after we started, we make it to a village.

"Here it is," Truong announces. *"This is Minh Luong Village."*

"I don't remember any village. Brick houses, markets. Where did all this come from? Where are the farms, the rice paddies?"

Twenty years have sprouted a village around Minh Luong. The compound itself has changed, too. None of the old structures survived. New blocky buildings and new fences everywhere. All gone, says Truong. The incarceration ended in the late eighties. I make him drive around the village and approach the compound from every direction, trying to look inside. Armed guards are posted around the institution. I make him do another circuit. And another. Nothing looks familiar. I feel stupid. Not knowing what else to do, I whip out my camera. Truong goes ballistic: *"What in the hell do you think you're doing? You want to get me killed? They'll jail and beat us both. What are you thinking? They're police. POLICE! Don't you understand? Anything, they can do anything they want. I don't want to spend another two goddamn years of my life in jail. Why are you so stupid!"*

He wrestles the camera from me and puts it in his pocket. I can tell he wants to give me a taste of his knuckles. He glares at me, then mounts his bike and revs up the engine. I hop on before he can change his mind. We pull away fast.

He parks us at a café far down the street, still within sight of the compound. I apologize and make it up to him with a round of beer and lunch. Truong drinks his beer in two long pulls. Stripped of his joviality, he looks like an old man, shriveled up, charred from too much punishment in the sun. Worn like an old leather bag. Empty now. Here is a man, the very sort, perhaps, the very *one* that my father had recruited when he was the Province Director of Propaganda. A sense of remorse opens my eyes to the old soldier–taxi driver, this remnant of my father's world looking back at me with tired eyes.

"Forget this place. Go see the world," Truong urges me. *"Everything has changed. Your roots here have turned to dust. Nothing here to bind you."*

Baptizing-Buddha

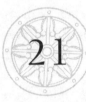 Grandpa Pham smelled of plum candy and Chinese medicine.

It was an odor that made me nauseous and hungry all at once.

His opium smoke.

I served as the footman of Grandpa's opiate dreams. As his family went through the process of closing doors, shutting windows, keeping the confidence, I knelt at the door of Grandpa Pham's study, a servant awaiting his wishes, witnessing the rite that came to be the center of his existence. In the seasons before Saigon fell, Grandpa was many years into his pipes, his grown children's wages keeping him in the habit. I brought him the accoutrements of his ceremony and he arranged them on the straw mat: an oil lamp, matches, crisp unwrinkled newspaper, a bowl with a spoonful of steamed rice, a kettle of lotus tea, porcelain cups, a water-smoke pot, and old-fashioned Chinese brick pillows. He produced a cough-drop tin rattling with loose nuggets of black opium.

He smoked with an old friend, both of them Hanoi expatriates so wizened and emaciated it was difficult to tell them apart in the gloom of their conspiracy—hovering over their opium, their instrument of sedition from the world. Those Nationalist bastards, one cheroot figure said to the other, sold nine American bullets out of ten, no wonder we are still fighting this war. The other figure protested, though without much passion, It's good for the economy, all the foreign money pouring in. Impotent to the world, they were still supreme patriarchs of their extended families. This, their War Room: two ancients sipping tea in cement air. Saigon is too hot, too corrupt, nothing but barbarians, said one. Yes, yes, Hanoi is the true soul of Vietnam, agreed the other. Shirtless in the heat, they sat on a handwoven straw mat, propping themselves with one arm locked at the elbow like a tent pole, a knee up near their chins. The room was bolted tight against ill winds. Their liver-spotted hide, the texture of week-old tofu-skin, did not sweat but drooped, flaccid on their chests and bellies, stretched taut over the ridges of their spines. The Americans are generous with their aid, but the French, they knew how to live well, one observed. True, the other nodded, true, they built the most beautiful mansions in Hanoi. The two jurors reached into a bowl, clawed a few grains of leftover rice, and wedged these between their gum and cheek like chewing tobacco. The newspaper was smoothed out, folded, and torn into two perfect squares. Starting with one corner, they rolled the papers into tapered pipes, overlapping the layers tightly. They took the moistened rice out of their mouths, pressed it into a paste, and glued the pipes. With tinker deftness, they fit the pipes to the water-smoke pot. Every practiced motion carried the serene precision of a ritual even as they talked. The Japanese were the true bastards, weren't they? All that killing and the famines. Yes, yes, but that was war and so is this. No, for the Northerners, it is war. For the Americans, it is politics. For the Southerners, it is business. A precious opium nugget was placed on the pot they shared. Ah, but wasn't Hanoi beautiful in winter? Yes, persimmon winters. They lay their bones down on the mat, on their sides facing each other, heads on brick pillows, the opium between them. Don't you remember that one hot summer, so hot catfish died and floated in the creek? Yes, but wasn't the monsoon wind blowing off Ha Long Bay magical? They worked themselves back through the years to the good memories, and when they were ready, they touched the flame to the opium and, with great sighs, began to feed from their paper pipes. They perfumed the air with opium sweetness, making it wet and soft, filling it with the watery gurgle of two old men drowning.

Once they slipped far into their refuge, a pair of goldfish dying on the floor, I moved the oil lamp out of the reach of their limbs and left them to their slumber. Their smoke swarmed the house, announcing that their spirits were temporarily on a journey, yet everyone tiptoed past the room as though fearful of waking a baby.

The First Baptist Church of Shreveport, Louisiana, was our bridge to America. They loaned us the airfares. They rented us one of the church properties, found Dad work, and generally took care of the family, making sure our transition to America was comfortable. We went to church three times a week: all morning Sunday, Wednesday night for Bible study and bowling, and Saturday night for church youth-group activities. Except for two trips to the movies, we never went anywhere in our nine Shreveport months except to church. It was the most magnificent place we had ever seen. It had huge white Roman columns, lofty marbled halls, great diamond chandeliers, walls of stained glass, miles upon miles of cardinal carpets, and velvet drapes that went almost to heaven.

When we boys weren't in church, we were in school. It was dull, particularly because we didn't speak English. The teachers couldn't talk to us and, not knowing what to do, they left us alone. A college student was sent down to work with us. He did flash cards and taught us how to tackle a guy carrying a football. I got into scrapes regularly with kids calling me Viet Cong. I fought with every boy who wanted to try kung fu with Bruce Lee. The teachers called home. Dad just shrugged and said I'd better keep up my grades. He had too much on his mind.

A few months into our immigrant lives, Uncle Hong in California called about a telegram from Vietnam: Grandpa Pham had passed away.

Dad hung up the phone and sat at the table, staring out the dark window unable to finish his dinner. We children, keen to his temper, knew something was wrong even before he told Mom. Without a word, she stood up, turned on the stove, and boiled a chicken. The glutinous rice was steamed. The expensive sheet of red silk was brought out and spread over the bookcase to let spirits know that this was the family altar. A framed photo of Grandpa, in black and white looking severely into the camera, was placed on the altar. Mom served the freshly cooked food to Grandpa's picture. Dad bowed before the altar, incense cupped in hands, and said his prayers, planting the sticks in a bowl of uncooked rice. While Dad went to their bedroom to sit alone, Mom started fashioning mourning bands, six-inch-wide pieces of black cloth, for the entire family. Wear them over your sleeve, and when someone asks, she instructed us, tell them you're grieving a death in the family. But I'm not grieving, I protested, I didn't even like him. Shhhhh! She put a finger over her lips. Don't let your dad hear you say that. You must wear this band for a month. Now go to the altar and pray!

During the night, it snowed a thin layer. Dad rose at his usual 5 a.m., made his lunch of ham and cheese on white—he preferred rice but wanted to fit in at work—and went to his janitorial job. I found his small, black footsteps mincing over fresh snow in the wintry stillness. I felt very sorry for him. He was so utterly alone in a foreign land, poor with the weight of the entire family to bear. There was no wake here for him to make his peace with Grandpa. No brother, sister, or friend to partake of his grief.

For Dad, life in America wasn't easy. In Vietnam, he was a teacher and an officer with two thousand men under his command. In Shreveport, he was a janitor in an industrial plant. It was physically demanding. His back was killing him. He'd injured it in the labor camp. And for Mom, America was a lonely, scary place. After she delivered Kay, Mom rarely left the house. She didn't know anyone and she didn't speak a word of English. The supermarket used to be her favorite destination. Dad got mad at her because she could never make up her mind. The choices were stupefying. After they strip-searched her for sampling a grape at the supermarket, she did her shopping only once a week, making Dad drive her to a different grocery store across town every Saturday.

Her fears of America abated significantly when Christmas came around. During that season of giving, the kindness and hospitality that the Southern folks showed our family—the only Asian family in town—warmed us to America. People started showing up at our door with presents, wishing us a merry Christmas. There were so many visitors Mom had us wear our good clothes all day. Mom fretted that she might run out of tea and sweets before she ran out of guests. Dad busied himself with taking names and addresses for thank-you cards. The doorbell kept ringing. Strangers, neighbors, and friends brought us presents, food, clothes, little things, big things to help us make a life in their town. The glittering piles of gifts grew steadily until it dwarfed the Christmas tree. Mom, wanting to make the Christmas spirit last as long as possible, suggested that each person open only one present a day, every day until the entire hoard of goodies was gone. This would have seen us through February. Fortunately, our sponsors, the Harrises and the Johnsons, stopped by and convinced her that all presents should be opened on Christmas Day.

Dad invited them to stay for dinner, but they were well aware that it was our very first turkey. The church ladies gave it to us for our holiday feast. Mom said it was the biggest and funniest-looking chicken she had ever seen. Everything in America is big, she said, marveling how she couldn't even hold up the "chicken" with one hand. For days, Mom and Dad had plotted the cooking of our Christmas dinner. Dad, a serious foodie, had saved a newspaper recipe. An excellent cook, Mom considered the "fat chicken" one of the greatest challenges of her kitchen life. On Christmas day, they orchestrated Operation Turkey. Dad translated the recipes and helped with the preparations. Convinced that nothing could taste good without fish-sauce, Mom liberally basted the turkey with it, adding a bit of soy sauce for coloring. When he wasn't looking, she gave the turkey stuffing a dose of oyster sauce. Dad quoted the recipe: five hours in the oven. Mom said that was ridiculous. They quibbled and Mom covertly fiddled with the oven when Dad took a nap. Between his interpretations and her improvisations, they produced a frightful thing that resembled a boiled hen dipped in honey. Dad, an atheist, said a prayer for form and started carving. In sections, the meat was raw.

Glances darted back and forth across the table. We boys were uncertain whether we wanted to eat this bloated yellow carcass with the strange brown stuffing oozing out its bottom. Huy asked Dad if he could just eat the candied yams and the cranberry sauce. Tien murmured that he was full. Auntie Dung, Chi, and I knew better and kept our mouths shut.

Pointing at the turkey, Hien shrilled, "It's bleeding!"

"Quiet!" Dad ordered. "Don't you know how lucky you are to have food to eat?"

We poked and nibbled the turkey. Our gushing enthusiasm riled Dad. He whacked the table with a yardstick and snarled, "EAT." We plowed into our food, keeping a close eye on the switch guarding the turkey. Mom mixed a side of chili-garlic fishsauce, hoping to make her bird more palatable. Dad launched into a lecture about the war-famine he had endured as a boy in Hanoi. I'm too lenient with you, Dad said. Your grandfather was strict. He would have whipped you and let you starve. By the time Dad went on to talk about the poor and unfortunate people back in Vietnam, we managed to sneak most of the turkey into our napkins. Dinner over, Dad reminded us to thank the church people the next time we saw them.

So when the minister inquired about saving our souls, we replied with a resounding Yes!

It was rude otherwise. And we wanted to thank them, to show our gratitude for everything, though, of course, we had no idea what baptism was. We didn't even know it involved water. In good Vietnamese etiquette, we smiled and bowed and were beckoned to the gates of heaven. The church folks made a special date. Our souls would be saved on a Sunday, before the entire congregation.

On the big day, we went to church without our jade Buddha pendants. They dressed us in white gowns and dimmed the lamps. We were lined up behind the spotlight trained on the baptismal pool set up high behind the pulpit. With the kind-faced minister leading, the congregation of maybe a thousand sang hymns, then prayed for us. The smiling men and women guided us one by one, barefoot, over the white marble to the holy water. They started with Dad and worked downward according to age. The minister prayed, pinched Dad's nose, and dipped him backward in the water. When it was my turn, I went without incident. I got wet but didn't feel any different. Huy came out coughing, water up his nose. They dragged Tien into the pool. Too cold, too cold, he spat in Vietnamese. The nice folks smiled, lifted Tien by his armpits, and delivered him to the minister.

I was thinking Grandpa Pham must be looking down on us and smashing his opium pot in fury. I told Huy and Tien this meant all our sins were forgiven, but they were jumping up and down, yelling, We're Americans! We're Americans! I was confused about the whole religion argument. I asked Auntie Dung why Americans go either up or down when they die, but Vietnamese go in a circle. We go up to the sky and stay there awhile—like Grandpa Pham—to watch over our children, then come back down again for another go on earth. Auntie said you have to believe in one or the other, not both. I said, Huh? But what about this sin thing? Now that we're Christians, can we really sin and all we have to do is pray for forgiveness and we're forgiven, just like that? Over and over? But if we were just Vietnamese, Mom said we collect our sins like stones in a bucket to be counted when we come full turn on earth again. Auntie said you have to pick one or the other, not both. I said I hope my bucket doesn't get too full because I don't want to be reincarnated as a pig and end up skewered on a spit. Auntie said, Don't be stupid. Still, I felt very lucky to be baptized because it seemed a really good deal.

After the splendid ceremony, the good folks shed tears of joy and lined up to embrace us. Dad was smiling broadly, shaking hands with everyone. He looked so congenial you'd never guess he was grieving for his father. The church ladies held a great feast to celebrate our salvation. The minister presented the whole family with new Bibles, big gilded tomes for Mom and Dad, lovely blue leather ones with gold tassels for Chi and Auntie, and sturdy picture Bibles for us boys. We shook hands, smiled, said thank you, took pictures with the important church people. They were ecstatic and we were very happy, glad that we could give them this token of gratitude for all their kindness.

We displayed the new Bibles above the fireplace. Chi kept hers and read it using a dictionary. Dad, expecting church visitors, had us relocate Grandpa's shrine from the living room to the master bedroom. Mom put a fresh pot of tea and a bowl of fruit on the altar. Dad had us take turns praying to Grandpa so we could commune with his spirit more intimately. I closed the door, lit my incense stick, and said to Grandpa that I hoped he wasn't too mad at our being baptized because it was the only polite thing we could do. I said I probably wouldn't see him in heaven since he was Vietnamese, but I hoped he didn't get reincarnated as a donkey. They say people who hit others too much will come back as donkeys so others can hit them back.

Deep in my gut, I knew a part of Grandpa lived on in Dad.

One day, not too long after our baptism, Dad took off his belt, bellowing, You lazy, disobedient child. I had lingered in front of the television too long when Dad summoned all us kids outside to help him bring in the groceries. My brothers and Chi went out. I was transfixed by Bugs Bunny fooling with Elmer Fudd. Dad came in howling, Where's An? Where's that disobedient boy? He found me in the den in front of the television. His hands strayed to his belt buckle. His arm rose and the belt snaked out of the loops. He started whipping me, shouting, I slave to feed you and you are too lazy to carry your own food into the house. The strip of leather chased heat across my arms, legs, chest, back, branding me. He lashed me from the den to the kitchen. I fell back from his onslaught, retreating, wanting to flee the house but too fearful of the consequences. His pale olive face bled with rage. The belt cut looping X's in the air, striking me, hitting the cabinets, the refrigerator, the dining table. He beat me into the laundry alcove. I balled into a corner between the washer and dryer. The blows fell like hot rain. The moment I thought I could not bear it anymore, something in the pit of my stomach found its pattern and came together, interlocking like a puzzle, creating a fortress. My legs straightened on their own, and I stood up, looking at him. Wind sounded in my ears. I did not cry. I just looked at him, taking the full brunt of his anger wherever it landed. I looked at him with eyes that had seen the phases of his inner beast beating us all. I saw the falsehood in his anger. I looked at him, pitting my mettle against his. My steel against his fire. His arms tired; the stroked slowed, then ceased. His face had gone purple as though he couldn't breathe. He huffed like a sprinter after a race. I looked him in the eyes. And he turned and walked away, never to raise a hand against me again. Eleven years old, I walked out the back door and into the winter afternoon, realizing abruptly that I had clenched my jaw so hard I couldn't open my mouth.

Grandpa Pham was a fair man, Son. He beat my brothers and me because he loved us. He wanted us to succeed.

Your father is unstable in the head, An. His father made him kneel all day in the summer sun. The sunstroke changed him. Made him violent.

I am violent, Mom.

A curse in my father's line.

The rage was passed on to another generation. A monster in me, for I am violent. A few years down the road, I cane Hien with a spark of Father's fury. And Hien, barely ten, comes back at me with a knife.

Foreign-Asians

The morning following my return to Vung Tau from Mekong Delta, I aim myself north toward Hanoi and start pedaling. After Minh Luong Prison, I took a day ride down the Mekong River on a banana boat, caught an all-night bus back to Saigon, then shuttled back to Vung Tau. Yesterday evening was spent tuning my rickety bike for what will probably be its last journey.

As usual, I leave early, quietly fading into the dawn. Today I am going to Phan Thiet, the place of my birth. Out on the road, I feel vulnerable, especially when passing through villages. Vietnam seems full of villages, squalid gatherings of dwellings and shops every two miles along any road. The road is busy with peasants commuting up to ten miles daily on the saddest-looking bicycles on the planet. I slip into an easy rhythm, conversing with other riders. On the recommendation of a stranger, I take a fork in the road, opting for the more scenic coastal route to Phan Thiet.

Around noon, a white sun broils the land. Even the road dust feels baking hot. I fry inside my helmet. The sun-block cream is inadequate, milking down my face with my sweat. By one in the afternoon, the red-brown skin on my arms is covered with tiny blisters like fine sprays of sweat. They pop watery when I scratch them. The sun burns my arms raw. I don't have any long-sleeve shirt except my sweatshirt and my rain jacket. I spot women sitting at sewing machines in thatched huts. They graciously cut up one of my T-shirts to make sleeves for the one I am wearing. Within minutes, I am handsomely outfitted with sleeves. They refuse payment, saying it is a gift. I thank them and get back on the road in better spirits, still thinking I can make Phan Thiet by nightfall.

The countryside opens up with an endless patchwork of four- or five-acre farms, the houses hidden among the willowy trees and banana palms. In the lightly wooded areas, herders, rangy men with broad-brimmed hats, dusty clothes, and long bamboo staves, move quietly, watching their cattle grazing. The land is rich, green shooting up everywhere—out of the paddies, along the river, between the cracks in the road. The asphalt ends abruptly without road signs, and I find myself struggling on a red dirt road, sandy and full of children trudging home from school. Every five or six miles, there is an abandoned guardhouse with a boom-gate which is no longer levered across the road but raised like a flagpole. These are relics from the dark decade following the War, when the new Communist government kept a firm lid on civilian movement. People had to apply for inter-provincial travel. Now children play in these guard stations and people pass through the gates without glancing at them. It seems as though, here in the backcountry, the government simply got bored and went back to the big cities. The only souls making a big racket out here are batches of twelve-year-olds riding two or three to a bicycle, going here and there, racing each other. I catch up with one large group. They are going to the local hot spring. They say they make the six-mile round-trip every other day. The way they twitter and yip, it sounds like the best way to bathe.

Although there are people everywhere, I am hesitant to ask for directions because everyone wants me to come in for tea. I manage to take several wrong turns. The hungry, curious way people gawk at me makes me feel spoiled, self-indulgent. I am also embarrassed to be "adventuring" through their homes, bedecked in outlandish gear they could never afford. At last, I summon enough courage to talk to a few poor peasants whose villages have only a handful of motorbikes

each. Many villagers haven't ventured farther than a day's bike distance from the place of their birth. No one seems to have a solid con-
cept of the distance to the next town, Ham Tan. Dusk is falling and I
know my shaky legs won't make it to Phan Thiet. My touring instinct
urges me to look for a suitable place to strike camp, but as far as I can
see in the weakening light, the land has been cut up into bite-sized
lots, each one devoid of trees and surrounded by pigsties, gardens,
and rice plots. The air is coarse with smoke from cooking fires.

Two hours after dark, I creak and bump to a commoner's inn in
Ham Tan village. It is a clean but run-down place that houses merchants and traveling peasants. Bolted to the concrete floor, plywood
partitions, three feet short of the ceiling, section the dormitory into
individual cubicles. I pay my three-dollar fee and turn my travel
papers over to the owner for processing with the local constable. Both
natives and foreigners must register every night. Bureaucrats still keep
a record of travelers.

Across from the inn is a corner diner, a corrugated-tin-and-
plywood-scrap place, its concrete floor an inch higher than the mud.
It has the looks of the shoddiest establishments in the old gold-rush
towns, where streets eternally switched between whipped mud and
dust fog. Dinner conversations die the moment I step inside, and the
only things blaring are the TV and my sixth sense. Raw-faced men
crowd four of the six tables, facing the television until I arrive. On
the tables are nests of empty beer bottles.

A woman looks out from the kitchen. She approaches guardedly,
twisting a rag in her hands. She eyes the men and asks me, *"What do
you want?"*

"Hello, Sister. Are you still serving dinner?" I nod toward the inn across
the street. *"I'm staying over there. The owner recommended your place."*

She hesitates, then flicks the rag at the back table near the kitchen.
I sit obediently, wondering yet again why Vietnamese prefer kindergarten furniture. I haven't acquired the penchant to sit with my butt
lower than my knees. With the tabletop so low, whenever I eat I feel
as though I am licking myself like a dog. A string of black ants
marches crumbs off the table. Houseflies buzz around my head.
People stare openly at me, so I try to keep myself from batting the

flies and squashing the ants. I play stoic and take immense interest in the Vietnamese soap opera playing on television.

"Oy! You," a man slurs in English. He sits up front and is obviously drunk and talking to me. I groan, pretending not to hear.

"OY! YOU!"

Oh, Lord. I show him my friendliest smile and nod, fingering my pocket for the tiny canister of pepper spray.

The speaker switches to Vietnamese, his English apparently at its limit. *"Brother, I want to ask you a question."*

"Please do."

"How is it you speak Viet so well?"

I grin. This is easy. *"I'm Vietnamese."*

He hitches up one corner of his mouth and blows out a note of disgust. His liquored eyes flicker over to his drinking partner, a shifty man with a knifish look—a perfect killer right out of some bad Chinese mafia movie. He mutters privately to Killer, who smirks in agreement. Pointing a grubby finger in my direction, my antagonist raises his voice: *"You're not Vietnamese. Where's your birth-roots?"*

"Phan Thiet."

"Say it again."

"Phan Thiet."

"Liar. You're not from Phan Thiet. You didn't pronounce it like a man from Phan Thiet."

"I've been in America a long time. My Viet isn't perfect."

"Liar. You're Korean, aren't you?"

"Chinese," offers Killer.

"Japanese," counters another.

I am the tallest one present, my skin the palest. My wire-rimmed eyeglasses make me look foreign. Worse, I have a closely cropped crew cut. My hair is straight and spiky. Vietnamese call it "nail hair," a style commonly seen on Korean expatriates working in Vietnam.

I should know better, but I insist, *"Really, I'm Vietnamese."*

The drunk bolts up in his seat, pounds the table, then points at his own nose with his index finger. He slur-screeches, *"Brother, you call me stupid?"*

"Oh, no, Brother. No," I blurt, thinking, Oh, shit. Oh, shit.

He starts spieling his body of knowledge on the matter: *"I've been to the City* [Saigon]. *I know what's going on in the world. All you foreigners come into the country to work. You go to the university, learning about . . . about mathematics, history, books . . . all that. You live in the City for a couple of years and you think you can pass as a Vietnamese. I know all about you foreign Asians. My brother-in-law lives in the City. I'm a poor villager, but I'm not dumb."* He encompasses the room with a sweep of his hand. *"We're not stupid!"*

Magically, his insult becomes theirs, and the whole rooms falls in behind him. A hostile grumble rises, amplified by the noisy television. Someone growls, *Motherfucker.* Another mumbles, *Bastard thinks he can come into our place and lie to our faces.* The whole affair has taken all of thirty seconds, and I realize with horrible dismay this is not how I want things to turn out at all. I'm here to learn about them, about my roots, about me—and they look like they want to cut me up. My pepper spray isn't going to handle this crowd. Damn! I haven't even eaten yet.

I raise an appeasing hand, smiling, making chuckling sounds. *"You're all right! I was just joking. Sorry. I am Korean. You're very sharp. Most people can't pick me out. I've been in the country three years. Studied Viet at the University. Pretty good, eh? So sorry. Beg your pardon."*

My tormentor seems happy at my concession to his intellect, but his friends appear even more riled. They cuss. I palm the canister beneath the table. A couple of mean-looking guys give me the eye as they mutter among themselves. This is definitely out of hand. I have seen three fights break out in Vietnamese bars over smaller issues than this. The last time, one drunk with a hatchet amputated a few fingers and hospitalized four men before he was subdued. I must get out quickly, but the exit is blocked by this hostile crowd.

BAM! I jump in my seat. The waitress is next to me, slamming down plates and bowls of food on my table so hard the whole room fixates on her. A huge plate of rice covered with stir-fried cabbage. A bowl of stewed pork and eggs. A bowl of squash soup. A saucer of pickled radish. A mug of hot tea. She glowers at them as she rearranges my meal.

I gape at the food I hadn't ordered.

She turns on the men, challenging them with her hot eyes. She speaks slowly, as though reprimanding boys who should know better: *"Let a man eat. Remember your manners."*

My foe says something under his breath. She whirls on him, fists cocked on hips, yelling: *"What, Lang?"*

He turns to the television. She pans the room for dissenters. When no one says a word, she marches back into the kitchen without looking in my direction. I lower my eyes to the food and dig into it cyclo style—chopsticks in one hand for picking up morsels, tablespoon in the other for shoveling rice. I eat *binh dan*—like a commoner—fast and hungry, sipping soup with the spoon once every three mouthfuls. I am shocked that they actually leave me to my rice. This is the last place I expect the observance of that old custom my father had taught me when I was a boy.

Father stocked bamboo canes around the house so that whenever I was due for a whacking, he could lay his hand on a wand-of-discipline quicker than I could flee the room. My sister Chi and I must have been rotten kids because he caned us regularly. The only time he didn't was during mealtimes. If the food had been put on the table, he would postpone the punishment till well after the meal. My mother said that hitting a person when he is eating was the cruelest, most uncivilized thing anyone could do. And that if you caused a person to cry into his rice—*souping rice with tears,* she said—you would be cursed with the bitterness he swallowed.

I figure I'm safe until the last bite. Lang and Killer are watching me, plotting something between themselves. The others argue over the pros and cons of Vietnam opening its market. Wondering if and when the waitress will return and bail me out again, I glance at the kitchen and notice a back door near where she washes dishes.

Halfway through my food—I am still hungry—the TV program switches over to news and everyone turns to the anchorman announcing the headline stories. In a blink, I breeze out of my chair, making for the kitchen. My mouth full, I hand the waitress a large bill and bolt through the back door, across the street.

The inn owner is sitting at the front door, smoking and chatting with a neighbor. He sees me running and asks if anything is wrong.

Abruptly, the waitress is at my elbow. I jump, startled. She hands me the change, unfamiliar with the custom of tipping. She briefs the old man on my dilemma. I stand by looking helpless. He cusses and hollers for his sons and the servants.

"Go inside. I'll take care of those dog-spawned. I'm sorry they bothered you. Go, go." His beatific face now thunderous with anger.

He doesn't need to tell me twice. Killer, Lang, and four men are coming toward the inn. By the time they cross the street, I am out of sight. Five of the inn's men run to the front with machetes. A shouting match ensues. Someone is dispatched to get the police. The bullies back off. I go back to my cubicle, lock the toy door, and crawl inside my mosquito netting.

Too jazzed with adrenaline to sleep, I count the geckos scrawling across the ceiling. I am inexplicably happy, thrilled not by my escape but by the goodness of my hosts. This is Vietnam. These are my people. Phan Thiet, the village of my childhood, and Mui Ne, the gateway of our family's flight from the fatherland, await me down the road, merely a day away.

Milk-Mother

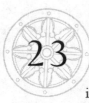 I wake full of hopes, aching to get going. Surely Phan Thiet, a puff of a fishing town, couldn't have changed much after two decades. Everything, all my good memories, had happened in this dusty town, on its sandy beaches and among the coconut groves.

I sneak out of Ham Tan before dawn, skipping breakfast to avoid a chance encounter with the mob. The road inland toward Highway 1 is quiet. Peasants are bringing their produce to market. A group of girls carrying huge baskets of home-fired coals on their shoulders greet me so cheerfully I dismount and walk my bike. They laugh and the air around them is perfumed with the scent of soap and river-washed hair. In their sun-bleached clothes, they smell and look far cleaner than me. They go to market twice a week. Their cargo varies seasonally, sometimes fish, other times vegetables and fruits. For this dry season, the men fire coal, and the women bring it to market, two baskets at a time.

I have a wild urge to marry them all, take them to America, give them American citizenship, and tell them they will never have to walk barefoot on hot asphalt again. But their laughter is so pure and rich that I quell my foolishness and simply enjoy their company until far down the road they board a Tuk-tuk for the next village.

On the main highway, a motley collection of dwellings on half-acre arid farm lots line the road. Mile after mile, children sprout out of the land like weeds. They tag each other down the road to school, sit and play cards right on the edge of the blacktop, paying no mind to the buses roaring by and spraying them with dirt. They hound me on bicycle, wanting candy, practicing their English. Elloo. Ow arrr uu? Fuk you. Fuk you. What yore nam? Where uu from? Bye-bye. They overrun the land like an infestation of locusts. Where is the food to feed all these mouths?

A scrap-metal collector blames it on the government. I meet him sometime after midday and ride with him all the way to Phan Thiet. He chain-smokes hand-rolled cigarettes and rides a rickety one-speed bicycle with a thirty-five-pound truck transmission casing tied to the rear rack.

"The government screwed up," he says, *"and they're trying to fix it, but it's too late. It was all the fighting—the War, then the skirmishes with Cambodia and China. For a long time the government said it was patriotic to get married and raise many children because all the young men had died in the War or were dying in battles against Cambodia. Their message was a big hit. Now they've got a country full of people and no war to thin out the population. The way we're breeding we could drain the country's resources in another generation."*

He was a struggling college student when the South Vietnamese government fell. The Communists drafted him, sent him to burn down the jungle for farming, then planted him on the border to fight Cambodians. Six years later, when it was all over, he returned to Saigon to finish his education at night, paying for it by working as a laborer and driving a cyclo. But it wasn't meant to be. He never got over the strange jungle sickness he contracted at the border, and no one could think straight in night class after twelve hours of hard labor. After a few years, he abandoned his academic pursuit, got married, and fathered a son. To support his family, he found himself riding his bicycle thirty miles a day, collecting and bartering in scrap metal and spare auto parts.

We part ways at the city line, him heading to the poor quarter of the city, me rolling down the main thoroughfare. Narrower than the average unmarked two-lane road, this dusty pipeline happens to be the national highway. No trees, just dirt, sand, and people. The first structure I recognize is the Catholic school Chi and I had attended before my French education days. The ghost tree is gone. It used to litter the street with tamarind pods, which, with sugar, made tasty treats, the Vietnamese equivalent of sourballs. We never dared touch them. The old folks said it had been a hanging tree when the French had the run of the land—ghosts of those unjustly killed haunted the branches and poisoned the fruit. The school is still there but the nuns are gone and the student population has increased tenfold. I dismount and meander through the series of rectangular one-story buildings. At the far end of the school yard, beyond the badminton nets, is a fence of red paper-flower bushes. Chi had rescued me from a pair of bullies there, the four of us standing ankle deep in leafy confetti redder than New Year's paint.

I ride on down the main artery. Houses come closer together as they reach higher toward the tangle of power lines. New structures are going up everywhere, piecemeal, like Lego blocks. Workers weave steel lattices and pour concrete into them to make columns. Shops have blossomed. A big-city intensity has found its way into Phan Thiet. The road expands into a four-lane boulevard to accommodate the commerce, then bridges over a river where the water is logjammed with wooden boats of all shapes and sizes, a living city on the river as far as I can see to the next bend nearly a mile off. Sampans loaded with colorful produce putter across spinach water. A boy perches on a wood piling, defecating into the river. Sitting against the railing at the crown of the bridge, a blind old woman clenches into herself, the whole of her no bigger than a fire hydrant, fitting into the shadow of her farmer's hat. An arm extended, stiff as a twig, a withered palm waiting for alms. I pedal on until I reach the other end of the city. I pay for a room at the edge of town and eat dinner. Feeling slightly under the weather, I turn in for the night.

First thing in the morning, I find my childhood home on the southern lip of the town. It is a motorcycle repair shop. Six greasy young men are sitting on their hams tinkering with engine parts. Oil and dirt cream the floor. The tenant is a man my age. I chat with him, and at my request he takes me to the backyard. The well still gives sweet water, he says. I tell him that as a boy, I had accidentally drowned three puppies by lowering them into the well for a bath. He walks me to the bedroom in back, partitioned from the shop with sheets of plywood. In the corner, exactly as I remember it, is the divan where I'd slept. It is dirt-stained. On this divan, my father had caned Chi until I took her by the hand to Grandma's house.

We are chatting amiably about the virtues of the house when our eyes meet—a strange moment—and we know we are holding a common thought: the transparency of our situations. Fate could have switched our destinies and no one would have been the wiser. I clear my throat and take demi-steps toward the front door. I thank him for showing me his home. The tides of traffic and horns disorient me as I step into the road short of breath. Feeling guilty, I am very thankful we had the money to escape Vietnam.

I trudge up and down the street but can't recognize Grandma's house. An old woman watches me from her hammock strung just inside her door. On my third or fourth pass, she comes to the door and waves me to her.

"What are you looking for?" she asks.

"Good morning. I'm the grandson of Mrs. Le—son of her daughter Anh. They used to live somewhere near here. I'm looking for the house."

"AAAAAA!" she cries, happily. *"I remember you! I'm Mrs. Sau-Quang. Do you remember me?"*

"Oh . . . I'm sorry. I don't." I can't place either her name or her seventy-year-old face, flabby, floppy like a Halloween pumpkin left out through November.

Mrs. Sau-Quang beckons me inside and serves me tea, welcoming me like a lost relative and introducing me to her nieces and nephews. She says she knew my grandmother from the day Grandma bought the house way back when. I sit long enough to be polite then beg her to take me to my grandmother's house.

We walk slowly along the drumming traffic and come to a dwelling ten doors down. It is a hovel more suitable for animals than people.

"This is your grandmother's house. Do you remember it?" she quizzes me with childish glee.

I shake my head. She flashes a toothless grin, encouraging me to dredge the recess of my memory, but I don't recognize the beggarly shelter where I had spent many lazy summer days.

"Where's the shop? My grandmother had a little store," I ask her.

"They knocked it down years ago and built this lean-to for storage."

"Where are all the trees? I remember walking from my house to Grandma's without stepping out of the shade."

"Seventy-seven. Everybody chopped them down for cooking fires in the summer of '77. Didn't even last the whole year."

"Does Hoa—the girl my age—still live next door?"

"No, she married a laborer ten or eleven years back and the whole family moved to Nha Trang. We neighbors-relatives lost touch with them."

Mrs. Sau-Quang raps the door with her cane and a short man in his late forties lets us in. She introduces me. Mr. Phi, the current owner of the house, agrees to give me a tour. Mr. Phi is a taxidermist and a hunter of wild game. A fetid odor pervades the house. Cages are stacked against walls of rotting plaster. Cobwebs mummify stuffed bobcats, tortoises, peacocks, monkeys, and other furry animals I don't recognize. The blue plaster remains, unwashed. Untouched for twenty years.

"May I see the backyard? I'd like to see the star-fruit tree," I ask Mr. Phi, feeling lost. Chi and I had climbed it, ate its fruit, and gazed at the stars.

"Ah, yes. But it is barren. No fruit."

We file through the house and find my tree out back. It is dying, bleeding sap. It reminds me of Grandma sitting in her sad American room, old and lonely, thousands of miles from her homeland. The tree is a season away from becoming firewood. Bricks barnacle the earth at its foot. No longer a geyser of leaves, it droops like an old woman napping in her seat. Like Grandma, wizened, gnarled, crusty, and crippled. I doubt its main limb could bear my weight now. On the branches two small monkeys flit back and forth, scolding us. They don't go far with the chains around their necks.

"Thank you. I've seen enough," I murmur. *"Forgive me, I must go now."*

I retreat to my room at the inn. Where is this place I am seeking? There is only ash. Secretly, I am thankful no one is witnessing this unearthing of my roots. It is true what Vietnamese say: Viet-kieu are the lottery winners. The payoff stretches forth through the ages. America has it all, owns it all. And nowhere else are we safer than in America. That much I suspect is true.

In this Vietnamese muck, I am too American. Too refined, too removed from my *que,* my birth village. The sight of my roots repulses me. And this shames me deeply.

I am awakened by a runner sent by Mrs. Sau-Quang. He brings word for me to come at once. Su is waiting at Mrs. Sau-Quang's house. I hop on my bike, glad that I had hired a motorbike runner to find Su, my nanny. I was too young to remember her, but my mother had told me Su was a kind woman who nursed me the first three years of my life. My milk-mother.

I bow deeply to Su. She bows in return. We sit across from each other in Mrs. Sau-Quang's front room, just staring and smiling. How are you? Well, and you, Auntie-friend? I get by, but are your parents well in America? Yes, they want to know how many children you have. Ten, two passed away, but we are fortunate to have eight obedient children.

The formal words trade back and forth between us. Over and over, she keeps repeating: *"Who would have guessed I would see you after so many years?"*

Su moved to the country fifteen years ago when Vietnam was in its deepest depression. Her family farmed, fished, raised pigs, and hired out its labor to whoever needed them. She remembers me but she also remembers other babies she had nurtured. She doesn't see why I'd come back to see her, but she is glad I came. I apologize for not having come for her myself. Mrs. Sau-Quang had told me to wait. It's best, Su says. The runner was lucky to find her, since there are no such things as addresses or road names out in the deep country. Most peasants don't read or write, so they go by name and word of mouth.

"Su has a very difficult life. Pity her. Look at her. Just skin and bone. Can you believe she is only forty-five? Why, she looks sixty. Pity her," says Mrs. Sau-Quang. She harps along this line the entire hour, edging in a few words about her own impoverishment as well.

"Do you remember my sister Chi?" I ask Su.

"Yes, she was a beautiful child. How is she? Is she married? How many children?"

"Chi passed away."

"So sorry. That is terrible," she says. *"What happened?"*

The answer has always been on my lips: *"An accident."*

That's what it must have been: An accident. Kind of like one of those calamitous highway pileups on a wide flat stretch of asphalt that would have been an easy, safe passage on any other day except that one foggy morning when everyone was going a little too fast to notice one car was having problems—each man too intent on his own purpose to notice the flashing hazard lights of the troubled driver.

"She became too American," Old Quan had said to me after Chi's suicide. An elderly Vietnamese American who had seen his share of horrors, Old Quan was, for a time, my good friend and mentor until I, too, became *too American* for him.

"Your sister Chi—too selfish, too into herself. She wants to be herself. That's wrong. All wrong. To live a good life, you live for others, not for yourself. Your parents bring you into this world so you be what they want. What do you think: I plant a tree for shade. I water it. I put fertilizer in soil. I wait and I work hard for tree, but when tree is big, tree don't give me shade. Maybe tree give me thorns. Is that good? What do you think?

"Your sister, she not know how to ignore desire. Not know how to accept herself. She not see her duty to parents. To her, desire is above—higher—than duty to parents . . . She not know sacrifice."

We always worked for those behind us, those who brought us into the world and pointed out the gate to the Empire beyond the barbed wire. Our father sacrificed for us as his father had sacrificed for him, each one of us racking up a debt so large we'd never dare to contemplate pursuing our own dreams. No, there are no independent visionaries in a line of sacrifices.

Since I met Su four days ago, I have been in bed, feverish and lonely, coming up empty-handed in the village of my birth. I am bedridden, waking up merely to sip broth and orange juice. And spewing my innards into the toilet. I am feverish. I am cold. My joints ache. Maybe it is a stomach flu. I don't know. I keep asking the innkeeper if Su has dropped by to see me. She hasn't. Having given Su much of my money as a gift, and wining and dining Mrs. Sau-Quang's sons as etiquette demanded, I cannot afford to go to the doctor. I am nearly out of cash. Phan Thiet doesn't have a large bank where I can dredge my bank account for my emergency funds. I will have to end the trip here and return to Saigon. I don't have the strength to go on. What is the point anyway?

It can't end here. I must beg my way north, crawl if I have to. It seems not only cowardly but selfish and dishonest to quit now. Not after all Chi went through. I rise from bed on the fifth morning. My fever breaks sometime in the night and my sinuses are clear. I know I am better as I wake. The stench drifting into my room from the sewer and the salt flat is just as bad as it was the first day I arrived. I pack my panniers and head to the door without breakfast.

"No. No!" Hai, the inn owner, beseeches me, hands flapping like crow wings. "You're not leaving today, are you? You, you are so sick. Are you crazy? You're weak. You'll catch an ill wind and you'll end up in the hospital."

"I'll be fine," I assure her, putting on my confident face. "I feel great. I get sick, but I recover fast." Two lies. I feel woozy and clammy. Recovery of any sort isn't my strong suit and I haven't been sick in years—not even a cold—until I set foot in Vietnam.

"Just one more night. How about it? I'll cook something special for dinner," Hai offers, smiling sweetly, practically begging.

The truth is I can't afford to stay here much longer anyway. Hai has been overcharging me blatantly, quadrupling the price of everything from orange juice to aspirin to laundry service to room fees. She is bleeding me to death financially and my unanticipated departure is something of a shock to her business plan.

"Thank you, Sister. But I have been looking forward to seeing Mui Ne for a very long time. You know, it's where my family escaped."

"Ah, your border-crossing point," she says appreciatively.

With that, I ride away, dropping vague promises to come back for a few nights if I make tracks through town again. I fight the bike into the sandy road, joining the light traffic of trucks, bicyclists, and motor scooters. I feel exhilarated to be back on my bike. The sea wind wipes away the bedridden fuzziness in my head, giving me a clean slate. A few miles out, the land turns arid. Over a couple of rises, I peek at blue water. The road hems the coast for a mile or two, perching lightly on a rocky lip not ten yards above the surf. Then, abruptly, the road sweeps down into a coconut forest and I remember it all, our walking down this road with my mother twenty years ago. It is plush, shady, and airy beneath the palm canopy. Between this green roof and the white sand carpeting there is only quiet air bathing the ropy trunks of the coconut palms. With only the soft hiss of the sea breeze, the silence is eerie.

Deeper in, I realize it isn't quite the same place I'd left. The forest now teems with people. They have thinned it out and built huts on one-acre lots. I leave my bike by the side of the road and plod across the sand to see if the forest is thoroughly perforated with dwellings. It is. An old man rises from his hammock nap to tell me not to waste my time. The whole peninsula is populated, he says. They migrated down from central Vietnam a decade ago. I sigh, thank him, and go on my way. There are too many children and the school system can't teach them all at once so there are two sessions, one in the morning, one in the evening. At the changeover during midday, hundreds, maybe thousands, of white-and-blue uniformed schoolchildren flood the road. Soon they shed their uniforms, and the sandy floor of the thinned-out coconut forest is alive with half-naked children playing, shouting, running. They trail me, smiling, waving, yelling, *"Tay! Tay!"*—Westerner, westerner.

I track the road, over and over, looking for the precise spot where my family had staged our escape, but it is hopeless. The landmarks are all gone. The locals say that for every house swept away in the last big storm several years ago, five more took its place. There are even restaurants, shops, and hotels right on the beach. One very fancy resort, featured in several travel magazines, hogs up a prime tract of beachfront land and boasts a manicured garden and South Pacific–style bungalows, protected behind a Cyclone fence, topped with barbed wire, besieged on all sides by ramshackle huts inhabited by skinny, half-naked people. Despite the fancy amenities, it reminds me of Minh Luong Prison. I avoid the commercial lodging and scout the area for a camping spot.

I climb the brow of a hill. Off in the distance, a mighty flotilla of wooden fishing vessels moors in the crescent cusp of the bay. Bobbing gently in the winter sea, nose to the beach, they are the color of driftwood save the bright, gaudy trimmings of eyes and dragon heads like those of the ancient Phoenician warships. The bay is rimmed by a village thriving like undergrowth beneath the palms. A fisherwoman, mending her strung-up net, suggests I go to the other side of the peninsula and camp on the back bay. It's more peaceful, she explains. The kids won't pester you there. "Pester" in context could mean anything, including stealing.

On the other side is a long, gorgeous stretch of near-white sand dunes lapped by three-foot swells. It is desolate in comparison. The fisherfolk switch bays by the season. Here, the late December wind whips onto the beach with a mild cut, just enough to chill someone bare-chested. Behind the dunes where the road ends is the most forlorn café I've ever seen. There is no structure save a couple of strings of lights and laundry lines. The sand, speckled with bits of ocean-splintered wood, is strewn with rusted lawn chairs, a few plastic tables, and six tattered sun umbrellas. The proprietor, a nervous Vietnamese man named Han, serves three Brits warm beers. I lean my bike against a tree and ask the man for permission to spend the night on one of his hammocks under the stars. He says that he'd welcome any company to help him guard the café against burglars. The Brits tell me, in their polite British way, that they think I am insane and leave in a car with their tour guide and driver.

In the middle of the night, a cop comes by on a motorbike and shines his flashlight in my face. Han tells the cop to fuck off. The cop tells Han to go fuck himself. I groan and pull my jacket over my face. They squabble, apparently friends. The cop wants Han to fry him some eggs. Han tells the cop to fuck off because he doesn't have any eggs. If you want eggs, you'll have to go down to one of the farms and tax them out of some eggs. I doze off and wake up a few minutes later to see them drinking rice wine and the cop eating a bowl of instant noodles. They tell tall tales under Christmas lights powered by a car battery.

Chi-Daughter

"In the end . . ." Grandma intoned, summoning the very words a Buddhist monk had composed for Chi on the day of her birth, *"in the end, it will be as if she had no brother or sister. No father or mother. Her life will be a difficult journey. She will die at thirty-two, alone of a broken heart. This child should be loved, for in the end she will have no one."*

A Vietnamese first son is worth his weight in gold, all his life. But I don't think that's why Chi wanted to be a boy. She was just never meant to be a girl. That simple. I had always known she was different. Unusual. A strong, quiet, and thoughtful first child, Chi carried herself in such an unassuming way that I instinctively looked to her as my older brother. Perhaps I even resented it as a child because I was the first son. While I reaped the prodigal privileges, I suspected they should have been her honor.

Nine months after we came to America, we weaned ourselves from the charity teats of the First Baptist Church of Shreveport, Louisiana. Mom couldn't handle being the only Asian family in town and Dad wanted to be closer to his brothers who had settled in California. A bunch of ingrates, we loaded a U-Haul with the secondhand loot the church had given us and said amen to the South. We bolted through

Texas, New Mexico, Arizona, and right into sunny California—as close to Vietnam as you can get, my uncle had claimed. With a couple of hundred dollars in his pocket, the only footing Dad could afford was in south San Jose, smack in a den of poverty, alcoholism, drugs, and domestic violence—a street where the cops came by daily, so regularly that the residents had a running joke: If you can't find cops at Winchell's Doughnuts, you'll find them on Locke Drive.

We lived in a gutter-level unit that flooded with every heavy rain. Barbed wire separated our backyard from no-man's-land, a desolate plain of bulldozed dirt, beyond which trickled a toxic creek weeded with trash. Standing at our front door, I could wing a rock over the chain-link fence of the city dump down the street. It was a colossal stadium of debris, four football fields wide and three stories deep, the sides treacherous ravines.

It wasn't as bad as it looked. Even though, on humid summer days, the stench stewing off the raw trash turned my stomach and made Mom sick, the tainted air became as familiar to us as our own body odors. Besides, it was a treasure land of odd trinkets and toys, and the creek provided a vast stomping ground infested with imaginary enemies and very real poison oak. Seagulls wheeled across the sky, making the dump look like beachfront property. My brothers and I became street urchins, lurking in empty lots, the creek, and the dump because the local kids—whites, blacks, and Mexicans—were out to kick our skinny Asian asses. Some of them routinely took potshots at us with BB guns. *Go home, Chinks!* Kids' style of picking fights was different in America. In the old country, kids took a running slug at the sight of a foe. Here, they squared off like cocks, traded insults, and shouldered each other for an eternity before the first blow landed. After a month of fighting, usually walking away with the heavier damage, we pocketed stones and slingshots whenever we left the house.

While we boys reveled in the family's poverty, Chi was largely confined to the house for chores and changing Kay's diapers. With the family on welfare, Dad, a worn-out man in his mid-forties with eight mouths to feed, studied eighteen hours a day, seven days a week for his Associate of Arts degree in computer programming, a two-year program which he was trying to cram into nine months. The migraine headaches and the malaria chills he picked up during his time in the Viet Cong prison plagued him. He merely clenched his jaws and chiseled away at the books. Mom, who hardly spoke any English, spread out a vinyl mat in the living room, put a swivel office chair in the middle, brought out the dresser with the mounted mirror, and was in business. She cut hair for the neighborhood children and permed fancy heads of the local ladies, many of whom were also in the dire strait of public assistance. Mom got the idea from looking around the neighborhood.

In the suburban slum of Locke Drive, hustling on the sidelines of welfare was serious business. Saving for the American dream was the immigrant's religion. The Lees, two doors down from us, ran a convenience store out of their one-car garage. The driveway of the Martínez house across the street hummed with the racket of their after-hours auto-repair business. Recent arrivals from Pueblo, Mexico, the Martínezes were in cahoots with the Lious, a Hong Kong Chinese family up the street, who turned their lawn into a used-car lot. Mrs. Nguyen next door took in tailoring work at night and ran a day-care center. Old Mrs. Chen, a Chinese-Vietnamese grandmother who lived with her children and collected social security, operated an underground catering business. Every day, she cooked dinner for some thirty neighbors who moonlighted at second jobs and didn't have time to fuss in the kitchen. Locke Drive was a busy place, a loud place, an industrious place—if you knew where to look.

One of our white neighbors, Mr. Slocum, once asked Dad, "Why are you people killing yourself working around the clock like that?"

Dad replied, "How can you kill yourself when you are already in heaven?"

But Dad was realistic because his heaven was full of traps. While Mom made friends with her egg rolls and fried rice, and Dad was the friendly neighbor who lent his tools as readily as he lent his back, they were telling us: We're different. Never forget that we are different. You are better than they. You must study harder, work harder, and be better than they in every way.

Remember, Dad said, behind every company CEO is a gang of janitors and a hive of worker bees. Don't ever think America is yours. It isn't.

We plotted and we schemed and we dug our escape tunnel in humble silence. No one was to know. We would leave them all behind. Leave them with the dump and the drugs and the cops and the incarceration statistics. Locke Drive wasn't home, but a minefield we had to cross to get to the real America where we could live in comfort, in anonymity. Away from this noisy place dangerous with the occasional frustrated husband a little done in with liquor. Vicious with young punks strutting wild on the taste of easy drug money. Redolent with ethnic cooking, stinky with the offal of the entire city. We would escape. That was the mantra of our daily lives. We were so certain we were above it all. We never thought our family might not make it through this minefield without a casualty.

We escaped it every other Sunday. Government food stamps were neither amusement-park tickets nor movie passes, so Dad took the family to the beach. Mom bought baguettes and made pungent Vietnamese sandwiches with margarine, cilantro, pickled carrots, onions, cucumber, black pepper, chili pepper, and a squirt of soy sauce mixed with rice vinegar—a concoction that reeked to American noses. Traditionally, the sandwiches got fattened with paté and cured ham, but that was expensive, so Mom substituted with homemade Vietnamese bologna, *cha*. Our family of eight sardined into our ancient Malibu sedan with beach balls, badminton rackets, towels, and coolers—flea-market treasures. On the way over the Santa Cruz mountains, Dad pulled over at the midpoint to the summit to cool off the engine. We sat in the car watching the traffic whizzing by, our windows down, the car smelling oddly addictive with a mixture of mountain pine, car exhaust, and Mom's spicy sandwiches.

Hien and Kay fidgeted in the front seat between Mom and Dad. In the back, Chi and I both got window seats because we had seniority over Huy and Tien. The Malibu's radio didn't work so Dad and Mom did most of the talking. It was interesting to hear Dad talking to Mom or his brothers, but he always sounded stiff when he talked to us. We had question-answer sessions that sounded like a poorly written script.

Dad: "How are your classes going?"

Me: "Great, Dad. I'm getting straight A's. A-plus in math and science."

Dad: "Are you still drawing?"

Me: "Not much. Just like you told me."

Dad: "Good. Artists never make any money. They always die poor. Huy, how about you, Son?"

Huy: "All A's except one B-plus, Dad."

Dad: "Tien?"

Tien: "Two B-pluses, Dad, and four A's."

Dad: "Hmm. You two should be more like your older brother. He has straight A's. I sacrifice so you can go to school. You must study hard and be the best."

Dad rarely asked Chi anything. On these trips, she was silent, laying her head on the door frame, eyes fixed on the mountain pines blurring by. I didn't know her like I used to when we were playmates. Now, she was toeing adulthood. Chi wasn't attractive. Handsome, strong, perhaps, but never cute or feminine. Her coarse black hair, cropped close, limped hopelessly around her unhappy face—*flat and big like a cutting board,* kids used to tease her. Some kids inherited the good parts of their parents. Chi got all the unflattering features of hers.

At sixteen, she was as tall as Dad and much stronger. The beam of her shoulders matched any boy's her age. Every morning, she hammered through her routine of fifty push-ups, a hundred sit-ups, and twenty pull-ups without breaking a sweat. Trained in martial arts since age eleven, she held the equivalent of a black belt. Her chest was flat but thick and tight. And only I knew why. Chi bandaged her chest, like someone with broken ribs, to hide her breasts. She had been doing it since puberty. Once in Saigon when Chi and I went swimming at a public pool, we were both in bathing trunks. The pool owner yanked us out of the water and pointed at her nubby twelve-year-old bee stings. *Cover that up with a bra or I'll kick both of you out.* She didn't have a bra, so he booted us and kept our money. The other kids laughed at Chi as we gathered our clothes and shuffled out. The chest bandaging followed soon after that.

Unlike the rest of us, Chi hated these beach outings. Dad always took us to Carmel, a posh beach town of wealthy retirees and movie stars. He didn't have much of a choice. The first time Mom saw it, she exclaimed, *"Ooooo! So pretty. It's almost like Nha Trang."* She repeated it many times, smiling at the memories. As newlyweds, Mom and Dad had often vacationed in Nha Trang, commemorating their budget excursions with lots of pictures.

So Dad took her to Carmel without fail. As soon as he landed the troops on the sand, Mom trudged off with him in tow to take pictures of her sitting on dunes, footing the surf, and leaning against wind-carved pines. We boys stripped to our shorts and charged into the waves and built sand castles. Chi stayed with baby Kay and the cooler. In 90-degree heat, she was clad in a pair of cutoff jeans and a dark T-shirt to hide her chest bandage. She didn't bring the bathing suit Mom bought her. No intention of ever wearing anything that betrayed the fact that she was a girl. When Mom and Dad returned, Chi grabbed a sandwich and an orange and vanished into the dunes. No one would see her until it was time to leave.

We picnicked out of brown paper bags, chomping on homemade sandwiches and drinking sodas in paper cups. It was not always a comfortable place. The good-looking people—tall blond folks of sandy, burnished skin, long legs, and jewel eyes, the locals—gave us a wide berth, and gave us the eye. Without being told, we boys knew, faces buried in smelly sandwiches, that we were playing in someone else's backyard.

Chi must have known her life would veer away from ours at some point. She must have stared at the dark ceilings for years, wondering what was wrong with her. Why was she so different? She must have known her unique orientation was in the eyes of her parents a per-version which they discounted as her troubling adolescence. She must have known the momentum of tradition would sunder her fragile world of secrets—her microcosm of one.

The first thing Chi did when we moved to California was throw away all her dresses and skirts. From her first day at high school, she wore men's clothing. Her teachers, misled by her confident male body language, instinctively classified her as a boy. One thing rear-ended another and suddenly it avalanched beyond her control. Whether she wanted it or not, Chi had a new identity. At school, she was a *he*. And she used the boys' locker room and competed in boys' sports. She didn't speak much English then, but what friends she had were all boys. She was one of them.

Things had gone quietly for a year and a half on Locke Drive until she had a row with Dad. He knew about her chest-bandaging and he tried to teach her how to be a normal girl. Chi, mirroring her father's stubbornness, had sassed him. So Dad schooled his child, measuring out his love, in the way his father had taught him. He caned her.

How our lives became unhinged in those three days, I can't recall precisely. Some of it happened while I was in school, and my parents never talked about it. And we kids never had the audacity or the bluntness to ask them.

After we came to America, Dad didn't whip us as frequently. He heard it was frowned upon here, but once in a while, when the pressure to survive was great and we were less than exemplary, he lit into us. He was a good man but there was much of his father in him, the rigid traditionalist who espoused discipline, pride, and honor. These things gave him the right footprint to set off the mines of Locke Drive. It was the sort of predatory place that had evolved to break his sort of man. One way or another, the price had to be paid. No family made it through unscathed.

Sometimes, I wondered why Chi's final days with us on Locke Drive did not take on a more explosive texture. I suspected it was because the flavors surrounding Dad's last quarrel with Chi were the very flavors of our lives in its absolute normalcy. It was the first time we were all under one roof living as a family, free from the appraising eyes of the church that sponsored us. Tossing in America without a net, we were learning English, we were learning about each other. Just beginning to weave the fabric of our family there in the tiny three-bedroom duplex, our halfway house to the promised land. What I remember most were the ingredients of the everyday—the smells, the sounds, the jars and hums of an immigrant family, new to being immigrants as well as being a family. I remember the nauseous perm chemicals of Mom's salon. The apartment's moldy carpet that knew more floods than any of us. The bulk meat stewing in fishsauce, Mom's attempt to save money. Incense burning eternally on the family altar, sending ever more prayers to heaven for yet another deliverance. Our eight bodies sweating without air-conditioning. The dump down the street sneaking into the house on a breeze. The convoy of dump trucks rumbling through the street. Mayo and bologna sandwiches. And homemade French fries leaving an oily, smoky tang on everything. The neighborhood shrill with heavy metal, yelling kids. The television warbling nonsense. Mom's incessant complaints. Us boys quarreling. Baby Kay crying.

Our house at times took on the grimy madness of a roadside diner halfway to hell. This was the context of our downfall.

Chi didn't come home from school that day, but the cops came for Dad after he returned from work. They had a warrant for his arrest. Showed it to him. Said his daughter Chi was in a detention center, a safe place. Handcuffed him in his own living room in front of his wife and children. Took him away in a patrol car flashing red lights, all the neighbors standing on the curb watching the spectacle the way we did when the cops came for them. Mom cried, yelling in Vietnamese, no idea what the cops were saying to her. Chi's high school teacher said bruises don't lie; Dad was a child beater.

Jungle - Station

Jungle shadows nip the heel of the day's last passenger train as it lumbers toward Muong Man Station. I fight down a surge of panic. Early in the morning, I ride back into Phan Thiet from Mui Ne and hop the peasant commuter train out to this way station. With $45 in my pocket, I know the train is my only chance of reaching Hanoi, some one thousand miles north. Several Vietnamese informed me the ticket was $30, but the Muong Man Station officials want $120 because I am a Vietnamese American, the porters want $10 for handling my bicycle because it has heavy luggage panniers, and the constable wants $40 because his salary is $25 a month. $170 in total.

"Where are your American papers?" demands the constable with a doughy face peppered with blackheads.

"I left them in Saigon with my relatives." A street-savvy friend had informed me of the brisk black-market trade in Vietnamese-American legal documents. After all these years, I sometimes feel as though my American skin is only as thick as my passport. This makes me very nervous about taking my "return ticket to America" on the road.

"Ho Chi Minh City, not Saigon!" he barks. *"Travel is not permitted without a passport. A photocopy is not acceptable."*

Inside the decaying way station, sweat steams in the heat. Sour. Workers' sandals flap on the dirt, powdering the air. Rust scabs the window's metal grilles. Door hinges dangle on doorless frames. I sit in the center of the office on a long bench surrounded by seven uniforms. The stationmaster, a thick joint of beef grizzled with graying black hair, lounges behind a desk with one leg cocked on an open drawer. The constable plants his hams against the edge of the desk and eyes my bicycle and the loaded panniers, no doubt appraising their value. Three conductors and a pair of deputies form the spectator gallery to my right. They scowl, not buying my pleas of poverty. Foreigners aren't poor. Can't be. Especially not Viet-kieu.

The underlings file out to meet the train, leaving me with the two honchos. Outside, the beggars, vendors, and peasants stir out of the shade onto the hot concrete, buzzing toward the ancient iron monster as it groans to rest. Healthy beggars abruptly develop the gaits of cripples. Vendors sing their wares, clawing at the passengers, jabbing sandwiches, bags of peanuts, pouches of sugarcane juice, T-shirts, straw mats, and tawdry gifts through the windows, pleading for a buyer. Peasants are frantic to get their baskets of produce aboard before the whistle blows again.

Four laborers haul pigs individually caged in woven baskets and drop them on the concrete. The pigs squeal, pissing terror, yellow urine running across the pavement. The stench wafts into the room on a hot breeze and infects me with the animals' fear.

"May I go now? That's my train." I manage a smile and inch to the edge of the bench. They have detained me in this room for two hours, causing me to miss one train already.

"Here, I'll help you out: $140 U.S. dollars," the station boss offers.

I carefully explain again that I have only enough for the regular fare. The constable frowns, orders me to stay in the room and goes out with the stationmaster, cursing cheap foreigners.

Alone, I watch the peeling strips of ceiling boards flex in the wind playing in the rafters. I am still hungry and weak from my bout of stomach flu. The minutes tick by. The stationmaster pokes his head into the room and says, *"The train's leaving in two minutes. Changed your mind? It's the last passenger train today. Do you want to pay now?"*

"*Go through my bags! If I've got any money in there, it's yours!*"

He shrugs and leaves. Two minutes. The whistle blasts twice. The train sighs northward without me. Practically broke and emotionally exhausted, I consider abandoning my bike trip altogether and retreating to the villa in Vung Tau until the fever and the diarrhea pass. Touring Vietnam isn't shaping up as I had hoped. This morning while I was eating breakfast, a pickpocket stole my pepper spray. Afterward, a minivan came within inches of hitting me head-on, my closest call yet after months of bike touring. I am miserable with flea and mosquito bites and, between bouts of diarrhea and unexplainable fevers, I haven't felt well since I stepped off the plane. Every Vietnamese I meet corrupts me with the certainty that I will die if I attempt to bicycle the country. Now the train officials strong-arm me: *No passport? Then you must stay here in this jungle.*

An hour later, still detained at the station on the constable's order, I watch the rail crew work.

"*Yes, that's what I said, you idiot!*" a conductor explodes into a telephone receiver.

Squatting on their hams in the dirt, four junior conductors, deep in a heated debate, don't even look up. They shuffle pebbles along a line drawn in the dirt. The station manager is testing them on train-car sequence management and track scheduling. With a single track, it is paramount to keep the northbound and the southbound trains from meeting.

The conductor bellows: "*The train left fifteen minutes ago, you idiot!*"

A roar of curses and victory whoops rolls out from the room behind. The laborers are gambling with the rest of the station staff, most of whom are relatives.

"*Yeah, you come out here,*" says the man, dripping each word into the receiver. "*Come out here and I'll cut off your balls.*"

A baby wails.

"*Your mother!*" He hammers the receiver into its cradle, lights a cigarette, and saunters over to inspect my bike. Finally, his curiosity gets the better of him. "*Hey!*" He turns to me. "*Hungry? You want to go for coffee?*"

A friendly gesture. Unsure if going for coffee means just coffee or a whole meal with plenty of drinking, I blurt, *"Sure. Thanks."*

He confers with the constable, then motions for me to follow him. I move to get the bike, but he says, *"Leave it. I'll have someone watch it for you."*

I swallow the lump in my throat. Trust him or insult him? Neither a winning choice. Oh, hell.

We stagger over the mounds of debris that ring the station, then tread around peasants sitting on the ground amid great baskets of produce waiting to load their goods on the next overnight cargo-only train. Red dirt, the color of half-baked clay, kicked up by foot traffic, drifts down on the houses, layering thick over the leafy trees and powdering the farm women's white shirts. On the side of the road, stooped grandmothers gather the cabbage they laid out this morning to dry in the sun. Dogs scat erratically, noses to the ground, pissing and defecating next to the vegetables.

At a kitchen-shack diner, an establishment held up by four posts and a motley collection of plywood, we sit on low bamboo chairs under a thatched awning. A stray mutt curls up at my feet and shares his fleas with my ankles.

My host orders each of us a liter of draft beer, rice, pork chops, vegetables, and chicken squash soup. The owner-waitress-cook calls a little boy from the street, fishes a greasy wad of money out of a blood-stained pocket, and peels him a five-cent bill. A minute later, he trots back with a lump of ice with a rind of dirt, juggling it between his hands like a hot potato. She wipes the ice with a rag, cracks it with a cleaver, drops the chunks into clear plastic mugs and pours our beer.

My host's name is Hoang and he wants to hear about my travels. He is a prolific reader of travel literature and magazines about exotic locales with strange names, but he has never been farther than two hundred miles from his home village. Hoang is thirty-five, married with three children. His family of five lives on his meager salary. He seems like a real nice guy, a dreamer of far places and quiet inner glory. For strangers like him, quiet souls who murmur, *I wish I could do what you're doing,* I dig deep into my bag of tricks—my tales of the road—and spin the best yarns within my power, casting a sheen on every detail. After my stories and several liters of beer run dry, a wistfulness comes into his eyes.

"*I remember the day before the North Army came in,*" he said. "*The whole village, those that hadn't fled already, gathered in the market for the news. A merchant who had just come back from Saigon to fetch his family was there, telling everyone that the Americans were taking refugees on their ships.*

"*My neighbor asked me if I wanted to come with his family. He was my best friend. They had two motorbikes; they got rich working for the local American army base. They rode out of the village that day with what they could put in their bags.*

"*I got a letter from my friend a couple of years ago. His family is in France and he is an engineer. He is married to a Frenchwoman. They live in a nice house outside of Paris.*"

"*Many people are still emigrating?*"

"*No. It's a dream . . . Even beggars come back rich.*" Breaking the mood with a broad grin, he asks me, "*So you really don't have money?*"

"*Forty-five dollars is all I have until I get to the Vietcom Bank in Hanoi.*"

"*That's six weeks' wages to me,*" he notes, eyeing me. "*Well, there may be another way to get you north.*"

"*How?*"

"*Hitchhike.*"

"*You mean on the road with my bike?*"

"*No, hitchhike a freight train. But you've got to pretend you're a Vietnamese. No one will dare take a Viet-kieu. I admire what you're doing. If I didn't have a family, I'd go with you. Leave it to me. I'll get you north . . . eventually.*" He grins, flourishes his hand like a street conjurer, and pats me on the shoulder, which makes me nervous.

"*But what about the constable? Your boss might fire you.*"

"*The constable: no problem. Once you're gone, you're out of his jurisdiction.*" He pauses, grinning. "*My boss, he's family—my uncle.*"

Hoang confirms my suspicions that the *big men* believed me when I failed to hock up the cash when the last train rolled out. According to him, I can't take the passenger train to Hanoi even if he sells me a civilian ticket, because I don't look native. The officials on the train are certain to give me trouble when I present a civilian ticket.

We stumble back to the station. Hoang suggests I sleep off the booze while he goes to his night class. Hoang and five other rail workers, all drunk, trudge off to their English class with notebooks and pencils in hand like schoolboys, chanting: *Times are changing, we must be ready for opportunity, we must learn English, the international language of commerce.* They stagger down the road. Hoang yells over his shoulder that I shouldn't worry, he'll have me on my way when he gets back.

Night falls. I retire to a broken divan in a dark room. The shredded straw mat reeks of stale beer and sweat. The walls bubble with zigzagging geckos. The air buzzes with crickets, one ricochets off my forehead. Mosquitoes assault my hands and face. Fleas sneak up my pant legs to ravish my calves. I am raw with bites, crazy with itches, hoping Hoang and his boys will come back for me but certain that they'll pass out drunk somewhere.

I give up on sleep and stroll into the village. It is 11 p.m. Nearly everyone is awake. In the shack-diner, a crowd watches Vietnamese soaps on a nineteen-inch Sony. Across the street, young men hang out at a two-table billiard hall, four posts holding up sheets of corrugated aluminum. Around midnight, I squat in the market square at one of the dozen single-basket food sellers and eat a late supper of rice porridge cooked in chicken stock and scallions.

By moonlight, I stray down to the disused section of the station. Broken, abandoned train cars crowd the rail yard. The dark masks the garbage, the coolness holds down the stink, the still air sick-sweet with a scent of urine and wet hay. Crickets sugar the night. Hammocks creaking. Soft words. Rhythmic breaths, gentle moans seep through caboose windows. Passion-rich this world of beggars, homeless.

Down at the main platform, vendors' oil lamps dot the dark cement islands between the tracks like fireflies. I am drawn to the lights. A beggar boy and a white-haired man sit on six-inch plastic blocks next to a girl selling hot soy milk from a tin pot. They smile, inviting me into their circle.

"Try some hot milk," the boy urges me. He looks about ten, naked save for a tattered pair of shorts and mismatched rubber thongs tied to his toeless feet. I saw him earlier hobbling about begging the train passengers and bantering, teasing the food vendors. Cheerful and roguish, he seems to forget his lameness though he dramatizes it well when he works the crowd.

"Egg-milk?" the girl queries. I nod. Smiling, she briskly whips an egg yolk with sugar in a cup with a fork for five minutes, then tops it off with a ladle of hot soy milk. It tastes foamy, sweet, and warm, just like what Great Granny used to give me when I couldn't sleep. I tell her as much and she blushes with pleasure.

The grandfather is on his way to see his grandchildren. He makes twenty dollars a month as a laborer, so hopping a freight train is the only way he can travel five hundred kilometers once every year to visit them. The beggar boy is waiting for a cargo train to take him into Phan Thiet, where he panhandles every morning in the fish market. He travels widely because beggars ride trains and buses for free. It is considered bad luck to turn them away.

"What about the cops?" I ask them.

Grandfather laughs. *"Those crooks?"*

"You, Big Brother, you watch out for them," warns the boy. *"The train cops are the meanest. They'll peel and gut you for everything you have."*

Grandfather and Milk-girl nod solemnly, murmuring for me to be careful. I tell them that in America the police are actually very honest, real good guys. *"It must be really nice in America,"* says the girl, her eyes dreamy with a young girl's infatuation.

"You must be able to eat whatever you want, as much as you want," chirps the beggar boy, swept up in the girl's emotion.

"But I heard work in America is very demanding, isn't it?" protests the old man. *"You can't go home for a nap during lunch, can you?"*

I shake my head. The girl hasn't heard a word anyone said. *"America is really big, isn't it? It must be so big that people can just disappear into it. So, so big. Fifty states, each as big as Vietnam,"* she exclaims, hands on her knees as though ready to take that leap into the thin air of America.

Her aunt's family has disappeared into the States. Their letters had arrived while they were in Thailand, but once they made it to California, nothing was heard from them. It has been almost a decade. What happened, she asks me over and over. It is too common, Viet-kieu severing ties with relatives in Vietnam. No matter what I say, it is hard for them to understand why relatives are so unwilling to help those left behind. How can people refuse to help when they are living in a country where a teenager can earn more money in a day than a Vietnamese teacher earns in a month?

I stay with them until near morning, when the girl's sister arrives to relieve her. She has two sisters, and each of them takes an eight-hour shift on the basket. Her sister brings a tin pot of soup with udon noodles, chopsticks, spoons, and bowls. Yielding the baskets and clay stove to her sister, she goes home with her empty pot.

During the night, three freight trains stop at the station, but Hoang, who came back on duty after his English class, can't secure me a passage. One look at me and the cargo supervisors all shake their heads; no one believes I am his cousin—a bona fide Vietnamese. Each mumbles something about getting caught with a Viet-kieu aboard—which could cost them a month's wage.

At 7 a.m. Hoang manages to press me onto the cargo train of a reluctant acquaintance who owes him a big favor, claiming I am his cousin. Hoang shakes my hand, escorts me to the train, placing a brotherly hand on my shoulder for show, and whispers through his grin, *"I wish I could go with you. Watch out for the cops. This guy, Tung, is not really a close friend of mine. After the train rolls, he'll negotiate your fare with you. It should be much less than what you have with you. Be careful, remember your Vietnamese alias. If he finds out that I lied to him, he'll dump you at the next station. Good luck, Brother!"*

Tung, the train's cargo supervisor, meets us at the caboose. He is thirty-seven years old and rail-thin with boiling-red drinker's eyes and withered smoker's teeth. Tung shows me to the caboose and tells me to stow my bike next to the pig and monkey cages in the rear compart-ment. The caboose is already packed with ten "unofficial passengers" and four cargo clerks who take an instant dislike to me because I am "imposed cargo." I introduce myself several times without success.

One of the clerks, a man with an angry crimson scar running from his forehead to his jaw, glares at me when I extend my hand. He seems intent on gutting me sometime in the immediate future.

After the train begins to roll, I wonder if this is a mistake. Red-eyed Tung shows me to a sleeping compartment reserved for the cargo clerks. Great! Me and Scarface are roomies. It has six hard bunks, three on each side with just enough standing room in the middle. We sit on the lower bunks and five other men file in to join us.

At Redeyes' suggestion, I introduce myself to this hard-bitten lot. Redeyes sums up my predicament to his compatriots. No one bothers to reciprocate my introduction, so I nickname them—to myself. Bugsy is a short fortyish man with pudgy cheeks and a pair of bunny teeth that pin down his bottom lip. Scarface is a twenty-something punk. Shyboy is a youthful mid-thirtyish man who speaks little and does most of the work. VC is a brawny and loud soldier, a stout military lifer in his late forties, returning from one of his frequent joyrides in liberal Saigon. Dealer is a paunchy hustler, cardsharp, and cigarette smuggler.

They confer and decide that they will take me to Nha Trang for ten dollars, and, perhaps, Hue for twenty dollars more. Hanoi isn't part of the negotiation yet. Redeyes doesn't buy Hoang's story that I am a Vietnamese national who spent years studying abroad in America. He makes it painfully apparent that he doesn't want to risk getting caught transporting a foreigner on a cargo train—not without adequate compensation. They aren't allowed to transport luggage, animals, or "unofficial" Vietnamese passengers in the caboose.

Redeyes asks me to stay in the compartment for my "protection." A couple of passengers are allowed to come in to talk to me. Most have questions about America and Europe, usually about towns where their relatives and friends have emigrated. A young woman named Mai stays with me for an hour asking about the places I have seen. When the train draws closer to Mai's village, she looks out the window at the rice fields and the huts squatting on the mud flats. *"Do you really think it's beautiful?"* she asks me, taking another hard look at the countryside, trying to fathom what is beautiful about poverty.

I reassure her that it is beautiful in its own way. American cities, I confide, are not too attractive. Lots of steel, glass, and concrete.

Concrete everywhere. You have to go to a park to see dirt. She giggles into her palm.

"How funny! Americans don't like concrete. We love it. It's special. It's great for floors. We don't have it, but my aunt does. Her sons bought her a concrete floor for her house. Concrete floors are very cool in the summer. Very nice for taking naps. In the rainy season, concrete floors are very clean, not like our dirt floor. Very easy to clean."

I have taken concrete for granted. I nod dumbly, looking at this young girl with new respect. She is seventeen but malnutrition has given her the body of a fourteen-year-old. Her fingers and nails are brown from the dye of the leather factory outside Saigon where she works with her older sister. She talks about her family's poverty frankly, with no shame and with just a touch of sadness that hints at the Asian way of accepting life.

I ask her whether the lifting of the American embargo is a good thing for Vietnam. She doesn't know, but it couldn't be bad since her boss is hiring more people, at $1.50 a day, to turn out more leather, which will be sent to Korea, then to America. She hopes to get her fourteen-year-old sister a job at the factory. Sharecropping on poor land isn't enough to feed a family of eight.

"I hope they take you all the way to Hanoi," says Mai as she leaves to help her sick mother off the train. Unaccustomed to traveling, they are all reeling with motion sickness. I am sick with the incongruity of our lives. I stare off into the countryside. We are separated by seas of rice paddies.

Suddenly, a barrage of rocks showers the train. One stone strikes the cabin wall near my head and bounces into the passage. More follow. I duck beneath the window and cover my head with my hands.

Scarface finds me crouching on the floor and laughs. *"The cow herders are pissed. Last week we hit one of their cattle that got onto the track. The herder wasn't around so we hacked off enough beef to last us all the way up to Hanoi."*

"Nowhere on earth—nowhere is there a steel road, an asphalt road, and a beach so close together. Ten paces between each! Fire-ship and ocean-ship right next to each other. Magnificent isn't it?"

Bugsy is howling his excitement in my face, both of us clinging precariously on the open door of the caboose, him throwing an arm wildly toward the ocean, me not wanting to diminish his fervor, nodding with the ready affirmation of a convert.

"The French built it to rape Vietnam. The Americans bombed it to divide Vietnam. We rebuilt it to reunify Vietnam!" Bugsy declares, and chops the air with his hand. It sounds suspiciously like a government slogan. I decide not to tell him that he's got it all mixed up. It was the Americans who tried to maintain the tracks and the North Vietnamese who were adept at bombing and hijacking trains. Maybe he is thinking about the national highway or the Ho Chi Minh Trail.

"Eight months, that's all it took to get the entire line working. This Reunification Express Train was inaugurated on 31 December 1976. In eight months, we repaired 1,334 bridges, 27 tunnels, 158 stations, and 1,370 switches! Eighteen goddamn thousand kilometers."

Flashing his crooked incisors, Soft-heart, one of the more congenial passengers to befriend me, pats me on the shoulder, encouraging me to take pride in this Vietnamese accomplishment. His brother, Eager-boy, is standing with us, flushing with pride at this national treasure. I am fond of them, wishing I could take them with me and show them all the tall mountains, the great rivers, the wonders I have seen. The national highway, paralleling the railroad, separates us and the surf crashing in on high tide. From the train, only a few yards above the water, it is a majestic view sweeping the expanse of the bay. We are edging, clacking, along the mountain's foothills. The wind whips off the water, warm and hard. I fancy we could in two hops splash into the ocean for a quick swim.

Abruptly, the train—our *fire-ship*—shunts into a tunnel. We are worming into the rocks, in the belly of a metallic night crawler speed-eating its way into the marrow of the mountain. An utterly complete darkness gulps us down. Chilled cavern air, earthy and moist, skirls around us like wraiths. A thousand teeth, the roar of metal on metal bites down.

I am in awe of this train, of this steel road laid by Vietnamese hands. I am in awe of the Vietnamese. I admire them. I respect them, but what I really want is to like them, to find them likable. Perhaps the former U.S. ambassador to Vietnam, Graham Martin, touched on something when he said in an interview given to author Larry Englemann long after the War: "I never really had any great attachment to the Vietnamese, North or South. I don't particularly like any of them." Maybe Vietnamese as a whole are not likable.

And what about Vietnamese Americans? What does that say about us?

I think we are, by our own closed-door admissions, a fractious, untrusting tribe unified only because we are besieged by larger forces.

Morning of my second day, Redeyes summons me into his cabin, where the inner sanctum of the caboose is holding court and presiding over bottles of rice wine. Redeyes invites me to drink with them and, seeing my hesitation, he declares, *"We are all friends here. Our lives are simple. We don't have much but we are friends. And friends drink and eat together. Are we your friends?"*

He need not say more. They are still debating whether to take me all the way to Hanoi and risk running afoul of the cops at the inspection station north of Hue. I need their friendship more than they need my money.

At thirty cents a liter of rice wine, friendship goes a long way. Scarface, Bugsy, Redeyes, Shyboy, VC, Dealer, and I cement our friendship with murky rice wine that tastes like a mixture of kerosene, vinegar, sugar, and bad sake. We waltz the bottle and the single shot glass around the table. Each man drinks, grimaces, pours another shot into the glass, hands it to the guy on his left, then eats something from the dishes on the table. If someone has something fatally contagious, we are all history.

In an alcoholic stupor, I confess that I'm actually a Viet-kieu who is indeed broke and needs to get to Hanoi. They look at me gravely. Scarface mutters that I must make amends. The rest of them agree. Redeyes says I must make it right with everyone present. How? I ask him. He grins and pours me a shot. I toss it down. Scarface pours me a shot. I toss that one down, too. I toss down a shot for every member of the party. They laugh and pound my back. It is a great joke.

Redeyes chuckles and says he knew I was lying the moment he set eyes on me, but, hey, what are friends for?

We drink, sitting together in the cabin, leaning on each other. They want to know about the West and about Western women. Sex before marriage, really? Sex on the first date, you serious? Sex in high school?!

"Does eating rice make Americans sick?"

"Is there such a thing as a ten-lane freeway in America?"

"Do you know O. J. Simpson?"

With them shoving gizzards, intestines, livers, and hearts at me as though I've never seen such delicacies before, I succumb to the peer pressure and swallow. When we finish, Bugsy brings out another party platter, piled high with snails, goat testicles, fish heads, goat blood pudding, pig brain, and some sort of sausage the color of wet ash and old blood. After four bottles of wine, they doze off happily. I retch out the window. They wake, chortle, and curse me for wasting good liquor. I sit like a dead man, watching the land scroll forward and away. It is chilly and a light drizzle softens the distance. On steep hillsides footing the mountains, peasants in plastic ponchos trudge up scraggly slopes, their backs bent under impossibly heavy loads of twigs and cords of firewood. They strain ever uphill, loose pants bunched at the knees, their lean muscular calves, bare, working like knots of rope. They are terribly strong these small, lithe hill people. My train clacks through a crust of shanties, its mournful greeting, then good-bye, belayed on a rush of wind as it crashes through without stopping. A little girl, barefoot in mud, clutches a wooden doll, her eyes stabbing mine, wonders on her face.

At dusk, Bugsy rouses me from my nap and escorts me to the front of the caboose, where fifteen people gather for dinner. This is an improvement over last night, when Scarface gave me rice cakes and bananas to eat alone on my bunk. In the light of a single oil lamp, I join them elbow to elbow, squatting on the rolling floor of the car. The passengers have cooked a meal of pork stew, steamed vegetables, cabbage soup, and rice. The man next to me hands over a large bowl of rice and a pair of bamboo chopsticks. In a gesture of hospitality and friendship, people within reach start putting morsels of food into my bowl.

I try a piece of pork and immediately fight down a fit of retching. Someone hadn't bothered to shave the pig before butchering it. The prickly hair scrapes the roof of my mouth. It feels as though I've bitten a chunk off a live pig; I can almost hear it squealing.

I avoid eating by regaling them with tales of Mexico, America, Japan, Hong Kong, and Indonesia. I tell them of the real world: Mexican Indians scratching a living off arid land, the slum dwellers of America with their concrete-and-bullet jungles, the unwanted Gypsies of Europe, the gentle homeless of Japan, the poor of Hong Kong who live in chicken pens, and the oppressed minorities of Indonesia. It helps them see that heaven really isn't just a place beyond Vietnam's borders.

Our freight train sighs into a way station high up in the hills. It is dark and the drizzle which first greeted us in Hue is still coming down. The gambling gang light their gas lanterns and trundle up and down the train checking wheels, junctions, cargo-car padlocks and generally pulling guard duty. A penny-ante card game is dealt among the women. A group of children squeaks a singsong chant outside. A white-haired old man who boarded at Nha Trang slides open the door, spilling light onto five young faces waiting in the mizzling darkness. They are holding plastic bowls, begging—not for money: *Uncles, Aunts, could you spare us your leftover rice, just a fist of leftover rice.*

Like any train hitchhiker, the old man is extremely poor, but he scratches his pocket for a thin roll of dime-bills. He passes them out to the little paupers. We follow his example. We give them the rice and the stewed pork leftovers from dinner. Their mothers come with torches, thank us, and fetch them home to huts not more than ten yards from the tracks. The children are giggling, happy, cartwheeling in the drizzle, by the orange light of the flames. I am wondering to what century this train has transported me. Maybe I am wrong about heaven not lying across the Pacific.

All the foulness I've forced down my throat makes the night pass badly. The toilet is a hole in a dark closet. Rail ties blur beneath. The thunderous noise of the old train punishes a hangover like nothing on this side of hell. By morning, I am groaning in my bunk when the train pulls into the inspection station. Scarface and Bugsy hurry into the cabin carrying luggage, fruit baskets, and blankets. They drape blankets over me, then pile on the luggage and more blankets.

"*Don't move,*" Bugsy says, his fingers closing around my arm like a vise. "*If the cops find you, pretend you're too sick to talk.*"

I don't need to pretend, although the thought of not being able to get to the toilet is disturbing. The last thing I need is jail time and soiled pants.

The cops board the caboose and begin their inspection. I can see them through a hole in the blanket. Slowly combing through every closet and compartment, they work like termites from one end of the caboose to the other. One cop enters my compartment. Redeyes trails him inside.

"*What's in those bags?*" asks the cop. I know he's looking at the piles of luggage covering me. My throat seizes. I am drenched in sweat. My heart beats in my ears. Every breath is a shout.

"*Nothing,*" Redeyes replies. "*Just some clothes, gifts for my family. Nothing important.*"

"*That's a lot of nothing.*"

A pause.

Redeyes' voice shifts into a banter. "*How's the weather here been lately? Cold? It's hot in Ho Chi Minh City. You've been eating, drinking well? Smoke?*" I hear him knocking cigarettes out of a pack. A lighter zips.

Redeyes is speaking again. "*Here's a little something, Brother.*" I hear him flicking bills out from a roll of money he keeps in the pocket of his slacks.

"*The weather has been lousy.*" The cop is amiable now. "*You know how it is.*"

They laugh at this insider's joke.

Five minutes later, the train rolls away from the station. I crawl out of my bunk, shivering in my own sweat. The gang gathers for their last round of drinks for the trip. I beg off and crawl into a hammock to sleep. When I wake up, we are chugging into the Hanoi cargo depot. I've been on the train for three days and two nights. Expressing my heartfelt thanks, I bid them all farewell and we pour a parting round of rice wine. VC, Shyboy, and Bugsy escort me to the last barrier: the station police.

VC plucks the glasses off my nose and jams them into my backpack. *"Don't look conspicuous."*

"Without my glasses, you know, I can't tell if the Chief is laughing at me." Chief Redeyes is leaning on the door ten feet from me.

They cackle as they always do at my frailty. A round of handshaking and backslapping ensues, with me at the center taking the brunt of it. Knowing that I eat bananas like a monkey, Bugsy presents me with a parting gift. Over the last two days, he took pains to buy me all five types of banana grown in Vietnam, carefully pointing out the virtues of each. He ties a bunch of *su* bananas, my favorite, to my backpack with a piece of twine. Scarface gives me a smile worth a fist of gold. For a moment, he is handsome and full of good wishes, neither ugly nor wine-happy. Redeyes drapes an arm around my shoulder and reminds me again, *"When you're sick of pushing that bike, just head to the closest train station and tell them you're my cousin. They'll let you ride the freight train as a favor to me."*

VC carries my panniers. Shyboy walks my bike. We cross the rail yard, duck behind the parked trains, and sneak to the station's rear gate. The coast is clear. We make a break for it.

"Halt!"

A policeman clomps out from the warehouse next to the gate, hand raised at us. Five more uniforms saunter behind him.

Night-Wind

There was a power outage the night Chi escaped from the juvenile detention center. A knock at the sliding glass door startled us. Chi shivered on the other side. I unlocked and opened the door but she wouldn't come in. It scared me seeing my sixteen-year-old sister lurking fearfully outside like a stranger.

"How did you get here?" I asked her.

"I jumped the fence. They kept me in a small room. It's really nice. I had my own TV. They fed me. The food is better than the school's."

"How did you find your way back?"

"I memorized the route the cops took and I asked people along the way. I made it back this morning. I've been hiding down by the creek."

Huy and Tien fetched Chi's sweater and jacket from her room. I scraped the leftover rice into a plastic bag along with the rest of Mom's cabbage soup, and took some oranges from the refrigerator. We gave her the food behind the garage.

"What are you going to do?"

"I don't know. Go somewhere for a while. I can't go back to school, everyone knows about me. I can't come back here. Dad will kill me."

She really believed that.

"Why don't you go back to that place where they kept you?"

"I can't. They'll put me into a foster home. Dad is in jail because of me. I'm scared."

She equated being around to putting Dad in jail. He was sitting in jail about to be tried for child abuse. Her testimony would put him away, and that would be the end of us all.

"Where are you going to sleep?" I asked her, reeling in the void that suddenly separated her world and mine.

"I don't know. Maybe I'll find some place in San Francisco." She had been there perhaps three times. I doubted she knew the way. Besides, her English was worse than ours. Two and a half years wasn't enough time to learn a new language.

"They'll find me here," she said. "There are more Asians in Chinatown."

True. It was her only chance.

"Here, take this." I handed her two dollars and change, the sum of our savings—Huy's, Tien's, and mine.

She pocketed our parting gift. "I care for you," she said, and I felt strange because we never say soft things like that.

She said she'd be back in a few days. I assured her we would have a package ready for her next time. A noise came from Mom's room and Chi knifed into the dark, a bag of rice soup sloshing in one hand.

The police released Dad. Things returned to normal. We went to school not fully grasping the gravity of Chi's situation. Dad went to work. Mom cooked and cut hair. No one talked about it, so pretending that nothing bad had happened was easy. Still, we assembled a survival bag for Chi and stayed up late waiting for her knuckles on our window, but she never returned. Maybe she'd died. Maybe she had gone far away and couldn't return.

It was during these nights that I started dreaming in English. Abruptly, I was walking in two camps, each distinct and vastly different from the other. I didn't feel it then, but one side was beginning to wither. In my sleep, English words gushed out of my mouth and poured into my ears naturally as though I were born with it. My thoughts formulated themselves in the new language. I dreamt Chi spoke to me in perfect English. She said America was scary.

I was afraid for her, though my fears diminished as the days dragged into months and Chi stopped visiting me in dreams. Secretly, I was glad that she didn't come back because the court dropped the charges and Dad didn't go to jail. We would survive. There was enough to eat and, if everything went well, we would be moving away from the dump soon.

When we did move and the months had stretched into years, we "forgot" Chi. She slipped away from us the way our birth-language slipped from our tongue, in bits, in nuances. The finer subtleties lost like shades of colors washed out under a harsh noon sun. Unused words dried up and faded away. Her name was not spoken. It became awkward and slow when we switched back and forth between English and Vietnamese. At the least, it was difficult and cumbersome to explain to new friends that we had a runaway sister who wanted to be a boy. Even Mom was trying to learn English and Dad no longer made us speak Vietnamese at home. Chi no longer existed and Kay grew up without knowing who the sad, angry stranger in the old family portrait was. Kay spoke a sweet, flawless English; her Vietnamese never escaped its infancy. In our deepening silence, we buried Chi into ourselves, locked her into the basements of our minds. We became embarrassed by our immigrant accent, something that sneaked up on us when we were excited, when we least expected it. Somehow, she became the family's big shame, as if we'd somehow failed—failed her as we'd failed ourselves.

Fallen-Leaves

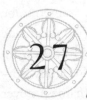An was five, his sister ten. They sat on a divan-bed in the dark, digging yesterday-rice from a pot. Fishsauce, old rice, spoons. Salty. The rice had gone crunchy. Nothing in the pantry. The maid had left with the grocery cash. Mom hadn't been home in days. She was away, business and money. Dad was away, army and money. An missed sitting on his father's lap for stories—a memory of beer breaths on which great voyages sailed. Chi missed the food her mother used to cook before she made the money that brought many quarrels into the house.

Outside it began to rain. They abandoned their meal to rush into the street with other children greeting the downpour. It descended in tiny wet fists. They turned their faces to the sky—though it could not be seen—and swallowed drops falling as fat and sweet as litchis. In the road, the red-brown water had gone knee-deep. Kids dragged each other upriver, up the street, in inner tubes. They jumped, they splashed. The roaring rain tickled. All young faces were grinning.

An pulled down his shorts and pissed into the river. Chi showed him that she could pee standing as well. No difference, she said to him. He looked at her dubiously. She peed farther than he. See? They laughed, white teeth like small lightning. Two sun-browned delights playing in a drowned gray.

In doorways, the old folks huddled, looking with old-folk envy on the children frolicking in the deluge, muttering the worn sentiment of a war poem: Monsoon rain falls like tears of grieving lovers; happiness comes easiest to the youngest.

Hanoi-Visage

28 At the sight of the policeman coming out of the warehouse, VC nods at Shyboy, who in one fluid motion, eases himself onto the saddle and pedals off without looking back. VC smiles tightly, *"Don't say anything. I'll talk to him."*

VC spins around, instantly jovial, laughing, hands outstretched. He strides into the cop's path, blocking his view of Shyboy's escape, duking, jiving like a chum. Shyboy glides beyond the corner and is gone. I trail VC, my face neutral, struggling hard to keep from squinting. Without my glasses, I can't even see the cop's face at ten paces, and this makes me extremely apprehensive.

"Brother! Is that you, Huynh? Yes, it is you. How have you been? In good health?" VC gushes as he tries to shake the cop's hand. The cop brushes past him, heading straight for me with the directness of a hound dog.

"Who are you?" he puts the question into my face. *"Where are you going?"*

At arm's length, I can see the displeasure in his face well. I nod politely, disconcerted at the cigarette sourness of his breath. VC answers for me, *"This is my cousin. I'm just giving him a tour."*

He glowers at VC. The cop looks absurdly small and nasty in his hat, the visor extending a good three inches beyond his nose.

"Come on, he's my cousin," says VC in a tone of mollification.

"He's Chinese."

"No, he's Vietnamese. What? I don't know my own cousin?"

"Then why doesn't he talk?"

"What do you want me to say? My cousin explained it to you already." I take care not to sound aggressive.

"You have an accent. It's not Northern or Southern." He looks me over carefully. *"Give me your identification."*

A small crowd begins to gather, two privates and a sergeant among the spectators. VC is waving, joking, apparently on familiar terms with most of them. I fumble with my pockets, pretending to look for my papers. If I show my visa and passport photocopy, VC's lie about my being his cousin is exposed. If I don't, this cop can arrest me. All Vietnamese are required to carry a photo ID and travel documents at all times. Law enforcement takes this rule seriously.

VC complains to the crowd, making it obvious that the cop is harassing us. He taps his chest, asking the cop: What's the problem? Don't you trust soldiers? The crowd's mood is shifting, but the cop remains adamant about seeing my ID.

I hand over all my papers. The cop peruses them, reading and rereading every word, then interrogates me. Why are you here? What is your purpose in Hanoi? How long will you be here? He is obviously doing the routine dance, fishing for a little grease. I'm not giving in, so the minutes squeak by awkwardly. VC grows more indignant at the delay and voices it to the crowd: Come on, he's one of us. Let him go on his way.

An older policeman approaches and the crowd parts for him. VC dips his head reverently to the man and backs away. Tall and lanky with a tinge of gray in his hair, the senior officer asks me where I've been. I tell him that I've traveled by bicycle across many countries to get here. We talk briefly, the crowd hanging on every word. His name is Thang and he is in charge of security at the station. I tell him of my intention to bicycle south back to Saigon. He smiles, saying that it is a good pursuit.

"Is your family from the South?" he asks me.

"Yes, sir, my mother's side. My father is from Hanoi."

"Ah, you're here to visit your father's roots," he observes, approving. Then, unexpectedly, he extends his open hand to me. *"It is all a new life for everyone, no? North Vietnamese, South Vietnamese, Viet-kieu, and Americans are all good people. It's all in the past. No ill feelings, no?"*

I accept his hand, my mouth hanging open. *"Yes, no ill feelings. Thank you, sir."*

"Welcome to Hanoi."

"Thank you. I'm glad to have made it."

He nods to his subordinate, who promptly returns my papers with smiles of goodwill. I bid them good-bye. VC and I walk out the gate. Shyboy is waiting for us around the corner. Shaking his head in disbelief, VC grins and sighs, *"Wow!"*

I shake hands with both of them and ride into my first Hanoi sunset.

The wide boulevard paralleling the tracks is full of Vietnamese men in army fatigues. Most are obviously no longer in the armed forces despite the fact that they are still in uniform. There are soldiers astride motorbike taxis. Soldiers pedaling cyclos. Soldiers sitting and drinking in cafés. Suddenly very nervous, I go directly to the first inn I see and take a room. I ask the owner about the soldiers in the street. She chuckles and says almost every male over sixteen has served in the army. Many wear their uniforms as a sign of patriotism, but mostly because the uniforms, often sold as army surplus, double well as durable work clothes. I heave a sigh of relief, amazed that there is still so much fear of the North Vietnamese Army in me. I drag my bike and luggage up three flights of stairs, toss them into the eight-by-six-foot room, lock the door, and beeline to the toilet. The organ meat and raw herbs I ate on the train are doing a number on me. At least I am off the train, I keep telling myself, as my innards faucet into the toilet.

My room, a deluxe suite, has "hot showers" provided by an electric heating tank, which takes half an hour to make three gallons of lukewarm water. It hangs from the ceiling like a water reservoir of an old-fashioned toilet with a long pull cord for flushing. Operating instructions are in Arabic. I take a shower fully clothed, a habit I picked up as I biked up the California and Oregon coasts. It is the fastest and most efficient way to get both body and clothes clean with the least amount of water. I soap the clothes, peel them off, soap myself, and as I shower I stomp on the dirty clothes. By the time I'm through, all I have to do is rinse out the laundry once, wring and hang it up to dry.

After dark, I wobble downstairs to the *com-phon* kitchen next door. *Com-phon* is the Northern style of "commoner's cafeteria." Down South, it is called *com-dia,* rice plates served with entrees on the side or "poured" over steamed rice. Here, a buffet table—a dozen plastic basins of food, some steaming, some cold—adorns the front entrance, announcing the day's bill of fare to the dusty street. A man fans away the flies with a piece of cardboard. I point out my dinner to him: bitter squash stuffed with ground pork and mushrooms, a small pan-fried trout, melon soup, a piece of fried soybean cake filled with eggplant. He notes my order on a pad, nods me inside, and scoops out servings onto little saucers.

I duck into the dark, dingy dining room. Sided by low benches, seven coffee tables form a single long board running the length of the corridor-like space illuminated by three dim light bulbs dripping from bare wires. A dark layer of grease and soot from cooking fires skins the wall. Leprous white patches glow where the plaster recently peeled off. The ceiling, stringy with cobwebs, sags ominously. It is early for the dinner crowd so only half of the seats are taken. I sit down at the end of one bench and cannot find the floor with my feet. Bones, napkins, cigarette butts, vegetables, and sticky rice cover the concrete. I nearly jump as a furry body brushes my leg—a small dog patrolling the ground for scraps. I'd heard these cat-sized dogs with the pointy muzzles are excellent mousers. They also make pretty good eating according to Bugsy.

The cook-waitress spreads out my meal before me and serves me a bowl of white rice and a cup of hot tea. The food is simple and good although not as fresh and hot as I'd like. I'm hoping it'll end my long bout of diarrhea.

Stuffed to the gills, I waddle back to my room, looking forward to a full night's sleep. I string up the mosquito net, flip on the ceiling fan, turn out the light, and go to bed, happy and thankful that I'd made it to my father's *que,* his birth village.

Hammering at my door pops me out of bed half an hour later.

"Open up!" cries a man outside. *"This is the police. Open up!"*

"One moment," I say, searching for my pants. I peek through the window shutter and, sure enough, a uniformed cop and the motel's receptionist stand at my door.

I unlock the padlock and open the door. *"Is something wrong, Officer?"*

"I'd like to invite you downstairs for a discussion."

"Huh?" It still hasn't occurred to me why he's here. *"Excuse me, Officer, but I'm very tired and I was sleeping. Can't this wait till tomorrow?"*

"I'd like to," he enunciates each word firmly, *"invite you downstairs for a talk. Please bring your papers."*

We sit down in the office with the hotel owner, a woman in her fifties. We wait uncomfortably while he inspects my visa, travel permits, and a passport photocopy.

"You cannot stay at this hotel," he says, returning my papers.

"Why?"

"You are a foreigner and it is unsafe for foreigners to stay here."

"No one told me that when I checked in and paid for the night's lodging."

The owner smiles apologetically. She speaks first to the cop in a sugary, submissive tone that surprises me: *"Officer, if I may explain . . ."* He nods and she continues, speaking as much to him as to me. *"We are ignorant of the rules. We never had any foreigners stay here before, and we thought that a Viet-kieu is just like a Vietnamese. We apologize for this inconvenience. We will refund your money."*

I can't believe what they are telling me. *"I was sleeping! You want to kick me out at this hour? Where am I going to go?"*

The cop seems unperturbed. *"I'd like to invite you to Hotel Cuu Long. It's not far."*

"The big hotel down the street? I can't afford it. I'm broke."

"It is not expensive," he assures me. According to the inn owner, a room at Hotel Cuu Long goes for at least fifty dollars. I am paying five dollars here.

"You will be safer and more comfortable there."

"I'm comfortable here!"

"The street here is very dangerous. Crimes are rampant in areas near the rail yard. We are ten kilometers from Hanoi. The streets here aren't as safe for foreigners."

"And you want me to go into the street at ten o'clock at night?" I scan his face to see if he is serious. *"I don't even have a map of the city."*

A smirk tugs the corner of his mouth, but his patience is wearing thin. A hard edge comes into his voice. Apparently, he isn't used to having his orders questioned.

"I order you to leave the premises. You will stay at the Cuu Long Hotel tonight."

"I'd really rather not."

"You must. If you don't, I will have my men remove you from your room," he says, meeting my eyes evenly.

We sit regarding each other for a minute. He rubs his hands together and rises to his feet. The matter is final. *"I will be back in half an hour with my men. You must be ready to leave the premises at that time. You will be escorted to Hotel Cuu Long."*

After he leaves, I ask the owner if the cop is serious. She sighs. *"Well, Brother. I'm very sorry for your troubles. Someone must have seen you going next door for dinner and reported you to the police."*

So the feeling of Big Brother watching me is justified after all. Suddenly, it feels Orwellian. A little claustrophobic.

"You see," she continues, *"he was expecting a little token of . . . cooperation—a few dollars."* She pauses, embarrassed at having to remind me of the mechanics of police protection. *"If you had given him a five-dollar tip to have him keep an eye on you, he would have let you stay. Since you didn't, he's going to make you stay at the expensive hotel. They'll pay him an 'introduction fee' for bringing them your business."*

"Thank you for telling me, Sister. I'm not sticking around so he can have his kickback."

In five minutes, I'm downstairs, packing my wet laundry into my panniers. The owner refunds my money and gives me directions to Hanoi. The streets are dangerous at this hour, she warns. Be careful. I thank her, flip on the headlight, and pedal to the city of my father's roots.

The wide boulevard is unevenly lit; burnt-out lampposts leave hundreds of yards between bright sections. Traffic trickles in both directions, as merchants and workers hurry home on bicycles without headlights. Grim-faced men in soldier uniforms laze in bars. I feel their eyes on me. People here do not wave, smile, or point as they do in Saigon. Northerners simply stare.

Up ahead across the street, a night alley market is in the final stage of shutting down, street sweepers combing the gutters, desperate merchants trying to sell the last of their perishable goods to bargain hunters. I cross over to the market. Maybe someone can direct me to an affordable inn. I ask two vendors for directions, but they don't know too much about the neighborhood. I pedal slowly down the wide alley, eyes peeled for trouble. People rush in and out of unlit stores, tidying up for the night. Their oil-lamp-cast shadows spook me. At this hour, these are the places where people are knifed for pocket change. It is almost pitch-black. Unnerved, I turn the bike around and hit a pushcart coming out of another alley. My cleat pedals jam and I keel over with a thunk.

They surround me pinned beneath my bike. Hands grabbing me. Two against one. They are masked like robbers. One arm up protecting my head, I jerk free.

A girl's voice pokes through my panic: *"Are you hurt?"*

I roll to my feet prepared for a fight. She loosens the scarf veiling her face. A street sweeper.

"I'm fine. Just a little scratch. No problem. My fault."

"Wash your elbow right away," says the taller girl. *"The street is very dirty. It'll get infected."*

"Thanks."

She wants to know why I am wandering around so late at night in the bad part of town. I explain and they offer to show me to an inn nearby. As we leave, she notices my concerned glance at the cart which they are leaving behind. She giggles, *"Nobody ever steals a garbage cart."*

Both girls are unmarried and in their late teens. They are a fun pair. We flirt as they escort me down the dark alleys, comfortable, at home, as though they own them. The taller girl teases: *"Brother, you have it all backward. You're looking for a room at an hour when other men are looking for roommates."*

I laugh. *"I'm too unattractive for any roommate. The only one that knocked on my door tonight was a cop who wanted some grease!"*

They cluck and giggle, perhaps thinking I am lying. *"This is the hotel,"* the shorter girl announces as they deliver me at the steps. *"Don't let them charge you over eight dollars."*

They hammer the metal sheet door with their fists and announce to the doorman that a guest needs a room. They smile and leave, the tall girl sassing me over her shoulder, *"Behave, Big Brother."*

The manager shows me my room. I shower away the market muck and go to bed. Just after I click off the light, someone raps the door gently. I answer it in my briefs, thinking it is the manager bringing the hot tea he promised. It's him all right. He is without the tea but smiling an ingratiating smile. Lined up behind him against the railing of the stairwell are six beautiful giggling girls.

"Brother," he says, *"I thought you might like the company of a sister . . . or two. Hanoi nights are chilly."*

Early in the morning, I puff my way down the wide and flat boulevard into Hanoi under a graying sky, pedal to pedal with ten thousand workers and students ebbing into the city on creaky bicycles. Here and there, a defiant red sweater bobs, like a maple leaf, in the churn of gray work clothes, olive army uniforms, and white school dresses. After a couple of miles, I see a woman sitting on the side of the road, between her legs a tray of brightly colored rice cakes, the size and shape of charcoal briquettes—I know what they are but have forgotten the name. For practice, I haggle with her awhile and at last, as I make the prospective buyer's exit, she calls me back and we agree on a price—thirty cents—though she seems fairly bitter about it: *"You Viet-kieu are even stingier than poor students. Even they pay me fifty cents."* I grin at her, but I'm thinking: Darn, I just want one of those cakes to nibble for old time's sake. Fifty cents she wanted. Heck, that's like a doughnut in the States. I am gloating over my victory when she bags me ten cakes and I realize that she was saying *"mot chuc,"* meaning ten, and I was saying *"mot cuc,"* meaning one lump. Too embarrassed to rectify the problem, I grab the prize and bike out to a park, hand the ill-gotten cakes to a beggar sleeping at the gate, keeping the one morsel for which I'd bargained. The park rings a small lake called Lake of Seven Colors. I sit on a waterfront bench to eat my cake. On a little island in the middle of the lake, a young guy is flying karate kicks, the sun rising over the pink mist behind him.

The one thing a solo traveler can count on finding in an area crawling with backpackers and expatriates is a bargain bed for the night. Usually, the food isn't bad either. I have no idea where Hanoi's tourist town is, so I buy a map and meander. It is an easy task since Hanoi is a more sedate city than Saigon. The traffic is much lighter, and in the cooler air under tree-shaded avenues, the smog is more tolerable. Hanoi lives on a scale more comprehensible than Saigon. The trees are smaller, more abundant, and not so tall and tropical like those of Saigon. I stroll along the fine mansions, taking in their faded, colonial French glories, their expressive arches, French windows, and wrought-iron balconies. Every structure holds itself up proudly in a state of elegant decay. At the north end of Hoan Kiem Lake, I find six young Caucasian travelers, lurking timidly on different street corners. Backpackers, baby-faced, flushed even in the tropic winter, treading about, wide eyes eating up all the sights, the details. Their pilgrim hands clench dog-eared copies of *The Lonely Planet Guide to Vietnam.* Alas, I have found my home for the next few weeks.

For tourists, everything that happens in Hanoi happens in the backpacker cafés. Anything that can be had, rented, chartered, borrowed, exchanged, and bought can be obtained or arranged in them. They sneak tourists illegally across the border into China for day jaunts, book hotel rooms, lodge people in-house, serve decent Western food, sell traveling supplies, fresh baguettes, and Laughing Cow cheese, which is the staple travel food for foreigners who fear stomach bugs. They book anything. Legal, illegal. You got the dollars, they can find your pleasure.

I bum around Hanoi with Australians, French, Danes, Brits, Germans, and Americans just soaking up the culture, exploring the urban sprawl one district at a time. The city is broken up into ridiculously distinct commercial sections, guild oriented, another French legacy. If you want to buy shoes, you go to the shoe district, where thirty or so adjacent stores sell only footwear, often the same style and brand. There is a part of town for every category of goods and services: clothing, poultry, silk, jewelry, and electronics. There is even an area with shops making headstones, where dust-covered men kneel on the sidewalk chipping names into slabs of granite. Our favorite is the street of *nem nuong* diners. Around dinnertime, straddling the sunset hour, the street is perfumed and grayed with the smoke of meat sizzling over coals. If you catch a whiff of this scent, you never forget it. It is a heady mixture of fishsauce marinade, burning scallions, caramelized sugar, pepper, chopped beef, and pork fat. Women sit on footstools grilling meats on hibachi-style barbecues. Aromatic, stomach-nipping smoke curls to the scrubby treetops and simply lingers, casting the avenue into an amber haze. When hungry folk flock from all over the city to this spot, they have only one thing on their mind. And the entire street, all its skills and resources, is geared to that singular satisfaction.

The days pass without difficulty. I am at last among friends of similar spirit, all non-Asian, not one of them Vietnamese. And I am happy, comfortable merely to be an interpreter. Every day, we troop off to some part of the city on sight-seeing missions. At night, we congregate for great bouts of drinking and barhopping. We splinter into smaller parties and sign up for organized boat tours in Ha Long Bay and ride rented motorcycles to the countryside. We joke, we romance each other with the wild abandon of strangers cohabiting in exotic moments. We ask about Hanoi and its people, we ask about each other. Bonding, trading addresses, and fervently believing that we will never lose touch.

Patriot-Repose

29 Uncle Ho was a Caucasian? This is news to me. But I find him encased in a glass box like Snow White. His white hair gleams with a blond tint. His face has that blushing freshness of an intoxicated Aryan. Well, maybe it is the light.

I gawk at him with the rest of the tourists, half of them foreigners decked out in Spandex, cutoff jeans, sports bras, and Birkenstock sandals, the other half Vietnamese, sweaty and hot, quietly suffering in their best Sunday outfits. For Uncle Ho's dignity, the officials don't charge admission to the Mausoleum, but the hourly event seethes with the subdued giddiness of a freak show. Lining the black granite corridor, scowling guards confiscate cameras and hush foreigners who seem to be in a wax-museum mood. An Australian boy, towing his father, chirps, "Are we going to see a dead man? Are we? Is he really dead?" Behind the kid, the Vietnamese visitors are doing a funeral march, barely breathing, heads bowed, not a word. Maybe they are ashamed that their leaders have put Uncle Ho on display in a ghastly tomb against his final wish to be cremated because "land is valuable and should be used for farming."

I think whatever Vietnamese—Northerners, Southerners, or Viet-kieu—feel about this man and his ideologies, they respect him as all the underdog countries of the world do. For here was a man of inconsequential beginnings who crept through the land of the white man as a menial laborer and returned to wrestle his homeland from empires. Founder of the Vietnamese Communist Party and President of the Democratic Republic of Vietnam from 1946 until his death in 1969, Ho Chi Minh was born Nguyen Sinh Cuong to a fiercely nationalistic scholar-official of humble means. He studied in Hue at the Quoc Hoc Secondary School, then migrated south to work as a teacher in Phan Thiet, my hometown, the very village where my father, eking out a living as a teacher, met my mother. At the age of twenty-one, Ho signed on to a French ship as a cook's apprentice, the first step of what would become a thirty-year journey that would take him to North America, Africa, and Europe. He settled in London, then Paris, earning a living as a gardener, snow sweeper, waiter, photo finisher, and mastered several languages, including English, French, German, and Mandarin. It was his tenure in the racially prejudiced Western world that led Ho to examine his roots and nurture his sense of patriotism.

How many "Yes, sir!" "Oui, oui, Monsieur!" "Yes, sahib!" did he utter, head bowed submissively? How many times did he long to stroll the cobbled byways of Paris and the marbled corridors of London as an equal of any Frenchman, any Englishman? How often did he gaze upon a white woman and wish for the pleasure of her company, the faintest possibility of her caress? Maybe patriotism has always been at the core of him. Maybe not. But I know; I've felt the patriotic urge. Walking in shoes vaguely similar to his, I know this deep-seated fire—this yearning for self-worth—fueled by the feelings of an unadoptable outsider, is nearly irresistible.

He changed his name to Nguyen Ai Quoc—Nguyen the Patriot—and began to write and debate the issue of Indochina's independence from France. At the green age of twenty-nine, he—an Indochinese laborer, a manservant—tried, without success, to present an independence plan for Vietnam to U.S. President Woodrow Wilson at the 1919 Versailles Peace Conference. The following year, disillusioned with Western intentions, he became a founding member of the French Communist Party. The Communist Internationals summoned him to Moscow for training in 1923 and later sent him to Guangzhou

(Canton) to found the Revolutionary Youth League of Vietnam, a stepping-stone for the later Indochinese Communist Party. The next decade and a half he shuttled back and forth between the U.S.S.R. and China, once landing in a Hong Kong jail.

At the ripe age of fifty-one, he finally returned, in 1941, to his homeland to help found the Viet Minh Front to extricate Vietnam from the yokes of French colonialism and Japanese occupation. He was arrested and imprisoned for a year, by the anti-Communist Nationalist Chinese. During its insurgency, his Viet Minh received funding and arms from the U.S. Office of Strategic Services (predecessor of the CIA). Immediately after the atomic bombing of Japan in August 1945, Ho Chi Minh unleashed an uprising called Cach Mang Thang Tam—the August Revolution. On September 2, 1945, at a rally in Hanoi's Ba Dinh Square, Uncle Ho, with OSS agents at his side, declared Vietnam's independence, reading a constitution he drafted that borrowed liberally from the American Declaration of Independence.

Uncle Ho died unmarried and without children. Maybe he was gay. Maybe he was in love with the loveliest of all females: Vietnam. They say Vietnam is like a beautiful woman wooed first by the Chinese, then the French, then the Japanese, then the Americans. The men always say this with undisguised pride—not anger or outrage—but pride, followed by a glint of zealousness when they say Vietnam is now ours. Ours. Though it is clear to me, *ours* doesn't include Viet-kieu.

Ours is those who believe in Uncle Ho. Those who believe in the thousands of photos of Uncle Ho preserved in museums throughout the country. His visage is old but strong and benevolent. Uncle Ho, the peasant irrigating rice paddies by hand. Uncle Ho, the teacher chalking history on the blackboard for his good students. Uncle Ho, the poet painting Chinese calligraphy. Uncle Ho, the worker shaping the earth with a shovel. Uncle Ho, the protector standing before children. Uncle Ho, your uncle and mine.

An odd, disorienting feeling tickles me as I study his gaunt face, thirty years preserved. I'd first seen that face over two decades ago, the day when Saigon fell. I remember peeping out of steel window shutters and seeing tanks and trucks growling through the street, Uncle Ho's victorious, grinning face emblazoned on their sides. I'd seen him on stamps, on the new currency of a unified Vietnam. And I had seen him smiling, looking on from the prison wall where they executed my fellow prisoners. I remember him grinning in my nightmares.

One of the four Imperial guards, supposedly as stoic and fearsome as a sphinx, shifts his weight, struggling mightily to stifle a yawn. The spell is broken. We shuffle out. The Australian boy pesters his father for another go around the mummy.

Down by the old section of Hanoi where the houses are nearing a century, a fifteen-year-old girl sitting on the sidewalk asks me if I'd like to buy a snack: rice dumpling with sugarcane syrup. Next to her are two baskets. Her feet are tucked beneath her at awkward angles. She is sitting with a friend, a twenty-something girl with two baskets of papayas, the smaller, green northern breed. They are thin, barefoot peasants from the countryside. I buy rice dumplings and a papaya on the condition that they help me eat the refreshments. Munching and chatting, we sit on the sidewalk, motorbikes sputtering in the narrow street, pedestrians walking around us.

Rice-girl wants to know how much an airplane ticket to America costs. A lot, I say, I had to save for a long time.

"*A hundred American dollars,*" Papaya-girl ventures, apparently noting what she considers to be an astronomical sum. I nod vaguely, having no heart for the truth.

"*Wow. Oh, my God. Can you imagine that? It would take us five years to save that much,*" murmurs Rice-girl. Her friend nods at the impossibility of saving such a sum.

"*You are good-looking,*" Rice-girl says to me, changing the topic.

"*Me? No, I am ugly. I have been traveling very long so I look like a vagrant. No haircut, no shave.*"

"No," she explains, "*you look good: you have nice clothes.*"

"*Ah, you mean my old jeans and T-shirt?*"

"*That's a nice T-shirt. You can't buy it here.*"

"*This orange-brown color?*"

"*No, that's a hugging T-shirt. There's no seam on the side. It's one whole tubular piece of cloth and it's pure cotton.*"

"Oh." I hadn't noticed. *"You are very pretty."*

"Silly man," chides Papaya-girl. *"We're not pretty. We're just peasant girls, selling papaya and rice cakes."*

"What's your name?" asks Rice-girl, clearly relishing a slice of papaya.

"Pham Xuan An."

"That's a nice name," says Papaya-girl, her friend nodding in agreement. *"Xuan An—peaceful spring—that's pretty."*

"It's girlish. My mother's idea. What's your name?"

"Mine is not so pretty," Rice-girl admits without shame, helping herself to more papaya. *"My family is poor and my parents never went to school."*

"Mine isn't pretty either," Papaya-girl admits.

"A name is just a name," I reassure them.

"Yes, but I don't have a real one. My parents call me Third Daughter."

"That's just a title, a nickname. Don't you have a real name?"

"No, my parents can't read or write. Don't you know it's shameful—bad luck—to give your children fancy names when you know they will live poor lives? How would it look if a farmer had a prettier name than a prince?"

They are from a village thirty miles outside of Hanoi. They walk to the highway and ride a three-wheeled Tuk-tuk to Hanoi four days a week. Rice-girl makes her own rice dumplings and Papaya-girl picks her fruit from the family orchard. Neither has enough merchandise for a stall at the market or makes enough to pay for a permit to sell on the street, so they go door-to-door.

A hubbub stirs the crowd at the other end of the street. The girls perk up, swiveling about like startled hares. Hastily, they pick up their plates and stools.

"Farewell, Big Brother. Thanks for talking with us. The cops are coming, we must go or they'll confiscate our baskets," Papaya-girl says, shouldering her staff, the pair of baskets tottering on either end like a balancing scale.

They bow and hurry away. Rice-girl is limping severely, walking on the outer edge of her deformed left foot. It is only noon. Hanoi is big.

No-name is a ten-year-old street boy. A deaf-mute who spends all of his time hanging around the foreign-tourist district. He befriends the tourists and tails them around town. His tourist friends don't know where he lives. No one on the streets seems to know anything about him. I could only trace his lineage as far back as a month before I met him. A German couple, on a brief three-day tour of Hanoi, had befriended him. They introduced him to a French girl who, before her departure, acquainted the boy with Steve, an Aussie. Steve took the boy to dinner with a group of tourists and introduced him as No-name. The name stuck. Steve bunked in the same dormitory as William. When Steve left on a train to Saigon, he entrusted a map of Hanoi and No-name into the care of William, who wanted desperately to know more about the wordless boy. So I came into the picture, the next foster brother.

No-name's gift is a room-splitting grin, his curse a continually runny nose which he drags on the sleeve of his sweater. He is the magic of the streets. You could be walking, shopping, dining anywhere within the ten city blocks of his stomping grounds, and, suddenly, he materializes out of nowhere walking beside you, standing at your elbow, or making faces at you through restaurant windows. He moves with you as though not a single beat has passed since you were last together. But he is no Oliver Twist who picks your pocket. He is much more dangerous. He steals your heart, and when you leave, your heart breaks as roundly as his.

I find myself lingering in Hanoi because of him. When I tour the city on my bicycle, he hops on the rear bike rack for a ride, laughing his mute laugh: *Ackackackack ack ack!* I carry him, my silly monkey, my little brother. We point to sights we know nothing about and smile at each other. Then he's off to some other part of his domain. Perhaps to visit another tourist. Perhaps to go home—wherever he lives.

He is a soloist, a pariah among the children in the area. A scrappy bright-eyed boy, the runt of the litter. Kids are cruel as only kids can be, and No-name always seems to be ducking from the pranks of one tormentor to the blows of another. They resent his easy camaraderie with the fair-skinned foreigners. These kids are decently dressed, fleshed out, and scrubbed clean, the stamp of children with homes and family. No-name is somewhere along the side, on the edge. He bears the earmark of a child relinquished into the care of a lone grandmother or a kind but poor aunt.

I zealously nurture a morning coffee habit and No-name often pays me a visit during my grumpiest hour. An orange juice for him. An espresso for me. Toast, butter, and cheese all around. He only lets me treat him half of the time. He pays his share with a greasy fist of dime-bills. The waitresses used to shoo him out, but once seven tourists, with me as their translator, assured the owner that if she ever mistreated No-name, we would never eat at her café again. Other tourists would hear about her cruelty. These businesses rely heavily on tourists' word of mouth and so she took the message to heart. Now, every other dawn, No-name sits next to me, contemplating the dust universe in the sunbeam angling through the window while I read the newspapers.

One morning, he signs me a question in his personal language. He doesn't read or write. Hands out, face turning about, looking; fingers touching hair, hands far apart; index finger to the sun; hands about knees, describing a garment: *Where's sun-bright long-hair girl?* I shake my head, fingers walking away. *Gone, gone,* I say, and he turns from me. I see tears rimming his eyes. He burrows his head into his folded arms on the table. When the waitress comes with his juice, he flees into the street, his breakfast untouched.

I know that when I go, I will leave as silently as Jen did. One morning he will come and I won't be there with my paper and my espresso. And some morning, somewhere a world away, I will look at the sun angling through a window and I will think of a boy called No-name.

Silence-Years

30 "We're gonna rumble tonight," Cu-Den told me after school at his house.

1985. A typical day. We were juniors in high school. Cu-Den, Manh, and I were digging around the refrigerator for leftovers. We were wearing shoes in Cu-Den's house because his mom wasn't home. When she was, we bowed, left our shoes at the door, and crept meekly around her house, a couple of acolytes new to the monastery. Usually, we had the run of Cu-Den's low-rent duplex because his mom and his older brother were at work. His brother paid the bills while his mother held down two jobs so she could bribe their father out of the Communist labor camp and bring him to the States.

"Who now?" I asked.

"The fucking Mexican *cholos,* man," said Manh, the craziest of the bunch, a natural athlete, lean and muscular but a bit on the short side, sporting the stereotypical coconut-bowl haircut. He had given up on hair spray, nothing could give life to his black mop.

"Again?" There were three major groups at school, white, Mexican, and Vietnamese. Each group claimed a different wing of the school. Fights broke out regularly.

"Yeah," Cu-Den said. "The rest of the gang is gonna meet us here. Six on six."

"What the fuck for?"

Manh cracked up laughing. "The *cholos* got blamed for the fucking gym job!"

A couple of nights earlier, Cu-Den and I had been watching TV when Manh exploded through the back door yelling, "Turn off the light! Turn off the fucking lights!"

The gang stormed in after him, huffing and puffing, sweating. All scraped up. They had jumped the backyard fence, which rimmed the school's soccer field. It was a six-foot chain-link fence with three strands of barbed wire.

"Hide these! The cops are coming!" Lee barreled through the door, a huge duffel bag on his lineman's shoulder. Tong and Thang trailed in, carrying similar loads.

We ran to the back-bedroom window. Lights flooded the school gym and the basketball courts. Police cars everywhere, spinning red-blue. Cops combed the field with their flashlights, walking the length of it and peeping into the fifty houses or so surrounding the school. We were lucky they didn't have dogs.

In the living room, Manh was beside himself, swaggering like a real bad boy. "We broke into the gym!"

"Got everything, man!" Lee exclaimed, twirling a crowbar like a baton. He was probably the biggest Vietnamese in America. Big, blindingly fast, and, in a fight, real mean. We called him The Thing and we never "rumbled" without him.

"Shiiiiiiit! You should have seen Lee, man," babbled Manh, grinning ear to ear. "Me and Thang were like pulling on the fucking bar forever and the damn door wouldn't even open a crack. Lee came up and went . . . gggrrrrrrrGGGGRRRAAHH!! . . . and—KRACK! Busted door, yeah. He ripped that thing off the fucking hinges!"

"It was totally cool!" Tong shouted, pumping his arm, gyrating his touchdown dance, a skinny, floppy marionette. "Man, you guys should have seen it."

"We cleaned the fucking place out," bragged Thang, the only one with enough facial hair for a mustache, which he fondled continually like a real Confucius. "All the best stuff!"

"WooooooooooooHooooooooo!"

"We're RICH!"

"YeeeeeeHaaaw!"

The gang had gone ahead with their plan when Cu-Den and I bowed out. They knew we were hoping to go to college and they didn't hold our "chickening out" against us. We were cool about things like that. They pulled the job because they needed the stuff. The adrenaline was good too, but at the bottom of it was the fact that any of us was lucky to have ten bucks in our pocket on any day.

Cu-Den and I gathered round to take a peek at their loot.

Socks, tennis balls, basketballs.

Cu-Den banged us a skillet of scrambled eggs, fried Spam, and steamed rice. It was all we could rake out of Cu-Den's sorriest-looking fridge on the planet. The thing was loaded with relish, horseradish, salad dressing, teriyaki sauce, mayonnaise, ketchup, mustard, and not a damn thing to slather the condiment galore on. We doused Cu-Den's special rice with fishsauce and chili paste and gobbled it up. We were going to need full stomachs to fight the Mexican homeboys who were a lot tougher than the redneck football players.

"When?" I asked Cu-Den.

"Ten tonight, behind the church."

"After work," Manh asserted.

We played tennis for the school, but we had to cut practice to make enough money to officially join the team. With the school's fiscal problems, athletes had to pay for their own uniforms, physical check-ups, and "team fees." When the season started and it looked like the school couldn't field a team, the principal and the tennis coach worked out a deal for the squad, which happened to be ninety-five percent Vietnamese American. Manh, Cu-Den, and I worked off a part of our fees by doing janitorial work in the classrooms after school. We still couldn't come up with the rest of the cash. Jobs, even flipping burgers, were scarce in our neighborhood. Too many poor immigrants. Manh's uncle owned an office-cleaning business. We were all underage, but his uncle said he could give us fifteen dollars each for four hours, if we promised not to "lift" anything on the job. Bloody damn generous, actually. Glad for the work, we cut practice and school to work for him whenever he could use us.

We hung around drinking Coke. Cu-Den did two hundred curls with a dumbbell, working only his right arm. He had been doing it for two years so he was as deformed as a one-pincered crawdad. His goal was to develop a powerful tennis forehand, even though Coach routinely yelled at him to keep the ball in the court—This ain't baseball, son! No homers, please! Manh divided his attention between MTV and a *Playboy* magazine he filched from a liquor store. I was on the phone sweet-talking Mai-Ly into letting us copy her chemistry lab report. We made a couple of stabs at our homework until Manh's uncle picked us up with his van.

I didn't mind the work. It was fun, clowning around with the guys and drinking sodas we stole from the workers' refrigerators. Though, of course, if my father knew I was cleaning offices instead of studying, he'd crap a load of bricks. He had levered us off welfare and bought a house, so money was really tight at home. Mom was constantly saving, cutting corners with the groceries. Sometimes, I felt like I had to get some meat in me or I was going to go crazy. I kept on telling her, *We're in America, Mom. You can't feed a whole family on eight ounces of beef.* And my father kept on telling me, *Don't think about material things. Hone your mind. Sacrifice now so you can have later.* He told me a slew of other stuff, too, but it didn't matter to me. I had made it a point not to talk to him, never asking anything and never giving any reply other than *yes, no,* and *I don't know.* Besides, I knew every word before it came out of his mouth. *I sacrifice so you can study and make a better life for yourself . . . blah . . . blah . . . blah . . .*

"Shiiiiiiiiiiiit! Check this out! Check this out!" Manh was rubbing himself all over the mahogany conference table. "This is like a whole fucking tree, man! Shit. I wanna work here—I wanna do Tammy Tran on this table." He bellied onto the gleaming wood and started humping the surface.

"I want Suzzie," Cu-Den said, and laughed his dirty poodle laugh—barely audible.

I put in my dibs: "Lan is my kinda woman."

"Naw, man. You get Mai-Ly, An." Manh started in with his girlie Mai-Ly voice: "You and me, An, we have chemistry."

"Guess who's gonna be doing his own chem lab."

"Oh, fuck. Okay, okay. Sorry, I take it back."

"Fuck," Cu-Den breathed, spinning dreamily in the chairman's seat. "This is gonna be my chair."

"Yeah, so you can watch me. OoooAaaaa! Yes, baby. Yes!" grunted Manh with the one-track mind. Kneeling on the table, he jizzed us with a bottle of cleaning ammonia.

"Manh, you sick son of a bitch!" Manh's uncle spat from the doorway. "Get off that table before you scuff the varnish!" Then he turned a wagging finger on us. "You want to be big men in big companies? And what are you doing?" He knew all about our sideline of misdemeanors and braggadocio. "You boys shouldn't be so dumb. Look at me, you think I got it good? Sure, I'm my own boss and I make good money, but I'm still a janitor. I clean up after the men who sit in those chairs. You boys want to be in those chairs, you study harder. You don't mess around. You listen to your fathers."

My father and I had had a falling-out a couple of years before I started hanging with Cu-Den and Manh. I was bossing my brothers around. They didn't like it, but, too bad, I was first son. It was my right. Occasionally, they balked and sassed me back, and I caned them to teach them respect. Once Huy and I got into a big fight. He disobeyed my order and couldn't stomach lying down so I could whack his butt with a yardstick. Huy wasn't much of a fighter so I pounded him blue. My father came home and cussed me out in front of all my brothers. He dressed me down good and I lost face. I hadn't talked much to him or the rest of the family since. And I didn't stop caning my brothers until last year when little Hien came at me with a knife and made me realize how screwed up we all were.

One day, we were driving across town, Father up front with Hien. Huy, Tien, cousin Hai, and me in the backseat. I was in seventh grade. Hai got into a scuffle with Huy and Tien. Father blew up. He thought it was me, but I wasn't a rat so I didn't squeal on Hai. He pulled over to the side of the road and told me to get out.

I shrugged and got out. No idea where I was. Maybe ten, fifteen miles from home. He drove off.

It took me all day to find my way home, but once there I kept on walking. I climbed an oak-studded hill on the edge of town and I thought about going away like Chi had.

For years after Chi ran away, I read the Bible and said a prayer every night. At first, I prayed for good grades for myself; good grades for my brothers; good health, happiness, and prosperity for Mom and Dad; good health for everybody, Grandma Le in Vietnam, too; world peace; and safety for Chi, wherever she was, if she was still alive. As time passed, I realized that I didn't get a lot of the things I asked for, so I narrowed my list. I shortened it, one item at a time, until all I prayed for every night was that Chi was all right, wherever she was, if she was still alive. But because we didn't hear anything from Chi, and because I was growing up, I stopped praying. I stopped hoping for miracles. I was reverting, starting to think of the Almighty—God, Buddha, whatever—the way I did when my childhood began to splinter, late in April of 1975.

It was a couple of days before Saigon fell. There was no school. The city was already beginning to crumble. People panicked in the streets. Everything had suddenly ground to a halt. Nothing for me to do. Even the book kiosks closed. I had a pocketful of change, but couldn't rent as much as a comic to read. I went out to catch tadpoles at a pond. There was no one in the park except me and a young woman. Standing on a green slope beside the water, she was very pretty in her white *ao dai* with her long black hair. She was very beautiful in her sadness. She asked me if I saw the lights in the sky. I said the sky is overcast. Look harder, Little Brother, can't you see the little lights, millions of them floating in the clouds? I didn't tell her that everyone saw lights if he stood up too fast or if he stared into a bright sky long enough. Look harder, Little Brother, do you see them now, the angels? Do you see them? She was desperate, I heard it in her voice, saw it in the way she turned her sad face to the sky, smiling. Smiling.

Where was He?

She needed the lights so I gave her her angels.

Now, on the verge of following in Chi's footsteps, I stood on the hilltop and looked at the gray sky. And I could not find it in me to give myself the angels.

When it was dark and I was numb with cold, I went home. All along I knew I was chickenshit, no guts at all.

We did the entire office floor, twenty rooms, four lobbies, and six toilets in four hours. Manh's uncle frisked us to make sure we hadn't light-fingered anything. On the way home, he swung us through the McDonald's drive-up window. We redeemed fists of McD Super Bowl game cards for fries, Cokes, and Big Macs—courtesy of Cu-Den's brother, who manned the grill at the Golden Arches. He had scored bags of game cards and set us all up with burgers for the whole year.

Manh's uncle dropped us off at Cu-Den's house and slapped us three fivers apiece. We bowed and thanked him like good Vietnamese boys. Cu-Den's mother was at her second job and his brother was out doing some girl. We cocked our dirty feet on the coffee table, chomped the Macs on the sofa, and smeared grease into the cushions. Cu-Den went to the stereo and cranked up "Eye of the Tiger," the theme from Sylvester Stallone's *Rocky,* to pump us up for the fight. We sat around eating and talking about girls and sex, talking trash because despite all the marginal stuff we did, we were still geeks. We cared about grades and girls who were too cool to date us because we didn't have as much as a jalopy to take them to the movies. Cu-Den's got the heat for Suzzie Nguyen: Suzzie's got big ones, doesn't she? Fuck yeah, Manh agreed, I get one, Cu-Den gets the other, and you can watch, An. Okay, sure, I'll run the videocam for you deviants.

Mouth around a bunch of fries, Cu-Den said, "I heard a couple years ago at our school, there was a girl who passed for a guy. She was Vietnamese, man."

"Yeah, yeah," Manh chirped in. "My brother told me about that. Fucking sick, man. Now, THAT'S a fucking deviant. She was like a guy or something. She went into the guys' locker room and all. Nobody knew."

Cu-Den asked me, "You heard about that, An?"

"Naw."

"You *anh lon,* ain't you, An?" Manh asked. None of my friends had been to my house or met my family. It was on the better side of town, theirs on the poor side of the toxic creek where we used to live.

"Yup, I'm the oldest in my family. Big Bro, Numero Uno, that's me."

"You never heard about this?" Cu-Den asked me again.

"No."

They were perplexed. It was the one big scandal that reverberated down the years at our school. The one dead horse everyone liked to beat. Manh said, "He—I mean she—was a trans, what-cha-call-it . . . a . . . a trans-sex, something like that."

"A transsexual," I told them, and threw away the rest of my Big Mac. I grabbed the baseball bat: "Rumble-time. Let's kick some ass!"

Blushing - Winter

This is a bad year for you, An, Mom told me. Nothing good will come of it. Don't go anywhere. Don't do anything. Keep your eyes out for omens. You're not American, you hear me? You're Vietnamese. You are not immune to the gods.

When I see the gravel truck driving on the wrong side of the road toward me and two dogs darting into the street, one chasing the other, I realize she may be right. I should have left Hanoi before dawn. I should have left days ago or, maybe, I should have stayed another week. I left today because my fear of Vietnam's Highway 1 has been ulcer-gnawing my gut ever since I left San Francisco.

This morning I woke, devoured a full breakfast, strapped the panniers onto the racks. Then I did the easy thing: I let my legs do what I've trained them to do—piston me right out of Hanoi. Traffic is not too heavy except when it funnels through villages, the national highway ripping through the middle and people crossing the road as casually as strolling across a courtyard. Even dogs have the same attitude about the street.

As the truck bears down on me, I am riding on the outer edge of a clutch of bicyclists and motorbikes. Everyone scatters like gnats before the oncoming truck. I try swerving off the two-lane road, but a group of children is playing in the dirt. I brake. The first dog scats clear of the oncoming truck. I see the wide eyes of the truck driver, a cigarette sticking out of the corner of his mouth. He doesn't brake, but instead hammers the horn. Doesn't swerve. Couldn't with the medley of villagers all around him. I plunge off the asphalt and hit a row of plastic chairs in front of a café. The second dog, the size of a golden retriever, abandons the chase and darts back to my side of the road. The trucker pounds the horn again. The scene strobes into slow motion: the beige dog, panicked by the horn, turns and tries to cross the road again. Too late. The truck's shadow swallows it at thirty miles an hour. It clears the first set of tires, then the undercarriage of the truck glances the back of the dog. It wobbles. Just when I think the dog will live, it changes direction, trying to get out from under the moving truck. The rear set of wheels, double mounted, catches the dog squarely. Thud. Without a yelp, the creature goes under the rubber—a flash of beige fur sucked beneath wheels. A loud wet crunch of snapping sinew and collapsing rib cage, a cracking, popping sound.

A great "AW" from the men in the café. The trucker never even slows. He keeps on rolling, and within seconds there is no trace of his passage but dust and a pile of bloody fur in the middle of the road. Across the street is a shack restaurant-bar, their specialty painted on a sign out front: a three-quarter view of a dog's head. Two men come out and drag the carcass into the diner.

I feel nauseous. I can almost smell roasting ginger and dog fat—the smoky arid edge of barbecued ribs dripping on hot coals. I remember my first taste of dog meat. My uncle had forced it down my throat when I was a kid in Saigon. The beerhouse smelled terrible, rancid if it weren't for the cigarette smoke and the grill. Red-faced men talk-shouted, tearing into dog ribs with their teeth and tossing the bones on the muddy floor. The owner, a mean-faced old woman, took my money and handed me a small plate of roasted dog meat, the pieces cut thin like nickels. One day, Uncle Hung was drunk and he ordered me to eat it. With him preparing to smack obedience into me, I put a slice into my mouth. It tasted gamy, almost like rabbit. The ginger killed most of the strange meat flavor. "Ha! Ha! Ha! You ate it! You know what this means? In your next life, you'll be reincarnated as a dog!" I tried to vomit without success and I bawled with fears only an adult could instill. Whenever she visited me, Chi would take pity and go in my place to fetch Uncle Hung's dog meat.

The land is green, every inch of it cultivated. Between the villages, the land becomes a sea of rice paddies, veined with dikes, stretching to the horizon so that the far-off mountains look like islands in the distance. Thatched huts and an occasional cinder-block house of a well-to-do peasant punctuate the rice-paddy ocean like fishing boats. And in stretches, there are the lumpy rock formations resembling those of Ha Long Bay, only here the ocean has been drained. They look like giant Hershey's kisses, five hundred feet tall, all moldy with vegetation and chipped jagged by the weather. The air smells of turned earth. Now and then, a whiff of smoke from a cooking fire.

"Lieng-Xo! Lieng-Xo!"—Russian! Russian!—the kids shout at me as they come rolling out of the school yard, a moving carpet of little black heads.

In America, I was a Jap, a Chink, a gook; in Vietnam, a Russian.

I wave back, slowing down to avoid squashing a six-year-old.

Ppht! A flying sandal misses my head. Then another. Laughing gleefully, the brats are running and flicking the sandals right off their feet. At me! Left. Right. One. Two. One. Two. Slippers shoot off their little feel like missiles. A hail of sandals smacks my bike. Bap! One hits me on the side of the head. Piss-angry, I swerve to a stop to smack some manners into the monsters. Thunk! Out of footwear ammo, they're chucking stones! I hammer the pedals and plow away fast without serious injury, save to my dignity.

I flee the village totally disconcerted. That is a new one. Mobbed by laughing elementary school children. This country never fails to surprise me. At the next school, ten miles down the road, I pick up speed and blow right by without giving the little monsters a chance to wave hello.

I arrive in Ninh Binh, a mid-sized industrial town sixty miles south of Hanoi, and take a room at the Star Hotel. The teenage bellhop, who is also the concierge, the handyman, the cook, and the room-service guy, encourages me to book a boat ride with him. Very beautiful, he says. The price he quotes is rather steep so I ride down to the river for a look. The city is a jumbled mess. Along the riverfront, the cops and government officials have a monopoly on the tourist trade bused down from Hanoi. They want six dollars for the boat ride and two dollars for parking my bike. I decline and go farther down the busy riverfront. A boatwoman smiles at me and waves from her boat. I return the greeting and she runs frantically after me. She guides me by my elbow to a café.

"Boat ride?" she asks, in accented English.

"How much?"

She holds up a victory sign: "Two dollars." She points to her skinny sampan.

"Okay."

I tell her I'm Vietnamese and she donkeys into an explosive laugh because she has never approached a Vietnamese before. We talk to the café owner, who lets me lock my bike to a post. The boatwoman crowns me with a conical peasant hat and secretes me down to the river. She doesn't want to be harassed by the cops, who would take a cut of her fee.

For two hours, she poles us downriver and across the wetland, carefully avoiding the more scenic route of the government-sanctioned tour. After the first half hour of chattering about the injustice of the local government, the woman senses that I am in a sight-seeing mood and falls silent. The stone formations here are very similar to those of Ha Long Bay—crumbs dropped when the gods were baking mountains—only smaller, five hundred feet wide, three hundred tall, and surrounded by rice paddies and shockingly green and lush swamp grass that makes the air smell sweet. I crack open a beer I brought with me and offer her one. She declines, saying it isn't right for women to drink, so she accepts it to take home to her husband. I sink low in the canoe, prop my sore feet up on the gunwale, and sip my Vietnamese brew. The world ceases to exist beyond the sweep of my eyes. It is silent but for insects in the reeds, the creaking of our single oar, and the watery swishing and dripping of our passage. We slip along the river, meandering through the green waterscape, coming close to homes and dirt roads, and it feels as though I am traveling through the Venice of Vietnam. Darkness is gathering, and somehow the splendor of the land blossoms into something even more palpable. The beer tastes wonderful and I am delirious in the cool air current, going downriver under a blushing sky.

Between the sheer blackened cliffs, the winter sun freezes, a soft pink violet in the misty sky, a painter's fancy, a moment thought impossible and forgotten upon passing. Moments stretching back through the ages. But they are here, the peasants flip-flopping down dirt roads, hoes and shovels on their shoulders. The pudding-rich earth at their feet lies like frosting on the land, good enough to eat. Field upon field of rice stretches out in the lowering light, quiet after the day's toil. An old man coughs, his feet dragging. A cluster of girls giggles, pealing clean, vibrant sounds over the whiskery glass of the paddies. A steer clops ponderously, a cart of earthenware creaking behind it. A boy naps on the back of a rare white water buffalo. A handsome young man herds ducks with a bamboo pole as long as a fishing rod.

I sit midstream, breathing softly, unreasonably fearful of this moment slipping away, wishing I could drink in this strange pink of evening. The beauty is so awfully sweet, I think I can taste it somewhere near the center of me.

Vietnamese-Karma

One crisp afternoon in late January 1989, my beat-up Toyota hiccuped back to San Jose. I was taking an unsanctioned religious holiday from UCLA, on my way to pick up Grandma Le for the greatest gathering of the clan since the first Pham set foot in America. We were observing the anniversary of Grandpa Pham's death. Technically, Grandma Le didn't have to attend, but she was lonely and wanted to mingle with the other side of the family. Strange how she couldn't bear to be within sight of *"that arrogant mud-footed prince"* when he was alive. A dozen years after he exhaled his last opiate breath, she was raring to go to the big party held in his honor and looking forward to gossiping with his widow, Grandma Pham, my father's stepmother.

I curbed the car and found her doing tai chi on the sidewalk, heron-stepping among the fallen leaves. Beneath her best maroon embroidered silk, she had double-packed herself in thermals and sweaters, hands in child-sized mitts, satin-slippered feet in three layers of hunter's socks. A black beanie swallowed most of her head, including her ears, and a brown wool scarf bandited her face. Her frost-rosy eyes winked at me. It was a marvel the neighbors had stopped staring at this crone doll who suddenly materialized amid their lower-middle-class suburban enclave two years ago, fresh off the plane from Vietnam. One day they woke up and found a four-foot-nine, eighty-five-year-old woman in black peasant pajamas doing Bruce Lee impressions in slow motion in front of their houses.

"Grandma!" I shouted, arms wide, walking right into her Rooster Sunrise stance for a hug.

She pulled down her scarf and grinned broadly, showing a silver front tooth, patting my arm, uncomfortable with the open affection but liking it. She squinted at me and said, *"Who are you? You look like An, but I can't remember what he looks like."*

"Grandma!"

"You haven't visited me in a month!" she squeaked. *"Bad grandson! Aiiya! Aiiya! Aiiya!"* And gave me a couple of karate chops to the arm. *"Aiiya! Aiiya!"* Two soft kicks to the shin.

I laughed and dropped an arm around her shoulder, nodding my chin on the top of her head. She smiled. She didn't laugh anymore. It took too much lung power.

"My school is four hundred miles away, Grandma. That's like driving from Phan Thiet to Da Nang."

"Hmm. Hmm," she mumbled, meaning I should have picked a college closer to home.

"Aha! Grandma, you're wearing makeup."

"Shuss! It's too cold here. I need some color in my cheeks." She pretended to push me away.

"It looks good. Maybe we can find you an elderly gentleman." I pinched her arm.

"Aiee! Don't be silly, you impudent boy."

"You're shy, Grandma."

"I'm not shy. A girl only needs one husband to lose her shyness. I had three, but I lose them like lizards lose tails."

Grandma used to be a real looker, with an attitude to boot. Back in Phan Thiet, she was the town's scandal with her history of three husbands. The first was an academic, her high school sweetheart. The second was a professional soccer star—my mother's father. The War claimed them both. The third, Auntie Dung's father, the fishsauce baron, was a polygamist with three wives. He was her true love and she always kept an altar for him. I had asked her why she still lit incense for him and put fruit on his altar year-round. She said he watched over the family. I teased that he couldn't possibly find her here in America, halfway around the world. She touched her chest: *In here, this place is the same.*

"Look what I have for you, Grandma." I flashed five Lotto scratch-off cards.

"Ah, good! Good grandson! Thank you. I never get enough of these." She inspected them for luck and slipped them into her silk jacket.

"Why do you like to play the lottery so much?" I asked her.

"I want to leave my grandchildren something," she answered matter-of-factly. She had given up everything, forfeiting land and business, to come to America and be with her children and grandchildren. I wondered how she felt not having her own place and needing to rely on her daughter, Auntie Dung, to take care of her. She had no idea her children and grandchildren were scattered and too wound up with American life to be with her daily.

"Auntie Dung and Uncle Hung aren't coming, Grandma?"

"No, they're afraid things might get difficult. You know, your mother and your father's brothers don't adore each other much."

Grandma still smoldered whenever she talked about how Dad's side of the family had mistreated her daughter. I didn't want her to get fired up, especially with today's festivities. I rubbed my belly and said we ought to get over to the party before they ate everything. I opened the door, ushered her into the passenger seat, and gingerly buckled her in. Grandma was brittle, broke her hip last year. She wanted to know why my car was full of stuff. I waved her off, claiming that I was moving. I didn't want her to know I was living out of my car because I couldn't pay the rent this month. It was still early in the term so the checks from my tutoring and grading jobs hadn't arrived yet. It had been pretty lean stretching a couple of packets of hot dogs an entire week. I had been salivating for days, thinking about this feast. On the backseat was my cooler. There ought to be plenty of leftovers.

That was the one good thing about the Pham women, in-laws included: They knew how to cook. Each had her own specialties.

During Tet, the Vietnamese New Year, they cooked up a warehouse of food and traded dishes around so that every household had the same feast though no one cooked more than one or two entrées. For the anniversary of Grandpa's death, all these treats would be crammed with forty-three hungry mouths into one rickety house in an old section of Cupertino where the neighborhood dated back to the fifties, when Americans had never heard of a place called Vietnam.

Grandma Pham lived with her married daughters and youngest son at the end of an oak-lined cul-de-sac with ruptured asphalt. All four of their cars were parked in the street, a dead pickup on the lawn. Untrimmed shrubs mustached the house. The garage door was holding up three bedrooms tacked together under an open-rafter roof. Stashed on the sides of the structure were curly sheets of discarded plywood, busted bookcases, rusted wheelbarrows, used car tires, and piles of aluminum cans. The balding back lawn was barely visible beneath worktables, sawhorses, mountains of paint cans, Formica sheets, neon machines, and toolboxes. Aunt Hanh's husband was a sign maker. They stayed in one of the bedrooms with their young daughter. Aunt Hang and her husband, both in their late thirties, were full-time college students, engineering hopefuls. They and their two children shared the master bedroom. Grandma Pham had her own room. Uncle Hau, the anchor of this household, lived in the converted garage space, using his professional-programmer income to supplement everyone else's. The economical arrangement cramped his bachelor lifestyle, but that was expected of a dutiful son. Besides, he only dated Vietnamese-American girls. They understood.

The party was in full cry when I walked Grandma through the door, last to arrive. The noisy house smelled of cooking food and too many people, definitely an Asian-house odor. My brothers and sister were drinking sodas and hanging out with our cousins. Grandma Pham, a sparrow of a woman, paired off with Grandma Le and, after brief greetings to everyone, they moused into the bedroom to drink tea and watch videos of Vietnamese soap operas. Mom was hovering in the kitchen with my aunts. She was blatantly avoiding Uncle Hun and Uncle Hong. When my father eloped with her, these two had come after him with handcuffs. I went around greeting my elders as was proper. It took the better part of an hour because my father had five brothers and three sisters and, with the exception of Uncle Hau, they were all married with children. I bowed and traded pleasantries with each.

Round-faced Uncle Hong, rosy with a beer in him, clapped me on the shoulder. *"How's school, An?"*

"Good. How are you?"

"Well. Strong. Engineering, right?"

"Yes, Uncle."

"Good, you'll make lots of money. Help your parents when they retire."

"Oh, yes, sure, of course."

I didn't have much in common with most of my uncles. I hated having to bow, grovel, and show them respect the whole nine yards like a ten-year-old schoolboy just because they were my elders. Uncle Hong was a natural entrepreneur, at the moment a real estate speculator. Uncle Hun was a lifelong technician, a classic worker ant. Slumlord Uncle Hoang was the only Pham nearing millionaire status. He used to have me paint his illegal apartments until I decided to charge him minimum hourly wages. His wife, a beauty queen who didn't get along with the rest of the family too well, didn't show up for the ceremony, causing fierce whispering among the wives-in-law.

After the aunts decorated the food and arranged it on Grandpa Pham's shrine, covering every square inch of the red silk tablecloth with meat and fruit, beer, tea, and rice wine, piling it on until the thing creaked ominously, Grandma Pham started the ceremony by lighting the first batch of incense on an altar candle. Head bowed deeply, she prayed to the same black-and-white photo of Grandpa that we had at home. The entire clan lined up for the procession to the altar, in descending hierarchy, oldest to youngest, sons to daughters, grandsons to granddaughters. There were so many of us that we dimmed the house with incense. The smoke detector panicked. Uncle Hun pulled its batteries, and the fire hazard continued unabated. Auntie Hang opened windows and turned on the oscillating fan. Grandma Le wasn't expected to pray to her old nemesis.

Mom was, but she boycotted by stirring the soup pot. I did my deed but filched a couple of egg rolls from the altar.

The clan sat around talking, mostly about money and investment, not a word about Grandpa, waiting for the joss sticks to burn down, which was about half an hour—the time it took for spirits to "eat" the offerings. The women fussed in the kitchen, setting the tables, putting on final touches, and readying pots and pans so they could warm up foods the instant the joss sticks died. Little cousins rioted all over the house, screaming in their cribs, playing tag, shooting space aliens on the television, bullying, pulling each other's hair, yelling, and crying. I couldn't remember all their names, each had two, one Vietnamese and one American. This country had been good to us Phams, we multiplied like rabbits.

By the time they moved the food from the altar to the tables, beer had been flowing steadily among the men for two hours. Spirits were high. Mom was the only woman who flouted tradition by drinking a whole can of beer. The men, none of whom were heavy drinkers, turned bright red, became more passionate and magnanimous with each toast. Jokes roared around the table. Uncle Hong, who was under strict doctor's orders to refrain from alcohol and red meat, threw caution to the wind, this his big once-a-year. My father, who never goes out even on weekends, became alive in the company of his brothers, venting his bottlenecked social needs. Uncle Hien, the former heroin addict and gangster, now married and in good grace with his family, bubbled over with raucous stories, slapping his older brothers on the back.

The uncles had saved me a seat at the table since I was an adult now, five months bordering engineer status. I begged off and roamed the buffet table. The spread was the sort I dreamed about. There were Peking duck with pillowy white buns to be eaten with scallion brushes and sweet plum sauce; roasted pig with cracker-crunchy skin to be savored on angel-hair rice noodles glistening with scallion oil; sweet pork spareribs complete with the three layers of good-fortune fat; several whole boiled chickens for dipping with lime, pepper, and salt; a tub of prawn salad tossed with rice vinegar and pickled carrots, great for making canapés with shrimp chips; green papaya salad with sugary chili-fishsauce; egg rolls made with ground pork, potato noodles, cat-ear mushrooms, and real crab meat; salad rolls with their translucent rice-paper skin showing slices of steamed pork, for dipping in hoisin sauce; yam and shrimp fritters; grilled lemongrass beef rolled like cigarettes and served on skewers; a whole sea bass steamed in a scallion soy sauce; hills of red sweet rice with drifts of coconut snow; a big pot of crab-and-asparagus soup thick with chicken and cloud-ear mushrooms; anchovy fried rice; scallops with chive dumplings; ginger stir-fried vegetables with watercress and young bamboo shoots; and vinegared beef served with sweet red onion and rice papers. I loaded up two plates, tucked a bottle of beer under one arm, and went into Uncle Hau's bedroom to watch football on the tube with my cousins and brothers.

Halfway through the meal, the conversation in the dining room grew loud. I went out for a third helping to see what was happening. Eating had slowed at the long table, no one reaching to refresh his bowl. My father was beet-faced and talking in a restrained manner. Aunt Huong and her husband looked irritated. Everyone else wore a silly, nervous grin, trying to make light of the tension.

It started with a discussion of how the Bay Area had changed so much in the last twelve years. When we first arrived, there were maybe two Vietnamese restaurants and one Vietnamese market, and people were excited when they met other Vietnamese. Now, they all agreed, there were too many Vietnamese in Silicon Valley. My uncles complained about the competition. Father said Vietnamese filled the ranks of the county social services with their friends and relatives, giving them special treatment, corrupting the whole system. It was his roundabout way of criticizing his sister, Huong, whom he felt relied too much on government subsidy. The comment riled his sister, and she wouldn't let it slide. After all, this wasn't Vietnam anymore.

My father said, *"You shouldn't abuse the system like that. There are people more needy than you."*

Indignation swelled her eyes. *"What do you mean I shouldn't? Who are you to talk?"*

Uncle Hun butted in: *"He's your big brother. You shouldn't talk to him in that tone."*

She wasn't listening, her eyes trained on my father. Her next shot came out slowly, drawing a careful bead on the mark. *"And did I ever say anything about how you made your money?"*

"No," Grandma Pham repeated, over and over but no one was listening. *"Things that went past shouldn't be called back. Let's not talk about it."*

"That's all right, Mom," Aunt Huong said. *"Let him talk. Let's get it out in the open."*

The eating stopped. Little cousins peeked in from the hallway, wondering what all the angry words were about. Grandma Pham shook her head in shame.

"We didn't judge you so don't judge us," sneered Aunt Huong.

Mom shrieked, *"What do you mean judge? And did your father have a problem with borrowing from us?"*

"Don't talk like that!" Uncle Hong growled, glaring at Mom. *"It's bad luck to speak harshly of the dead. Big Brother Thong, teach your wife not to talk like that."*

Mom whirled on Uncle Hong. *"Don't you stick your nose in where it doesn't belong. My business is my business, my family is my family."*

"Oh, yes. It certainly wasn't our sort of business."

"Ah, then why don't you pay back the money you all owe me. Pay back the money your father owes me."

Half-veiled accusations were flung back and forth. Somehow I had the feeling that they were holding back because all of us, nephews and nieces, were present. The uncles and aunts seemed to think that our family's dysfunctionality was karmic payback for whatever my parents did way back in Vietnam. And Chi, our main casualty, was the one person no one mentioned even in the heat of it. Tien looked at me and shrugged, then melted out with Kay, Huy, and Hien, not saying good-bye to the relatives.

"You and I are through!" Mom lay into her in-laws like a curse, slicing the air with the edge of her hand. *"Don't telephone. Don't bring your face to my door again. Ever!"* she spat, the steel coming into her. For a moment, I saw my mother, the same woman who faced down a mutinous fishermen crew who wanted to take us to Thailand. She stormed out the door and drove home by herself.

The clan gathering was now short two wives-in-law, my mother and Aunt Chau, Uncle Hoang's wife. Uncle Hong started in by drawing a parallel between my mother's disrespect for Grandpa Pham's spirit and Aunt Chau's attitude toward the family.

"*If you don't teach your wives manners,*" said Uncle Hong in general, but directing his comment to his younger brother Hoang, "*soon we'll be doing this whole ceremony by ourselves. Cooking, washing dishes, and all.*"

"*Maybe,*" Uncle Hoang said, "*you should do what Sister Anh said and mind your own business.*"

"*I did and look at what sort of a woman you married.*"

"*You shut up!*" Uncle Hoang barked.

"*You dare tell me, your big brother, to shut up?*"

"*Big Brother, say that about my wife again and I'll tell you to shut up again.*"

"*You disrespectful bastard!*" Uncle Hong grunted, staggering to his feet.

Uncle Hoang stood. They looked as though they were about to trade blows. My father was still glaring, talking heatedly with his sister. The other aunts, Uncle Hien, and Uncle Hau tried to smooth things out, their placation adding to the din. I stopped listening. Grandma Le and Grandma Pham whispered, holding each other's forearms, offering apologies and condolences. Grandma Le moved to the door. No one seemed to notice. I put down my plate.

I walked Grandma out and helped her into the car. We could hear the ruckus from three houses away. Things sounded as though they had just accelerated. Uncle Hoang came out the front door and slammed it behind him. His two older brothers, Hong and Hun, tailed him outside, yelling at him, pointing fingers.

Halfway down the driveway, Uncle Hoang whirled around and shook his fist at them. Voice cracking, he yelled, "*Leave me alone. You have no right talking bad about my wife. You can't tell me what to do. Leave me alone!*"

"*I'm your goddamn older brother. I tell you what I feel like telling you. You shut your mouth and listen, stupid younger brother!*"

"*Hey!*" Uncle Hun shouted. "*Where are you going? Don't you walk away when your older brothers are talking to you!*"

"What have you done for me? Father beat me. You beat me!"

"We taught you to be a better person then. And we're going to do it now! Come back here this instant!"

Uncle Hoang roared, his voice breaking into a shrill, shunting him thirty years back into his adolescence. He snatched rocks on the ground and hurled them at his brothers, screaming *"Fuck you! Fuck you! Goddamn you! Leave me alone!"*

The rocks, wildly thrown, thunked into the garage, bounced off the roof, ricocheted off the wood sidings. Uncle Hun and Uncle Hong stopped short on the porch, wearing stupid expressions, not believing that their younger brother, whom they had whipped so many times, was stoning them.

By the time their senses came to them, Uncle Hoang was getting his range and started whizzing projectiles closer to his targets. A stone skipped off the cement and nailed Uncle Hong in the knee. Another went high and wide—BUP!—taking out the porch light in a shower of glass. Uncle Hun ducked back into the house, Uncle Hong hobbling in right behind him. The door slammed. Uncle Hoang was still hurling rocks like a pitching machine gone berserk shooting at an empty batter cage. His flurry bounced off the door with the sounds of gunshots.

When he stopped, there was complete silence, as though none of it had ever happened. No one looked out the windows. All quiet inside. The pale streetlamps lit Uncle Hoang's face. It was wet. He was breathing hard, shaking. In disjointed motions—an old man uncertain of his bearings—Uncle Hoang found his feet and moved slowly toward his Mercedes convertible, not seeing me standing in front of my car two driveways down. He fumbled with his pockets, got the keys, lowered himself inside, turned on the ignition, the headlights. He flipped on the turn signal to the empty cul-de-sac, pulled quietly from the curb, and went to his mansion alone.

Surprisingly, the neighbors hadn't lined the street to watch our spectacle. I coaxed the engine to life, realizing I probably would never come back. This was my last tribute to Grandpa Pham.

"What was Aunt Huong talking about? What was she saying about my parents?" I asked Grandma as I drove her home.

"You know what I miss about Vietnam, An?" she asked quietly. I could never tell whether she was changing the topic or she was just old.

"You miss your house, your neighbors?"

"Oh, yes, a little, but most of them are dead now." She took a pensive moment, staring out the window, the back of her head to me. *"I miss the rainwater I used to catch from my roof. It was so sweet. Cool and sweet."*

I nursed the Toyota through the neighborhood. Grandma threw up at any speed over thirty miles an hour.

"You should go back and finish the meal. Play with your cousins. Get to know your relatives. Sooner you forget about their arguments the better. Don't let the older folks' quarrels change your friendship with your cousins."

"No, I'm tired. I don't need them anyway."

"If you don't need your family-relatives, who do you need?"

"Nobody. I'll work hard. Make a fortune. Travel the world. Marry a beautiful Americanized Vietnamese girl."

"Ah, I know you, An. You're too dreamy. Be careful what you do. Choose your life with your head, not your heart. You are like a butterfly. Beautiful. Quick to die."

Spooked, I forced a chuckle. We drove the rest of the way in silence.

Auntie Dung and Uncle Hung had gone out dancing. Grandma said she was exhausted and wanted to go to bed. I brewed her a mug of bedtime tea and brought it to her room. Grandma was pulling the silver pins from her hair, the tall bun unscrolled, her mane of too much salt and not enough pepper rolling down to her ankles. She hadn't cut it since she was a slip of a girl, when her first husband passed away. All her stories, her sorrows, her happiness had chalked their marks in her hair, this lifelong rosary I'd seen down maybe four times in my life.

"Grandma—those things they were saying about us . . ."

"Sit, sit. Here on the bed, next to me. Have tea with Grandma. You want some candied coconut? Your aunt's friend gave some to me, but I can't eat them with my teeth."

"Grandma! There is something I don't know. Those things the relatives scorned."

"What about them? Doesn't matter what people say."

"I know, I know. Tell me anyway. Tell me about my parents."

She considered and reconsidered my request slowly, until I sighed in resignation and moved to leave. The porcelain lid of the mug rattled as she put her tea on the nightstand. Grandma took my hands. I had a strange feeling I was holding the jigsaw pieces and she was about to help me put them together.

Grandma paused, straightening her back a moment, the gesture of an elderly woman taking a deep breath, and began, *"This is what happened . . ."*

Ill-Wind

I know they are up to no good when they pull alongside me, giggling madly like three imps. That and
their red faces. A red-faced Vietnamese is a drunk
Vietnamese. And three drunk Vietnamese scooting
along on one motorbike spells trouble. I tell myself,
Avoid. AVOID. But the road bowls straight into the horizon, banked
on both sides by rice paddies as far as the eye can see. Few travelers.
Oh, great.

For the umpteenth time, I wish I still had my pepper spray. I slow
down, they slow down. I speed up, they speed up. They cut in front of
me and slam on the brakes. I swerve, missing them by inches. They
bark with mirth. Then they are behind me. As they pass, one of them
kicks my rear pannier and sends me wobbling to the side of the road.
As quickly as they came, they pull away. I heave a sigh of relief. A
mile up ahead of me, they have stopped by the side of the road. I am
thinking: Ambush. I slow down, considering my options. For once,
Highway 1 is deserted. I can't outrun them on a loaded bike. In any
case, I am in no mood for retreat. Pedaling slowly, I unzip the bag
mounted on the front rack, and loosen the eight-inch fillet knife.

They are standing on the side of the road. I jump on the pedals
to pick up speed. Maybe I can ram them. Knock them down. But

something isn't right with the picture. I choke on my laughter: they are pissing into the rice paddies. The driver of the motorbike shouts something unintelligible to me as I blow past. I look back and see them hastily tucking themselves in and piling on the motorbike. I ease off the pedals. There is no sense trying to outrun a motorbike, even one with three clowns on it. My old schoolmate, who had turned professional Vietnamese-American gangster, used to advise me, his bookish friend, "If trouble is coming, don't turn your back, because that's where it's gonna stab. Best to meet it with a grin. That way, you can see what's coming."

I pull over and wait for them, my hand next to the open bag with the knife. They stop a couple of yards from me.

I wear my biggest grin. *"Hello, Brothers!"*

"Fuck, it's a Viet-kieu!" yelps the round-faced driver as though he'd come across a rat.

"I told you he looked like a Viet-kieu."

"But he looks like a Japanese. I don't like Japanese. Maybe he's a half-and-half," argues a short man with a shoe-brush mustache. *"Oy, you. Are you a half-and-half?"*

"Nope. Whole undiluted fishsauce, I am." I sniff my armpit, wrinkle my nose, and nod. *"Aiee! Pure concentrate."*

They bellow at the joke, warming to me. We strike up a conversation. They want to know where I rode from. The skinny guy asks me, *"Aren't you afraid?"*

"No," I lie, grinning enthusiastically. *"In America, they have a saying: If you die, you die."* I shrug.

"Haven't people attacked you?"

I nod.

"What did you do?"

I take out my knife, smiling, totally faking it.

"Mean like a tiger," says the leader. He chuckles and the others follow suit.

I grin. *"Either that or stay home and watch TV."*

They roar in appreciation. Sensing the shift in their mood, I slip the knife back into the bag. I tap cigarettes out of a pack of Marlboros

I'd saved for occasions like these. I offer one to the leader. His eyes catch the logo. I almost sigh aloud when he puts it between his lips. His compatriots follow suit. I don't smoke but I light up with them to keep things going smoothly. Soon we are sitting on a dike, feet dangling over water, blowing smoke out over the young rice stalks, talking about how people live in America.

Their alcoholic buzz has subsided by the time we finish the pack of Marlboros. They invite me to join them on their next round. *"Bier-om!"*—hugging beer—exclaims the leader. His chums hoot in agreement. Vietnamese men spend a great deal of money at these hostess-bars where pretty girls sit on a patron's lap as he drinks his beer. The "frisking" limits, if any, vary, depending on the depth of the patron's pocket. I decline and we part on handshakes.

I push on alone, feeling suddenly very tired and feverish. Just barely oozing down the road. I haven't eaten much all day. Breakfast was a lump of sweet rice and peanut crumbs wrapped in banana leaves. After chipping one of my molars on a pebble, I tossed the rice to the birds. Lunch was a bowl of beef noodle soup I couldn't eat because the meat, carved off a fly-encrusted lump, was rancid. I am exhausted. I've eaten nearly all my emergency rations: three Hershey chocolate bars, a snack-sized pack of Oreos, and six little cheese wedges. The last bar of chocolate in my bag is squishy like toothpaste, and my mouth is so cottony I can't bring myself to lick the chocolate from the wrapper. It is blistering hot and the sun is melting into the horizon like a scoop of orange sherbet. I am salivating. Haven't had ice cream since I arrived in Vietnam. Didn't dare. If I weren't already drier than a shingle of beef jerky, drool would be dripping down my chin. Funny, a scoop of orange sherbet was all I could wrap my mind around. Not even the faintest hankering for double cheeseburgers, French fries, chocolate milkshakes, apple pie à la mode, anchovy pizzas, Polish sausage, and fresh-baked croissants. I have no appetite and feel a bit dizzy. The fifteen miles to Ky Anh village seem like a hundred.

Up ahead a cattle-drawn cart—without a driver—labors along the side of the road, oblivious to the occasional truck thundering past.

Closer, I see that the dark lump on top of the load of bricks is the sleeping driver, hat shading his face. He is sleeping at the reins, trusting his bovine to keep both of them from turning into roadkill. I have stumbled on the quintessential portrait of Vietnamese industry. In Saigon, a white American tourist had asked me, "Don't take this the wrong way, but why are so many Vietnamese men lounging around all day—don't they have to go to work or something?"

I could see tour buses passing this cart all day and foreign tourists shaking their heads at this evidence of Vietnamese work ethics. I burst out laughing, waking the napping driver. His startled face melts into delight when he sees I am a cyclist.

"Aa-LO! Ow arr you? Wherre you prrom?" he shouts, pushing his army pith helmet back on his head.

"*Viet-kieu, Brother,*" I reply. He looks a little crestfallen.

I grab onto the cart, giving the poor cow my extra weight. "*Brother, where are you going?*"

"*Home. Where did you bike from?*"

I ask him about his load of bricks. Couldn't sell them, he says. His family made bricks by hand. This is a poor batch the builders rejected, so he is taking them back home. Maybe farmers will buy them at a discount.

A cyclist draws up alongside us. I see his silver hair and bow in greeting, then looking down, I nearly fall out of my seat. He has only one leg. His right leg ends above the knee, the dark nub sticks out of his shorts like a big salami. A crutch hangs on the bike frame. His left leg churns the crank in a jerking rhythm, hard on the downstroke, gliding with the momentum on the upstroke, a two-stroke engine running marvelously on one.

"*Uncle, that's amazing!*" I blubber. "*I've never seen a one-legged man ride a bike before.*"

He slows down and latches up to the cart next to me. "*Oy!*" he exclaims, very pleased for some reason. "*You speak Viet!*"

"*Yes, Uncle. I'm a Viet-kieu,*" I confess, and brace for his face to fall, but it doesn't. "*How far can you go on a bike?*"

"*Once I biked all the way to Ky Anh and back, twenty kilometers each way. But usually I only ride to the market, that's twelve kilometers round-trip.*"

His handlebar basket sags with packets of instant ramen, a bottle of what looks to be kerosene or rice wine, a can of condensed milk, and a tin of tea.

"This Viet-kieu is going to Ky Anh," the ox driver tells the old man.

"Ky Anh?" repeats the old man in a tone I don't find encouraging. *"There's nothing out there except a government-run motel. It's actually a barracks, but they'll overcharge you ten times for a bed."*

"I'm overcharged all the time," I point out nonchalantly. *"How far is it?"*

"An hour and a half. It'll be dark soon," the old man says, gauging the sky. He looks me over, apparently having come to a decision. *"Come with me, Nephew. I'll put you up for the night. I live by myself. There's plenty of room and you're welcome to hang your hammock."*

Over two months in Vietnam, it's the first time someone's invited me home without his hands out. I accept the old man's generosity, bowing deeply.

"It is nothing." He waves off my thanks. *"Good, good. You'll like my beautiful villa."*

Uncle Tu's home is a hut. In the burlap-textured dusk, it rises above the rambling vegetable garden like a big bale of hay. It sits near a lake, fifteen minutes from the road. He leads me into his plot of heaven, going down well-tended rows of vegetables, poking at this and that the way people open windows and turn on lights. He palms the tomatoes ripening on the vines, prods the earth with his crutch, clicks his tongue, squashes a snail, and fingers the fat string beans dripping off the vines. In the provinces, both hut and garden are required to make a home. Land is too precious to feed weeds.

The hut's thatched walls and roof are supported by four stout corner posts. The twelve-by-twelve-foot packed dirt floor is swept so clean it resembles hardened clay. The old man sits me down on a crude wooden stool and fusses with a coal stove to brew the traditional welcoming-tea. First, he produces some twigs and wood shavings and arranges them carefully in the stove, which is essentially an eight-inch clay planting pot. He lights the starter pile with one match and places a block of coal, the shape of a chocolate cake, into the stove. We have our tea in no time. He hops over to the pantry cabinet, an end table with long legs, its feet set in bowls of water to keep the ants off. He takes out a clay pot and holds it up tenderly like a bottle of wine.

"Clay-pot catfish, you like it?"

"Of course."

He glows with pleasure. It is impossible to travel in Vietnam without encountering clay-pot catfish. If Vietnam ever got around to declaring a national fish, the catfish would be it. Vietnam's rivers and lakes teem with this hardy creature. Peasants raise catfish in family ponds as they raise chicken in their yards.

"Three days old, very, very tasty," he croons, smacking his lips as he sets it on the stove. He adds a bit of water and a dash of fishsauce. Then both of us settle down to watch it come to a boil. My mouth waters in anticipation.

That is the most wonderful thing about clay-pot catfish. It keeps well for weeks without refrigeration. The older the dish, the deeper the flavors, the more evenly the fish fat blends with the sauce of caramelized palm sugar, cracked pepper, and chili. In Uncle Tu's pot, I see he has splurged and added diced pork fat, whole red chilis, and scallions. The best thing about this dish is that even when all the fish is gone, the dredging is rich enough, especially if the fish head is saved, to be stewed again and poured over rice to make a poor man's meal— something I did many times when I was a boy.

"Uncle, where is your family? I rarely see old folks living by themselves."

"All gone, Nephew. Lost them in the War, wife and son."

"Do you have relatives nearby?"

"No. I have my relatives-neighbors. That's plenty. They are good people, I'm a lucky man."

"Where are they?"

He hobbles to the door and bellows: *"Sonny! Sonny! Sonny!"*

A small boy materializes at the door. He sees me, glances at Uncle Tu, then, remembering his manners, he bows to us both. Uncle Tu tousles the boy's hair and gives him two packets of instant noodles.

"Take this home to your mom, Sonny." The boy bows and runs home. Uncle Tu smiles after him. *"See,"* he says to me. *"I have family, my relatives-neighbors. Not so lonely."*

He spreads the food on an end table, scoops out the rice into bowls for both of us. *"Nephew, please eat,"* he says, formally starting the meal.

"Thank you, Uncle Tu. Please eat," I reply in kind.

We wolf down our plebeian meal of catfish, rice, pickled fire-cracker eggplant with shrimp paste, and steamed string beans from his garden, polishing off every morsel. It is without a doubt one of the best meals I've had in Vietnam. For dessert, we drink more tea and nibble on my gooey Hershey bar. He strings up an extra hammock for me. Our fabric beds now crisscross the hut, making diagonals, mine above his since I am more limber. He blows out the oil lamp and we go to bed. Uncle Tu doesn't stop talking. He has an insatiable appetite for details about the rest of the world. How do they live? What do Americans do every day? Is driving a car scary? How do cellular phones work?

In the middle of the night, Uncle Tu makes a racket as he claws his way out of his hammock. I ask him where he is going. *"Going out for a piss,"* he moans. *"My worm isn't as strong as it used to be. Have to pee twice every night."*

"Wait. I'll come, too."

He urinates on the trunk of a tree. I go to the latrine down by the lake. Behind a clutch of brambles, a catwalk bridges out to the latrine platform built over the water, fifteen feet from shore. Since I came back to Vietnam, I have been able to avoid using these fishpond-latrines. I mount the steps and take care of business. Through the latrine-hole cut into the planks, I see the dark water beginning to churn, coming alive, coiling on itself. It is unnerving. The catfish come to feed.

I wake up, cotton-mouthed, with a searing fever. Uncle Tu pours me a bowl of strong tea for breakfast, feels my forehead, and, without a word, starts hanging blankets over the door and the single window. I complain that it's too stuffy. Keep out the ill wind and evil spirits, he explains. He calls "Sonny" next door and sends him off to find the village's silver coin. The boy scours the area, following the trail of illness from farm to farm. The silver coin is part talisman, part medicinal tool, Uncle Tu says, an heirloom handed down from generation to generation. No one knows who it really belonged to, although everyone uses it when he takes ill. Most of the peasants are too poor to own a silver coin, and those who can afford one don't buy one, preferring the heirloom coin for its legendary healing power. In an hour, the boy returns with the coin. Uncle Tu sends him back out with some money to buy heat-oil, a mentholated herbal oil that makes one's skin feel hot.

I tell Uncle Tu I don't believe "scraping the bad wind" is an effective way to break my fever. He hands me the coin as though an inspection of it would clear my doubts. I unwrap a scrap of crimson velvet, worn smooth and slick with mentholated oil, and pick up the silver coin, which is larger than a silver dollar. Decades of extended use have worn the faces smooth, leaving just a telltale Chinese character.

"It has healed many, many people. Very powerful," Uncle Tu says in a tone of benediction. He is very worried about me. *"You must have caught an ill wind out on the pond last night. That's very bad, water spirits are strongest at night."* He starts rambling about folklore and superstitions, something about the land having power over things that come from it. I tell him that besides spooking me, he isn't doing me any favor by talking nonsense. *"It's not good,"* he repeats to himself. I give in, rationalizing that it doesn't hurt to be sure. When I was a child, my mother used this folk remedy on me and the worst thing I got was a dozen bruises that weren't as nasty as they looked.

Taking off my shirt, I sit hunched over on a stool. Uncle Tu rubs the ointment on my back. His hands are bony and rough like tree bark, but his touch is kind and gentle. I am embarrassed at this physical contact. My father and I have never shaken hands. We do not embrace. I cannot recall our skin ever touching. On rare occasions, we placed a hand on each other's shoulder in congratulations. But here is Uncle Tu, a stranger-once-enemy, drawing on all his skills to heal me with his hands, skin on skin. It is oddly comforting, and I am almost ashamed to admit that much to myself. When the oil is hot on my skin, he begins to coin-scrape my back with a vengeance, making crimson welts six inches long. Then he proceeds to do the same on my neck and chest. Half an hour later, my upper body is tattooed with bruises, my skin tingling with the heat oil. I roll back into my hammock, feeling strangely better. For good measure, I sneak a double dose of aspirin and doze off. When I wake up, Uncle Tu is hovering nearby. We slurp down a supper of rice porridge sprinkled with diced scallions and *ruoc ga*, shredded chicken jerky, and talk about the War.

"No, I do not hate the American soldiers. Who are they? They were boys, as I was. They were themselves, but also part of a greater creature—the government. As was I. I can no more blame them than a fish I eat can be blamed for what I do.

"You see, their pond is America. Here, in these hills, in this jungle, they are food.

"Me, I am in my land. I am in my water. These hills where I've killed Vietnamese and Americans. I see these hills every day. I can make my peace with them. For Americans, it was an alien place then as it is an alien place to them now. These hills were the land of their nightmares then as they are now. The land took their spirit. I eat what grows out of this land and someday I will return all that I have taken from it. Here is my home, my birthland and my grave.

"Tell your friend Tyle. There is nothing to forgive. There is no hate in this land. No hate in my heart. I am a poor man, my home is a hut with a dirt floor, but he is welcome here. Come and I shall drink tea with him, welcome him like a brother."

War-Survivors

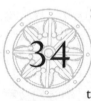 Seventeen years after the fall of Saigon, Colonel Van of the Vietnamese Nationalist Army was suffering a bitter exile in San Jose, California. Despite his poverty, he had thickened into a burly man, a diesel-powered tank, with M-16 fingers and a grenade of a nose from which he was squeezing out the blackheads. Stringy yellow stubble grassed from his pores as he hunched over a hand mirror on the kitchen table. Sedentary suburbia had fat-armored his five-foot-three structure to two hundred pounds. Muscles shelved his shoulders, sloping to the dome mountain that was his head of baling-wire hair, a galvanized gray. His boulderish face bunched and twitched with excitement over his plot for resurrecting a Nationalist army. He wanted to overthrow the Vietnamese Communist government and reclaim what was rightly his. The Colonel looked up and commanded his proposition to me in attack terms: "SOLAR POWER!"

I choked on a mouthful of spinach. My girlfriend, Trieu, and I were having our weekly dinner with her father—the Colonel—and his second wife. He puffed on his cigarette and scanned my face for reaction. I made a show of coughing on the smoke and reached to crack open the window. Instantly, the pregnant silence melted as the Friday night traffic of Chicanos low-riding the boulevard filled the room. Windowpanes quivered under the parade of thumping mega-bass speakers. Down at the corner gas station and the liquor store, cop cars packed the intersection, besieged up and down the blocks by Latinos, Chicanos, *cholos,* and even a number of Vietnamese—the new Americans—strutting, parading like war heroes. Everybody was out sweet on the night except us.

"Brilliant idea! I'd never thought of it," I exclaimed, pumping in more enthusiasm than I felt. I was taking classes for my advanced degree and working at the Company, becoming a full-fledged suit and walking immigrant-success story, putting in a hard week so I could listen to the Colonel's mad plans on my precious Friday nights.

Sitting next to him at the kitchen table, Trieu struggled with her face as she ate rice one grain at a time and did her best not to look at him and his nose. Having known her father less than a year, she was still adjusting to his rough country manners. The Colonel had put her up for adoption when they first came to the States. She was a toddler and her mother was lost—*disappeared*—during the turmoil of the War. (It was a forced/arranged marriage.) He said he didn't know how to take care of her. A Caucasian couple adopted Trieu and raised her in Georgia. Now that she had matured into a true Southern belle in her third year of college, Trieu found her biological father to be something of a barbarian. But she never said a word because she had moved across the country to live with him for a year to get to know her roots—him. She averted her eyes from the Colonel, who was mowing his blackheads with a fingernail and wiping them on a paper towel, his yield collecting like globs of mung-bean paste.

"Solar power," the Colonel repeated, pleased but suspicious of my zest. Then, noticing Trieu's studious distraction, he commented to me in Vietnamese, *"She doesn't like it when I do that. I'm teaching her."*

What? I didn't dare ask. She was twenty-one with an I.Q. of 140. My stomach jellied with grave foreboding about my prospective father-in-law. My grandma's karmic predictions bounced around my head like Ping-Pong balls in a dark room. I had real bad feelings about the Colonel, but I couldn't ditch him without losing Trieu.

She smiled adoringly at the Colonel, not understanding a word of Vietnamese. "Daddy, are you talking about me again?"

"Ha-ha-ha. Nooooo! Daddy said you are good girl. Here, Trieu, eat fish. I pick meat for you. No bones." His killer fingers displayed amazing chopsticks dexterity, stripping the fried fish, dipping it in garlic-chili fishsauce, and placing the morsels in her rice bowl.

"Oh, Daddy," she purred into his shoulder.

It shouldn't have made me jealous, but I knew too much. I tried not to begrudge her this small joy even though I despised the way the Colonel was manipulating her for his own gain. He hadn't given up trying to marry Trieu to her rich ex-boyfriend. There was also something discomforting about the way he gazed at her, calculating, maybe, but I kept telling myself it was my dislike for him talking. I pulled a grin and reminded myself there were enough bad things in her past that I didn't need to add the Colonel to it.

I had met Trieu on a double date, blind for both of us, who were riding shotgun to bolster our respective friends' courage. On sight, I knew she was the type of girl that wobbled men's knees and fogged their heads—the kind that set off all my alarms. Because I had decided to run the other way, my detachment opened her to me and her melancholy tumbled out in mysterious bits. Happiness, sorrow, and abuse were mixed up like vegetables in a soup—the broth, her essence from moment to moment. Yet I was held not so much by her tragedy as by a single gesture—the way she knitted her long hair, sheets upon sheets of fine caramel webs, with two fingers and tossed it back from her face. It was a gentle, careless motion, the way I supposed she pushed the sadness back from her brown eyes.

She was aristocratic, though with a nasty inclination for sharp humor, which suited me. There was inherent grace in her features, definitely something from her mother's line. Her father couldn't have given her those huge eyes, that delicate nose, the rosy alabaster skin, not of a tropical Vietnam, I didn't believe. The curves of her face fitted the cup of my hand like a sweetening mango. Those high cheekbones I had seen somewhere, on jade statues. Full lips, generous yet silent. But of course, it was her flawless English with its honeyed Southern twists that shackled me. She was Vietnamese and American in all the right measures, something I had aspired to without knowing.

We had been together almost a year. Day before yesterday, the Colonel told me bluntly not to drop by after work because Trieu would be busy. Just this afternoon, she said the Colonel had invited her rich ex-boyfriend to dinner in my absence. And here I was watching them showering each other with fatherly-daughterly affection, faking my admiration for him.

The Colonel turned back to me, all business again: *"We sell solar panels with inverters and rice cookers to farmers. Imagine what a great invention that is. They won't have to worry about gathering firewood or buying coal for cooking."*

I mumbled conciliatory consent. It was obvious why he targeted peasants. Who else would take up arms for the Colonel and his cronies' fantasy about liberating South Vietnam? It was the same song and dance my father played when he was recruiting soldiers. Lend them a hand, give them a present, then ask for their lives in the name of Liberty, Justice, and Freedom.

The Colonel laid out my role in his master plan. I was supposed to put up the initial capital and design a prototype. The Colonel and his cronies would take care of the test. I nodded vague encouragement while Trieu and Mrs. Van did the dishes. I sipped my jasmine tea. The Colonel wove his grandiose dreams. His wife smiled indulgently, wiping her hands on a flour-sack apron. Trieu hovered close over my shoulder. I smelled the honeysuckle fragrance in her hair. The moment was surreal enough for me to banish my doubts, forget the bad things, and pretend this was a normal family. I had learned from my own that if I didn't listen to the words too carefully or focus on the details too closely, everything seemed innocuous.

Then Mr. Beckett started screaming from his bed in the living room.

The Colonel and his wife were live-in caretakers for Mr. Beckett, who was obese, bed-ridden, and suffering from advanced Alzheimer's. Old Mr. Beckett started bellowing that he had to use the bathroom and would someone help him. Mrs. Van pushed herself away from the dinner table and hurried out front. The light clicked on.

"Oh, God! He did it again," she moaned, her tired surrender reaching us clearly from the living room. "Mr. Beckett, how many times do I have to tell you? Please don't wet the bed."

"Who wetted the bed?" the old man's reedy voice returned full of surprise. A couple of months ago he had stopped recognizing his live-in caretakers.

"You peed in your bed, Mr. Beckett. After we take you to the toilet, we'll have to give you a bath."

"No. NO! NO! I don't want no bath! I tell you I don't want no bath!"

"I'm sorry, Mr. Beckett. I'm giving you a bath."

"NO! I tell you I don't want no bath! Somebody help me!"

We went to see the fuss. The poor man suffered the indignity of waiting out his last days in the living room because it was the center of the house, accessible from every part, and closest to the bathroom. Most of the time he had no idea where he was, waking up babbling, Where am I? What have you done with my son? Where's my wife? I want my wife!

No one told Mr. Beckett his wife had passed away three years ago and his son, who lived in the adjacent county, hadn't stopped by for a visit since. An ungrateful son-of-a-bitch was what Mrs. Van called Mr. Beckett's only offspring, but once in a while when Mr. Beckett tripped into one of his half-lucid ramblings about how he used to whip his disrespectful son, she would shake her head and mumble that the wicked old man had this misery coming to him. We usually told Mr. Beckett his son was on his way. A little traffic delay. Your wife is out for groceries. She'll be back any moment. Go back to sleep, Mr. Beckett.

The poor man had let out a gusher and it was dribbling onto the carpet, infusing the musty clapboard house with the saccharine reek of medicated urine. Without a word, we rolled up our sleeves. Although the Colonel and Mrs. Van usually managed on their own—how I didn't know—it took four of us to stagger Mr. Beckett down the hallway of blistered wallpaper and into the bathroom. The old man winced and grunted with pain the whole five yards. His hospital scrub left exposed his saggy white buttocks, moon-cratered with purple-black bedsores, lumpy as though he had grapes under his skin. The Colonel held Mr. Beckett upright while Mrs. Van sponge-bathed him. Mr. Beckett's senses came back and he realized what he had done. He hung his head and sat dejectedly, mumbling apologies as Mrs. Van soaped between his legs.

When Mr. Beckett was snoring in a clean bed, we were back in the kitchen for dessert. The Colonel thanked Trieu and she plowed into his ribs for a hug. I sat there unable to make heads or tails of it all. A vanquished commander, formerly of great wealth, power, and corruption, now bathed an old man. A father who gave away his daughter because he didn't want to take care of her, now wanted to give away her hand in marriage for his own purposes. A young American woman shedding her identity to learn love from her biological father. I didn't fit in this puzzle. Sometimes I thought it would be best for both of them if I weren't in the picture.

I lost my appetite, but I gulped down the flan quickly, not wanting to insult their poverty with my waste. The Colonel lit another cigarette and plunged onward with his beloved war stories. White-faced with exhaustion, Mrs. Van slouched at the table and took her tea as though it were medication. Trieu folded her hands in her lap, a dutiful, attentive daughter, listening to her father's stream of words she didn't understand. I tried to translate, but the Colonel was irritated at having his oration interrupted.

The Colonel's mean streak came out in his stories. He relished the gory details of battle. How he killed a Viet Cong with a single blow of his paw. How he sacked an enemy camp that outnumbered his forces five to one. How Saigon politicians, businessmen, and mobsters feared him and paid him "respect" money. The one long-running practical joke he enjoyed most was the one he played on American GIs, particularly the green ones fresh off the plane.

"Those pitiful Americans," he said without remorse as he stroked the brush that was his sideburn. *"They were too big to jungle-march for weeks eating rice like Vietnamese. They couldn't get enough energy from rice and they wilted like flowers. The Viet Cong killed the young ones like flies."*

He loved breaking in his green Americans on the first mission by foxholing them three times a night. As usual, the mixed company of American and Vietnamese soldiers struck camp on the frontline by digging foxholes. The Vietnamese knew the Colonel's intentions, so they dug shallow pits or none at all while their American counterparts dug honest, good-sized holes. In the meantime, the Colonel sneaked off into the jungle for dinner with his lieutenants. After his meal and dessert smoke, the Colonel returned and ordered the men to abandon camp because the enemy had "spied" their position. Ambush was imminent. He marched them in circles for an hour to another spot and had them dig in again. Employing this tactic three times a night, a couple of nights in a row, he turned the green foreigners into a ragged, jangling mess. Upon returning to base, even the veteran American officers begged to be reassigned to other Vietnamese commanders, which was fine with the Colonel. He said the Viet Minh fought harder for American casualties, and he didn't care to be around GIs when the heavy fire came.

I listened to him with open amazement, wondering if he realized the irony of his current situation or the karmic disaster he was heaping onto his daughter. Sins of the father must be redeemed by his children. Maybe that was why our dead ancestors watched over us: guilt.

The Colonel smoked the last cigarette of his daily two packs at 2 a.m. and we wrapped up for the night. As I picked up my coat in the darkened living room where Mr. Beckett was wheezing in his sleep, Trieu kissed me good night and whispered, Stay tonight, please. An, I don't feel safe. I was startled, coat in hand, the Colonel waiting expectantly at the door. I squeezed her hand and bowed to the Colonel. Disturbed and confused, I reparked my new sports car a couple of blocks away and waited for the Colonel to go to bed before walking back. I jumped the fence on the side of the house, catted round the back porch, and climbed through Trieu's bedroom window, which she had left unlatched for me.

She woke and nestled her head into the hollow below my collarbone. I said that I couldn't keep sneaking around like this. It was too risky. I wanted her to move into my apartment. Soon, she promised, baffling me. She explained her sudden change of heart casually, as though she was brushing away a strand of hair from her face.

"Dad touched me in the car today."

Her words burned like a slow fuse. Then the meaning firecrackered in my ears. I went rigid. Oh, Jesus.

She felt anger coiling in me and withdrew instinctively. "Don't worry about it. I can handle myself. Nothing happened. I didn't let him. Go to sleep, hon," she whispered impatiently, already shutting down. Something terrible in her past froze her up in the face of anger. She rolled to her other side, away from me. A grainy stillness shifted between us. Trieu feigned sleep.

The room was cold, but I burned and could not breathe. There was something wild inside me. How could *it* be so little to her? And she so indifferent? This was sick. The anger wanted to rise out of my rib-cage and rip the room apart. My head was exploding. The tension ratcheted my gut. I wrestled against blaming her complicity for not seeing *it* coming. For not running out the door with me this moment. What did he do? What did you do? Has this happened before? A year passed for me in five minutes.

"An, you still awake?"

"Yeah."

She turned back on her side to face me. I could see the gloss of her eyes. She shelled her hands around mine and held them to her chest. "An, I knew I couldn't tell you."

"Trieu . . . How can you be so calm? Why didn't you tell me earlier? How can you pretend through dinner like nothing happened?" I fought to keep my voice level.

She replied with a child's simplicity, "He's my father . . ."

"No, no, no, no, no. No father does that." He was a goddamn pig. I wanted to tell her I wanted him locked up. I wished I could fold myself around her and sponge away the pain. I wanted to rage, but what do I know about abuse? I was weak to her vulnerability. What did I know about loss, pain, betrayal? She had been through an adoption gone terribly wrong only to find a worse truth. I wished I were wiser.

At last I asked her what I should have said first: "How do you feel?"

A long pause. Her eyes closed.

"I'm . . . I'm disappointed."

I felt my soul down on one knee before her, pledging my eternal fealty, for I could not understand her courage to continue the charade.

She needed him in ways I could not comprehend, and the finality of judging her father was a condemnation she had to make by herself. I touched my lips to her hands.

"Do you know what I like about you, An?"

I did. But I said, "No, what do you like about me?"

"You're good. You're different. One in a million."

It was her favorite cliché, one she wished to believe. It seemed so easy to go along with her, but the words sat in my throat. Someday I would have to tell her the truth. She made me strive to be something better, but at the heart of it I was no better than the next guy. I tried to be decent because she needed it.

"Can we go to sleep now?" she said. "I have to work early tomorrow."

"Sure, sure. Everything will turn out all right."

She turned and backed into me so that we were curving around each other on the twin bed. I draped an arm around her and she held my hand. Sorrow burrowed down my throat to roost in my ribs. Like a child wakened by a nightmare, she was fast asleep again, preserved by her ability to make dandelions of her tragedies. A breath, a wish. Away into the wind.

I had kept telling her—and myself—that I took her as she was. The past did not matter. I never suspected that it was not my decision to make, but a mutual consent we had to negotiate. We were both walking thin ledges, always at cross-purposes, just out of each other's reach. I stared at the darkness all night, keeping vigil over her, watching her sleep, her skin as pale as driftwood. There was an elegant slightness to Trieu I had always fancied I could sketch in three fluid lines, and if I got them right, I would know the whole of her with or without her leave.

I turned off my watch alarm before it rang. I sat on the bed as long as I dared, listening to her even breathing. The Colonel woke early so I had to get out. I should have left. Instead, I stood under the tree outside the Colonel's window and stared, balling my fists. In two steps, I could step through the window and snuff out his life. Garrote him with my necktie. No, he did not deserve that mercy. He needed to know what he meant to his daughter. I wanted him to taste her bitter disappointment. Then I'd gouge out his eyes, trim his fingers, one knuckle at a time.

A silent night. A coruscating blaze behind my eyes. Night flowers powdered the air, a whitish fragrance. A sickle moon splattered me through the bough of the tree. The lace curtain shifted as if by a breeze, but the air was not moving. In the window, a flame exploded—a match waking a cigarette. Cold wires cycloned into my skin. The Colonel was at the window, looking out into the yard. He drew a deep one, the fat balls of his cheeks, his hooded eyes, glowing in the tobacco's flare. Troll in the window. A Kitchen God gone bad. A monstrosity brought back from the War.

Smelling the smoke that was in his lungs, I was the sniper in the shadow. We were at war all over again, me on the other side.

"Hey! Somebody there! Stop!" Red embers flew from his cigarette.

I heard him bulling down the hallway to get out the back door. A drawer slammed. He was going for his guns. If he discovered me, he'd kill both Trieu and me. I crashed across the yard, vaulted over the fence, and sprinted down the sidewalk. I ran, skimmed, flew across the balance of the night, the pavement a streaking hardness. Glazing orange streetlamps could not hold me. I needed to be away from the twisted vestiges of Vietnam-America, wishing an escape to some distant normal place, an America at large.

Harlot-Heroine

35 I don't know why I climb into his cyclo. It must be his reversed Hitler mustache—the little tuft located below his lower lip instead of above his upper lip. My cyclo driver must either be on the cutting edge of facial-hair fashion or he is plainly a nerd. In any case, as I was mesmerized by it, wondering what sort of fool would cultivate such a ridiculous-looking thing, he talked me into going for a free tour around Hue, the former imperial city of Vietnam. *There isn't much business at this hour anyway, so let's just cruise the city. No charge.* I suggest we go for *che,* late-night snacks of sweet beans and coconut milk.

He is pedaling me around the city in a budget-rental cyclo so cheap it doesn't have brakes. To stop, Tin jumps off and, with both hands locked on the seat post for dear life, drags himself behind the vehicle, shredding his plastic sandals on the asphalt. On a steep downhill, he shouts a warning and I bail out of the cab to help him haul the cyclo against gravity. On even a moderate incline, Tin lacks the muscle power, so the both of us huff and puff to push it to the top. Of course, once there, we're fighting to keep it from barreling down the other side and crippling bystanders. We eat *che* on the side of the road at a four-stool kiosk. Then I insist on taking my turn at the pedals with him in the passenger seat. He wants me to meet his uncle, who has been like a father to him since his father died some ten years ago. Tin tells me he has a wife and three young ones. Near his house, his neighbors and cyclo buddies are hollering: *What the heck?* Surprised to see him in the cab—and me in the saddle. Tin shrugs and tells them that I am a foreigner, which seems to satisfy everyone since you never can tell what bizarre things a foreigner might be lusting after. We have tea with his uncle and they make me feel like part of the family. His uncle narrates his nephew's misfortunes. *So young with so many responsibilities and so little money. Talk to him. Maybe you can have some good influence on him. Inspire him.*

When Tin drops me off at my hotel, I demand he take something home for his wife and children. He declines, so I press enough money into his hand to make tonight one of his better ones. He takes the cash and tells me that money isn't necessary between friends. I tell him to swing by tomorrow morning, hoping to hire him on as a guide.

I am having breakfast when a tour bus pulls over and parks in front of the café. Road-dazed foreigners totter off the bus and into the hotel across the street. The driver, a young guy, takes a cigarette break in front of the bus. Before his third drag, the police materialize from nowhere, swaggering in their drab olive uniforms and vinyl belts. The pair beelines to the bus, one whipping out a citation pad, the other swinging his nightstick in short, impatient arcs. The driver's jaw drops. He nearly swallows his cigarette, knowing that he and his tour company are going to suffer huge fines.

"This is a no-parking zone!" barks the cop loud enough for everyone in the café to hear. There is no sign and the space is just an empty dirt lot.

"I'm sorry, Officers!" the driver squeaks, smiling apologetically, placating. *"I'll move it right away."*

"Too late," snorts the other cop, barring the driver from the door with his nightstick. *"It'll have to be towed."*

The driver disintegrates into pure panic. They want to see his license and the papers for the vehicle, so reams of multihued permits and authorizations exchange hands. The owner of the café, from where I am sitting, sends her son to the hotel across the street to warn the hotel owner and the tour operator. In seconds, two older well-dressed men emerge, wearing big friendly smiles. They approach with hands extended, each deftly steering one cop to a different end of the bus. Divide and subdue. Seeing now that they are in the presence of money and power, the cops adopt grave, almost serene countenances. A flock of spectators watch the proceedings from a wary distance—this here the only event where onlookers aren't practically trampling on what they're watching.

I turn to the café owners. *"All this for a parking violation?"*

She nods. *"Big fines."*

"Lunch fines?"

She chuckles and looks at me with interest. *"You know the way, eh?"*

I shrug.

Within minutes everything is resolved. The big men never stop smiling and the cops never crack as much as a grin. The driver takes the bus across the street into the hotel's courtyard. The big men stroll into the café, each draping an affectionate arm over his cop. The foursome take a table next to mine. The owner rushes to their elbows for the orders: espresso, Coke, beer, omelets, steaks, and four packs of Marlboros, two packs apiece for the cops. Small talk and a few American cigarettes, the ice is broken and they are chatting like old friends. Afterward, the big men show the cops into the hotel. Additional mollification required.

The café patrons, all white foreigners, observe the entire extortion with great amusement, marveling at the brazenness of the transaction.

Tin meets me at the café and pedals us down the river in his rented cyclo. The sky is overcast and the city smells wet and moldy. A sprawl of one- and two-story buildings, ancient Hue seems natural in its state of eternal dreariness. Mud slicks the roads. People slop through it, paying no heed to the sludge the way they did in the heyday of Midwestern oil shantytowns. Their feet are covered with it, slimy like grease. The buildings are crumbly, block after block of moss-furred cement and rained-out plaster. The weather wearing them out more quickly than the dwellers can repair them.

As I requested yesterday, Tin arranges for a woman to take us down the Perfume River in her canoe. I swallow hard at the sight of our vessel, a leaky tin tube, cut in half lengthwise and end-riveted to form a semblance of bow and stern. It's safe, she assures me, as they struggle to keep the canoe from tipping over while I board. I take the bow, Tin the middle, and the woman the stern. All loaded, we glide into the waterway with about four inches of freeboard. If one of us sneezes, we're all going into the river. She navigates us into the channel with the only paddle. Tin is bailing water with the vessel's sole plastic cup. I'm holding my breath.

We slide across the flat liquid face, the color of old moss, upriver to see the boat people. Around Hue, the Perfume River smells. From a distance, the riffraff of boats looks like a mess of daddy longlegs scrawling the water. The boats are uniformly slender with narrow beams and sweeping bows and sterns, a house set amidships. Most boast decent waterlines of at least thirty feet. Whole families live on these boats, eight to twelve people, with just enough room to unroll a sleeping mat. Yet they are a livelier crowd than the folks landlocked in mud-splattered shacks on stilts along the riverbanks of rich red clay. People bathe, wash, and defecate in the river. A barge crosses the water and nearly drowns us in its wake. The concrete sky begins to spit and Tin can't bail fast enough. I call it a day. Both the woman and Tin look visibly relieved.

I pay the boatwoman and Tin, tipping enough to bulge their eyes. I know Tin is trying to enroll his oldest son in school, so I give him a little extra. For your family, I insist, and Tin tells me the gift means much to him. Wet and covered in muck, I go back to the hotel for a bath. Tin and I agree tentatively to meet up around dinnertime. After cleaning up, I amble down to the market by the river to buy bags of candies, which I have come to enjoy giving to the beggar children. I bump into Tin's aunt and invite her to join me for a bowl of noodles.

"That boy Tin is so lazy. His cousin just graduated from college. His sister is a teacher and his brother has a motorbike repair business," she whines over

the pungent steam rising from her bowl. *"He's twenty-five already and he hasn't even begun to apply himself."*

"I thought he was twenty-eight," I say. Tin told me yesterday he was twenty-eight.

"No. He's twenty-five. Not even married yet. If he waits any longer, no girl is going to want him because he won't be just old. He'll be old and poor."

I leave Tin's aunt bitching with other patrons on their menfolk's paucity of character. I stroll along the riverfront, sightseeing, wearing the lost and wary demeanor of a jilted stranger, just another chump tourist.

Sometimes it is as though every Vietnamese is seeking a godfather, a sugar daddy, a saint. In the stark neediness of their lives, dignity doesn't ride shotgun to opportunism. But again they learned to separate both eons ago. And by this, I am not referring to the Saigon alley kids who shout in the foreigners' faces. Gimme a dollar. Gimme ten dollar. Gimme camera. Gimme sun cream. You number one. U.S. number one. Fuck you. You best. You go with my sister, you gimme U.S. dollar. You take me to America. Go home, pigs. Fuck you. Fuck you.

Vietnamese have a saying: *"A thousand years of Chinese rule, a hundred years of French subjugation, and ten years of American domination, but we survived, unified."*

Survive. That's the word. Survive at any cost.

"What does it imply," Professor Khai asks me, *"about the national psyche when its national literary heroine is a prostitute?"*

"Vietnam's national heroine is a prostitute?" I am alarmed, no idea how such a thing could have escaped my attention all these years.

It is raining. We are sitting in a royal box overlooking a pond situated in the center of an Emperor's palace. Other tourists have left and the curators fall to gambling with the guards, so we have free run of the museum grounds. I sit on the throne, playing the part of the prince, Professor Khai at my feet, deep in historical discourse. The weeping sky textures the pond, painting its lily-speckled face with a matted finish. The air smells washed, fresh. If I squint through the smallest cracks of my eyes, I can almost see a ghost retinue of some long-dead prince who sat on this very throne, his entourage, his wise men, his literati at his feet reciting poetry. That was the age when the literati and intellectuals were court ministers, politicians, noblemen, and ambassadors.

Taking great pains to fill the gaps in my education, the Professor explains that *The Tale of Kieu* is a story about a prostitute named Kieu, a melodramatic tragicomic poem of 3,254 verses written by an aristo-cratic scholar named Nguyen Du and published two hundred years ago. Every Vietnamese has read or heard at least parts of this story taught at various levels in school. As the Professor sinks deeper into his narration, he uses big words I don't understand. I interrupt him for definitions so frequently that his initial surprise at my ignorance begins to give way to impatience.

I sit back and grin, having struck a gold mine at last with the Professor. I made his acquaintance on a street corner. He was astride his Honda motorbike, wheels for hire. He speaks English and French and once taught history at the University thirty years ago. His one-time association with Americans resulted in his name's permanent residency on the government's blacklist. He can't get a license to work as a tour guide. So for five dollars, he is giving me a tour of Hue's countryside on his Honda, lectures included.

"It says everything about the Vietnamese, understand-no?" says the Pro-fessor in his lilting pedantic rambling. *"She is a prostitute. The things she has done are not commendable, great deeds. But don't you see, it is the reasons why she does these things. They are selfless acts. Sacrifices. Everything is there. You must read it."*

I promise him I will.

"It is also her dignity, her sense of humor that makes her the fundamen-tal Vietnamese heroine. Endears her to all Vietnamese. People aspire to her nobility."

I refrain from telling him that Western scholars describe the Viet-namese as a people who view themselves as victims, punished for a crime they neither understand nor know they have committed. I think there is truth in that, but suspect there are deeper things. I believe they think they are talented but they wonder why they can't forge a lasting, fruitful peace. I think they have struggled for so long, endured so many horrors, committed innumerable sins, which they've justified, rationalized for their survival. Perhaps, I think, they have lost themselves. Capitalism is still new to the Vietnamese. They are only beginning to discover themselves within it.

After Tin's paid-for friendship, something in me dissipates. I simply let myself flow along, not caring that I ought to seek out more Vietnamese, meet as many of them as I can, to learn all our differences and similarities. I immerse myself in the company of other tourists, and when a Vietnamese assumes that I am Japanese or Korean, I don't bother to make the correction.

In Saigon, I avoided other Western tourists, believing it would color my homecoming in shades less than true. I became lonely and infected with Vietnamese fears of traveling on the open road. In Hanoi, I thrived on the camaraderie and the adventurous spirit of other Western tourists, comfortable in my role of translator, a cultural go-between.

A group of us meet at the DMZ Bar to party. Most of them either have just returned from touring the De-Militarized Zone or are booked for the next day's tour. Hue is a major destination for many Vietnam vets because of the DMZ. Even those who weren't stationed there come to see it. It also holds some significance for the families of Americans who have lost fathers, brothers, and sons here.

During the evening, I meet Cao, one of the DMZ tour guides.

"It is very sad. I see them come here," Cao says, shaking his head. *"They get very emotional. They cry. Sometimes they just walk around as though they are lost. Lost their soul, you know. I feel very sorry for them. Maybe they aren't as tough as we are. They are big and strong but they have soft hearts."*

"Do you see many Viet-kieu taking the DMZ tour?"

"Very, very few. It's more for the Westerners."

"Why do you think Vietnamese soldiers can forget more easily than American soldiers?"

He pulls a half-grin. It is a question he must have contemplated many times. *"We live here. They don't. It's like, say, you and me falling in love with the same girl. We both had good and bad times courting her, maybe she hurt us both. I win and marry her. You go home to your country far away. After twenty years, all you have of her are memories, both the good and the bad. Me, I live with her for twenty years. I see her at her best and at her worse. We make peace with each other. We build our lives, have children, and make new history together. Twenty years and you have only memories. It is not the forgetting but the new history with the girl that is the difference between you and me."*

After working the tour for nearly two years, Cao seems to have developed great empathy for aging American veterans on pilgrimages for inner peace. He resents the script the government forces him to read on the tour. It is too harsh against Americans, he says. The war is over, there is no need to mock. He wants to know about Vietnam veterans in America, so I tell him about Tyle and Big Jake.

Big Jake and I crossed paths in a coffee shop along the California coast, near Eureka. I had pulled into a café for breakfast, waiting out a storm. He came in, poured his pockets into his hand, and counted out a cup of coffee in a manner that made me think that he was either very frugal or extremely poor. The harried waitress said, "How you doin' today, Big Jake?" He touched the bill of his weathered baseball cap the way they did in the old days, saying, "Sue," the corners of his mouth cracking behind the graying beard, showing what might have passed for a friendly grin in this dying lumber town. Beneath the counter, she had saved him a piece of cherry pie, explaining that they couldn't sell it anyway. And looked the other way as he secreted a dollop of something from a paper bag into his coffee.

He straddled the stool next to me. Two loners starved for conversation, we started to talk, gruffly at first. Crappy weather, ain't it? Yeah, the Old Man's pissing a barrel today! But as always with Vietnam vets, he asks me where I was from *originally.*

"I tell you, what we did to your people was a tragedy. A fucking disaster. I'm too fucked up now to say whether we should have gone in there in the first place. I just wish I didn't." He was still wrangling with himself about America and its fight against the spread of Communism.

Big Jake had college aspirations before Vietnam. Now he pined for the occasional salvaging jobs, looking forward to heaving his six-foot-four frame of two hundred fifty pounds up and down torched mountains, toting a chain saw among widow makers. "I'm not half as strong as I used to be and some of these young guys worry about having me along." When he wasn't working, he wrote. It gave him great pleasure. It was cathartic.

"No, I don't hate you. I always figured you people hated me more. We went into your house and tried to do our good deed. You see, if we'd succeeded, we would have gotten all the glory. And I suppose, since we failed, we gotta take the blame as well. It's only right.

"What I hate is this goddamned country, all the fucking politicians and the wishy-washy conservatives. I'm like the guy that was sent over to a stranger's house to sort it out, you know? I'm in the house settling shit that should have been between brothers. I come back, and my family takes off. They hate me. I ain't nobody. Still can't get a decent job and I'm all fucked up in the head. I picked up some disease over there and the fucking bureaucrats want me to fill out forms to prove that what I did for them made me sick. Fuck. This world is fucked up."

He reeled away toward the door, mumbling to himself. I, the yellow-skinned devil, had chased him from his half-eaten pie. Then he swerved back around, his hand extended to me: "Good luck."

Fallen-Leaves

An was four. Sitting in a cave of sheets. Cowboys and Indians.

36 *The great house of concrete floor, plywood walls, and tin roof was no place for a lone boy among strange adults.*

He had no friends. He carried a cricket in a matchbox in his pocket.

A plastic six-shooter in hand, he was hiding from red-Indians. The cave was a big table with a thin mattress on top, too high for him to climb. A white cotton sheet draped over the sides, coming almost to the ground. He was sitting on the floor. The plywood air was hot, the concrete cool.

A woman came into the room. He could only see her feet, her red high heels, but he recognized her voice. A man came in after her. Big, black soldier boots, dark-green pants. They were laughing, speaking a language An did not understand. They closed the door. He was trapped, in trouble because he knew he wasn't supposed to be in this room.

The boots stood close to the high heels, woman giggling, man laughing roughly. Wet mouth sounds. Perfume. Clothes going boneless to the floor. Bare feet stepping on each other. Skinny woman legs. Blond hair man legs. Giggling.

An knew this was bad—Dad would beat him. He was told not to come here.

They got on top of the table and the world began to rock and creak and the white sheet fluttered and they made noise and the table shuddered and An was scared and everything was moving and it was very loud.

Gaping-Fish

 I leave Hue with some trepidation for the day's ride. Every Vietnamese I'd ever talked to made such a huge deal of Hai Van Pass that by the time I get there it is anticlimactic. It is all jungle out there, they said, nothing to see. Trees and more trees—a bandit behind every bush. Many people died there. Watch out for snipers. You might not make it up in one day. Just hitch a ride on a bus.

I come to the foothills around noon and lunch at a riverside café. A shantytown has sprung up to cater to the bus traffic going over the pass. The sky is overcast and the air is humid. At the foot of the climb, a bicyclist is pissing on the shoulder of the road, holding himself with one hand and giving me the thumbs up with the other: Okay! Okay! I click into first gear and granny up the mountain. From half a mile up, the sweep of the bay is stunning. No time to rest, I snap a picture and continue upward. The road scales the cliff above the sea. I can't see much ahead. A scrim of fog melting into the steep green slopes hides anything beyond thirty yards. I have a sensation of climbing toward heaven. The breeze is sweet. It is uncannily quiet save for the sporadic bus traffic and the surf huffing far below. For the first time since leaving Hanoi, I go for five minutes at a time without seeing a soul. I am the only cyclist. I stop on the side of the road to have a cup of tea with a group of workers who paint concrete blocks, petite retaining walls that could only prevent motorbikes, not buses, from going over the cliffs. I am looking everywhere: There are no bandits unless the wood gatherers and the family tending a way station moonlight as outlaws. The vista is lush, grand, reminding me of the Northern California coast. With all the horror stories hounding me, I top the mountain in about an hour. A couple of cafés cling to the rocky peak along with a few abandoned munitions bunkers. Two dozen children selling postcards, candies, and beer lie in ambush. The sun washes the other side of the mountain range. Gentle hills undulate away to the hem of the sky. A large lake glimmers far inland. Warm sun on my back, I plow down the mountain, racing buses, passing them, enjoying great shouts and cheers from the passengers.

In the late afternoon, I take a small fork toward the ocean, heading out to an ancient town called Hoi An. Around a bend, a crowd gathers over a woman who has fainted on her back in the middle of the dirt road. The men sacking rice in a milling barn nearby come out to gawk. I linger, but being an outsider, I don't want to intervene. They can't shake her awake so they carry her to the side of the road out of traffic. Everyone is talking and no one appears particularly concerned, although some obviously know her. A man explains that she lives in a small hamlet six miles away and has been looking for work and begging at the market. She was on her way home when she fainted. As the woman comes to, someone floats an idea that one of the young men with motorbikes take her home. They refuse, saying it is too far. The woman attempts to stand up and passes out again. The sun is going down and no one is helping her up. I approach the oldest man present, a senior miller. I hand him some money and ask him to hire a motorbike driver to take her home and buy her some rice and medicine. Instantly, several young men step forward saying they are for hire. A merchant woman returning from market offers to sell her food at a discount.

It is twilight when I get lodging in Hoi An. I dump my gear, shower, and strike out for dinner. Picking a restaurant is no easy task in a city famous for its food. Closer to the riverfront, the houses stand true and strong, well-preserved specimens of antiquity, dating to well over a century and looking like a "spaghetti Eastern" Hong Kong movie set. Weather-stained and aged black, the great beams and wooden awnings of these humble structures were framed together without metal fasteners by long-dead master craftsmen. Row after row of carefully kept homes line the newly paved road like dignified old poets. The inhabitants seem more gentle and happy than in any other Vietnamese town I've yet seen. Just about every house has set up shop selling something, but the air of competition pervasive elsewhere is absent here.

I sniff my way into a restaurant that wafts wonderful, seductive aromas. I take a table next to a lone diner, a German man. As solo travelers often do, we start with a nod, a grin and wind up sharing a table just to talk. Dressed in pressed khaki, expedition grade, he has the looks of a corporate gentleman on safari: grayed hair conservatively but impeccably trimmed; large, soft, pink hands; shrewd, appraising eyes, hazel-gray; substantial girth that suggests good living. He is a wealthy consultant and published writer on corporate management, a lively retiree who is globe-trotting to compile a list of must-see wonders. His local destinations are the Cham ruins not far from town. We gripe about the business ethics of Vietnamese over a seven-course dinner. Foreign companies are required to have Vietnamese partners to do business in Vietnam. The combination of bureaucratic red tape and corruption kills most enterprises within a year. Many small companies find themselves swindled by their own Vietnamese business partners. One foreign businessman I met in Saigon estimated that besides the big conglomerates, nine out of ten joint ventures—not one out of three according to the official government figures—collapse or fail to meet business projections within three years.

As we polish off the meal with fruit tart, flan, and coffee, our twenty-five-year-old chef joins us. He tries to convince us to return, promising exotic creations worthy of our distinguished palates. The local cuisine, of which he is a recognized practitioner, is a strange mix of French, Chinese, and Vietnamese.

"Please, you must come back and try my specialty—Gaping Fish," he bubbles, with barely enough patience for me to translate to my companion, the German epicure. *"It is a dish I learned from a great Chinese*

chef when I went to Canton to study. I can make it with any sauce you want, garlic-lemon-butter, French tomato and mushrooms, or Chinese sweet-and-sour. Anything."

The epicure suggests that I inquire what kind of animal is a gaping fish.

Our chef claps his hands grandly like a magician: *"Any fish you want!"*

"So, it's a recipe?" I ask.

"Yes! Big secret. You see, it's very hard to make. First, I must tell the fisherman that I need the fish alive so he'll keep it in a bucket for me. I take two bamboo sticks that I cut myself. They must be the right thickness and length," he explains, holding his hands eight inches apart. *"I stick them into the fish's mouth, piercing its brain just so. This paralyzes the fish. It is alive but it cannot move. I don't gut it. I heat up oil just right. I put fish in hot oil, vertically so that the head is not in the oil. If the head gets in the oil, the fish dies right away. The fish is paralyzed so it doesn't flip around and splash oil. I don't want to get burned,"* he adds, grinning.

I motion for him to slow down so I can translate. He repeats the sequence again for my benefit, grabbing my arm, reminding me to interpret it correctly. The German epicure looks like he's holding down a hiccup: *Echt? Nein! Wirklich?*

"I cook fish just right. If the oil is too hot, the fish dies too soon. If the oil is not hot enough, not all the meat will be cooked," our chef plows on, mistaking the German's gasps for amazement. *"That's the real hard part. You must know when that is. You must be able to tell if it is about to die. You don't want it to die. Some species of fish are tougher than others, and every fish is different. You must take everything into consideration: How big? When was it caught? Young fish or old fish?"*

"Really? But how can you tell when it's about to die?" I ask, trying not to let my macabre curiosity show. *"It's not flopping around. It's probably not breathing either, once you've put it in the oil."*

"Ah-ha!" he exclaims, poking himself in the eyes. *"You watch the eyes!"*

The epicure and I look at each other, speechless.

Our brilliant chef pauses for effect, one hand poised, a conductor about to plunge into the grand finale. *"I put it on a plate covered with fresh lettuce, pour the sauce of your choice on top."* He pantomimes the act. *"Bring it to your table myself. Then I take the bamboo sticks out. And if the fish doesn't gape,"*—he mouths the gaping part, making O's with his lips—*"if it's dead, you don't pay. Free. On the house. I guarantee you that as you eat the cooked flesh of the fish, it is still alive! Alive and gaping!"*

The epicure's eyes balloon. He's about to hurl all seven courses back onto the table. The chef takes this as an incredulous but interested look, and begins to elaborate on which organs of the fish will be cooked and edible. With a little luck, there might even be a tasty sack of eggs. I clam up. The German crowbars himself out of his seat and declares the evening's revelry at an end. I tell him I might see him out at the Cham ruins tomorrow. A group of young backpackers are sweeping down the street looking for a pub. I wave hello and they invite me along. There are eight of us, but within minutes we double in number. Most of us have seen one another around in other cities. Vietnam is a small country. Tourists keep meeting up with friends they've made along the way. We randomly pick a watering hole and drink all night. The lucky owner is beside himself with joy.

In the morning, I rent a motorbike and ride out thirty miles to My Son to look at the Cham ruins. Six of last night's party join me for the trip. When we get to the village, we immediately discover that a gang of brutes has a vise grip on the tourist trade. They say we are required to pay hefty parking charges and a "foreigners" admission price. We must also hire their tour guide. Fees paid, we are driven by a group of motorbike taxis half a mile to a refreshment concession stand where the drivers dump us and instruct us to purchase overpriced sodas. The vendors take me for a Japanese, so I eavesdrop on them and find out that the gate to the Cham ruins is a hundred yards down the road. I lead the whole group to the gate. Our three "tour guides" follow sheepishly. At the entrance, a gatekeeper tries to extort more from each person.

I find my German epicure sitting on weeded-over stones. He grimaces, greatly vexed by his tour guides. He had paid them a hundred dollars to rent him a car. They took his money, told him at the last minute that the car had broken down, motored him out here on the back of a motorbike. "A worthless pile of brick surrounded by extortionists. The Cham ruins in Thailand are a thousand times better," my German friend grumbles as he stomps off to find his driver for the bumpy hour ride back to town. Our own tour guide doesn't speak more than a dozen words of English. He reads from a notebook every time we come to the remnants of a building. His thick accent is impossible to understand. We split up and wander off on our own. There isn't much left on the two-acre lot, just a few tombs with walls a yard thick to commemorate a historical period spanning a thousand years.

As we leave, we cross another group of tourists coming in, the last group for the day. The gatekeepers are giving them an extraordinarily hard time. A couple of them think it grossly unfair to pay to bring in their cameras even though they promised not to take any pictures. The gatekeepers demand that the photo equipment, in total worth several thousand dollars, must be left at the gate with them. The tourists balk at this suspicious scenario. Six of them, mostly college students, are sitting on the ground eating their sandwiches because the guards demanded fees for food carried past the gate. One Italian girl broke down sobbing at the harassment. I intervene without success. When our group heads back, we take the Italian girl with us. After the drivers drop us back at the diner where we had left our rented motorbikes, they demand tips—this in a country where tipping is an unheard-of notion.

I meet up with Carolyn, an Australian friend I made in Hue. We shack up in the same dormitory and spend a couple of days together touring the town. I rent a 100cc Russian Minsk and roar off with her on the backseat. We zoom around the countryside, trying to get lost, watching peasants work, me serving as her translator. They think we are married. I like touring with Carolyn because she is so openly enamored of the people, choosing to overlook their foibles much more readily than I do. In her company, I like the country more. We go to the beach every day to hang out with the flock of children selling fruit and sodas. They infest the beach like sand fleas and descend in a selling frenzy on every visitor except us, whom they count as friends.

"Vietnamese are so sweet. This country is so rustic. So beautiful," Carolyn sighs, sunbathing on one of Vietnam's most pristine beaches, bemoaning the fact that the country is changing so fast.

I tell her I think most of Vietnam looks in pretty bad shape, like every Third World country.

She disagrees. "We should help them preserve their culture."

"We don't preserve our own culture. We can't. It is a changing thing."

"It's natural to want to preserve beautiful things. I think Vietnam is beautiful."

"Perhaps," I say, "that's because your images are not wearing their rags."

C h i - M i n h

38 Chi survived fourteen years on the street. Once a battered teenage runaway, Chi came home at thirty-one,
a post-operative transsexual. She was a man and his
name was Minh. Everyone was surprised, but no
one was shocked. Minh had called ahead and Mom
arranged for all of us to be home for his reception. Huy came home
from Berkeley, Tien from San Jose State University, Hien from UC
San Diego, me from my crosstown studio, where I was living with my
girlfriend, Trieu.

"I remember you bigger. Taller," I said to Minh when he came
home, our arms about each other trying unsuccessfully for a hug.

He laughed, a husky man-laugh, his voice deeper than mine. "The
last time I saw you, An, you were a head shorter than me. Now you're
half a head taller than me."

We duked, jived, joking, hiding the strangeness inside us. I tried
looking him in the eyes, but it was hard. His maleness blocked my
view. Talking around his void of history, which we were too willing
to oblige, he seemed no more than a stout, easygoing guy with a real
blue-collar aura about him that I liked. A potbelly in the making kept
him adjusting his pants. His fleshy digits, labor callused, said he was
very nervous, tapping rhythm, wiping the thighs of his slacks.

"Oh, God. It's been so long," I said, but meaning I missed you for so long I'd forgotten you existed.

"You're a big engineer now, An," he said with genuine admiration.

I searched his face for jealousy, but found nothing unkind. He harbored no grudge against me, who had stayed and benefited. I was an undeserving runner-up who won the trophy due to a technicality. He was the true winner, who conceded the prize with the greatest of grace.

"And you, Huy," he said, grabbing him by the shoulder. "You're going to be a lawyer. Tien and Hien are going to be doctors. What are you going to be, Kay?"

She smiled shyly, having no recollection of this stranger-sibling who had changed her diapers. "Don't know. I'm only a freshman. Maybe advertising or something."

I sat back watching, wondering why it sounded so corny—everything uttered. The awkward patting, friendly shoulder slugs exchanged in place of embraces. Why are we spieling these empty words? Where are the tears of joy? Isn't there something important we're leaving out? I can feel it and if we don't say it now, it will never be said. We were filling all those vanished years with small talk.

Mom and Father were on the sofa, supervising. On the coffee table, a pot of tea and biscuits attended this halting family reunion, formalizing the role of each party. What is the proper etiquette for welcoming home a lost son–daughter?

Mom was smiling, and so was Father, except he had his puzzled, hurt look in his eyes. I thought I also saw a touch of pride in his demeanor. They were talking to Minh in Vietnamese. Although Minh was recently laid off in the massive aerospace and defense industry downsizing, Father must have been pleased that his runaway was now a professional welder with a home. Minh had told Mom over the phone that he was married and that his wife didn't know about his sex change. Their marriage had been on the rocks since his layoff. It was inevitable: She wanted children. They were getting a divorce. Everyone seemed accepting if not entirely comfortable with Minh in place of Chi, but no one knew what to make of his troubled marriage and the secret at its heart.

"I'm glad I came home," Minh said. But we all should have known that home was one place to which no one could return, not after so many empty years.

And now, with Minh gone from us, my greatest regret is our failure to make sense of those missing years. While he was with us, we left his personal history dormant, boxed in this new shell, this new being we didn't comprehend. Minh didn't like going into the details of his life as a runaway and a transient, and, only too gladly, we didn't press him. The vague sketch of Minh's life I gleaned during my brief time with him seems trivial, more a testament to my stony core than anything attributable to him.

After Chi escaped the juvenile detention center, she ran away to San Francisco and reverted to her true self. A man. He traveled as Minh, sleeping on the street and eating out of Dumpsters until a Chinese family took him in and fed him. They found him work in a Chinatown sweatshop among illegal Chinese aliens. Wages were dismal, and underground life was marginal and harsh. There was the constant fear of being caught. When Minh was eighteen, he hit the road, this time as a migrant worker. Seasons later, he arrived in Montana, where he earned a living as a ranch hand, doing whatever he could find. Moving among America's illegal workforce, he learned to buy false papers and eventually bribed himself into an assembly-line job in Detroit's auto industry.

After two years, he was laid off. Jobless and alone, he found himself pining for companionship, someone to whom he could relate. His halting English and double identity isolated him more than the color of his skin. He heard there was a place in California where many Vietnamese congregated, a mini-city where a Vietnamese could live and work without ever having to speak a single word of English. He packed up and migrated south to the smoggy sun of Orange County.

While working as a welder for an aerospace company in Long Beach, California, he fell in love with a Vietnamese-American woman. Minh introduced himself as a man. Soon a love blossomed and it became too precious for Minh, who knew loneliness all too well to risk telling her the truth. It was too late. Minh's life, whether by necessity or circumstances, had been a chain of deception, and the truth could not emerge from him. With his well-paid job and loans, Minh bought a house and finally went under the knife for a sex-change operation—a secret that his soon-to-be bride never discovered. He was now, in all respects, a man. They got married—without the blessings of her family, who deemed Minh's station, a welder, beneath their long line of physicians and degreed professionals. True to the in-laws' dire predictions, Minh couldn't find employment when he lost his job in the massive aerospace belly-up. Their new house rolled onto its second mortgage and the bills piled up on top of the secret Minh was hiding from his wife.

They sold the house, settled outstanding debts, and finalized their divorce. Minh came home to his lost family and plunked down five thousand dollars to enroll at a cosmetology school, seeking to make sense of his life. Six months later, Grandma Le leaked, *"He's not showing up in class. Every day, he goes to those Vietnamese cafés and spends all his money tipping pretty waitresses."*

Minh was lonely. The fanfare of his homecoming petered out quickly. Huy and Hien were away in college. Tien was living at home, overloaded with a full college courseload and work. I was across town, too engrossed in my own life to be any good to anyone. There was no one to help him patch the holes in his life.

"Minh's a Tiger!" exclaimed Mom, as though it explained all the difficulties. *"Her father is a Rat. I am a Dragon. Air, Water, and Fire in one house is bad. Her living here will bring trouble. It will be the undoing of our house. I cannot allow that. I cannot allow it."*

For the second time in his life, Minh went to live with Grandma Le, who had come to America with Uncle Hung and his wife, all sponsored by Auntie Dung. Grandma was living on the goodwill of her son and daughter-in-law. Minh soon fell into disfavor with Uncle Hung and his wife. After a season, Minh moved into a boarding-house. During these listless months, he called his ex-wife in an attempt to reconcile. He went on binges and flew down to Southern California to find her, but she was through with him. Her family shielded her, boarding her with relatives whenever he came back in town.

"I don't know. I'm just trying to get things together," Minh said in the weeks before Christmas. In retrospect, all the signs of his imminent suicide were there in front of us, but we chose to ignore them. He'll weather this storm, we kept reassuring ourselves. He's Vietnamese, a survivor. He must walk through this fire alone. It'll make him a better person for it.

After receiving some money as Christmas presents, Minh took a taxi to San Jose Airport and flew to Orange County to find his ex-wife. He lingered until his money ran out. It was his last attempt and it failed. Broke and brokenhearted, he returned on New Year's Eve to Grandma's, where his uncle and aunt put him up temporarily in the spare room. Three days later, Minh took his life with a yellow nylon rope tied to the bedroom rafters. At thirty-two, he died the most Vietnamese of deaths, a brokenhearted suicide. His father cut him down from the ceiling while his mother and grandmother wept. And his family, who could not love him while he lived, grieved his passing. His ashes were scattered on the sea he never finished crossing.

Fever-Ride

39 Predawn. My stomach feels queasy, gray like fungus. I lie in bed drowning at the prospect of starting the longest ride of my life. The sheet is soaked with sweat, chilly in spots. I'm a little feverish. From what, I don't know. Maybe I caught something here. This is the dirtiest, foulest dump I've ever seen.

Last night, I tossed the blanket, a cigarette-pocked rag, into the bathroom, a partitioned corner with a floor drain. I was cold, but the blanket reeked so badly I was tempted to burn it. Some drunk must have vomited on it. It was crusty like a dirty old sock. The ceiling fan, however, made certain that air circulated evenly throughout the room. At last, when I could no longer bear it, I threw the blanket and the pancaked pillow into the hallway. I lay down in two layers of clothes, my head on a jacket, and listened to the couple in the next room "thrashing rice stalks." I could smell her sugary perfume. The dividing wall fell a foot short of the ceiling and air passed back and forth like breaths between mouths of lovers. I squashed an urge to stand on a chair and have a peek. In the middle of the night, my bowels started doing the tango. I raced down the hallway, flashlight in one hand, roll of toilet paper in the other. The latrine—an eight-inch hole in a slab of concrete—was hidden deep behind a series of corridors and two flights of stairs. This, after all, was Hotel No. 1 of Quang Ngai City.

It was a raw deal, considering last evening I was dead certain that I was to be an honored guest in a traditional Vietnamese home, my hosts two college students. It seemed very promising because, as usual, the grandest building I saw when I passed through town belonged to the Tax Bureau and the two students I met on the road told me their father was a tax official. As they motored alongside me, we struck up a lively conversation over fifteen miles and they insisted that I spend the night at their home. Hosting foreigners was a big hassle for Vietnamese. The host was required to take his guest's identification to the nearest constable, who might not be very near. The registration process could take hours and might also need a little monetary lubrication. So I asked them if they were sure. They were, and we went seven miles beyond the city, most of it off-road. I earned the entire distance, miserably churning through red mud. It was a beautiful, rustic hamlet. We drank tea and waited until twilight when their father came home. During the formal chat required between host and guest, I had a feeling he didn't want a Viet-kieu in his house because it might not look proper to his colleagues. It took him half an hour to say so, but he said it at last: *"I'm sorry, but I think you will be happier in a hotel. It is much trouble—the paperwork, you see—for you to stay here."* To which I replied, through a cordial smile, *"Ah, but, you see, Uncle, I'm not very happy riding ten kilometers back to town in the dark."* As I expected, he put on his official face, the stony eyes: *"Really, Brother, I insist the hotels in town are better for you. There is no room here for you to sleep."*

And this was very rude because, customarily, Vietnamese are the greatest hosts. They would sell the family's pig to feed a guest. The entire family would sooner sleep on the ground than let their guest go without a good blanket. This was not lost on the two young men, who sat silently, their gazes downcast in great shame, a deep flush burning their faces. Their father started to name the hotels in town. Hungry and tired, I felt an uncharitable urge to piss him off. I could have gone on, but for their sake I didn't. I thanked their father and left. They trailed after me, begging pardon profusely under their breath. I clasped their shoulders. *"It is all right, my friends. I understand. I know when you are older, when you become established, your world will be different. Thank you for the invitation. It was your kindness that counts. Maybe we will meet again."*

The ride back to town was tortuous and the night passed badly in this cheap hotel.

I get out of bed, stumble downstairs, order a bowl of noodles, a shot of Vietnamese dripped espresso, and four egg sandwiches. I buy sweet rice from a woman selling breakfast from a basket. Then I'm off in the metal-gray dawn, jazzed at the challenge of 110 miles of hilly roads to Qui Nhon.

In Oregon, I'd hauled 90 mountainous coastal miles against a 20 m.p.h. head wind with a fully loaded bike. In Japan, I'd climbed and descended mountains in freezing rain. The distance didn't worry me; however, the combination of a sore crotch, roiling intestines, a mild fever, a hemorrhoid-in-the-making, and a quickly thinning pocket-book does wonders for my confidence.

I crunch through the morning, taking a ten-minute break every hour-and-a-half in the saddle. The scene zooms by without my taking much stock because the road, looping over rolling hills, is god-awful with potholes. Scattered every few miles on the side of the road are thatched lean-tos, roughly the size of a desk propped up by two front legs. A boy, sometimes a man, curls up like a dog, out of the sun's fury, selling live crabs tied up in bunches like bananas. Occasionally, he dips the crabs into the water of the rice paddies to keep them alive. In the most arid part of the country, where the soil is chalky, the peasants turn to *tep* farming, transforming the landscape into a surreal grid of rectangular ditches, a quarter of an acre each, maybe ten feet deep, filled with muddy gray water. Men drag fine nylon nets through these ponds for tiny, translucent shrimp no larger than newsprint. Women spread the catch out along the side of the road—the national highway—to dry in the sun and to mix freely with dirt, bugs, and dung. The masses of shrimp smell strangely sweet and briny, looking like giant sheets of lint from laundry dryers. Once dried, the shrimp are fermented into a paste with an unbelievably offensive odor. People use it for cooking. A powerfully pungent condiment, a tablespoon of this paste is sufficient to flavor a two-gallon pot of soup.

It is a visually engaging country, but in my sorry state, I have little mind for sight-seeing. I merely hunch down and chug at the pedals. Around noon, a half-inch nail pops my thorn-resistant inner tube. I push the bike onto a three-foot-wide levy dividing two rice paddies and start patching the puncture when my stomach cramps up. Nearby a peasant woman, well into the third trimester of her pregnancy, is wading calf-deep in the paddy and fertilizing the young stalks by hand, a basket of manure wedged against one hip. She sees my pained, urgent look and the roll of toilet paper in my hand. She gestures at a clutch of bushes a hundred yards off. I wave thanks and hobble away. As I squat, a group of children materialize out of nowhere—something I encountered unfailingly the length of the country. They gather around me at a disrespectful distance and just watch. The expectant mother chases them off.

I try eating another egg sandwich, retch, and throw the rest of it to the birds. To stabilize my digestive tract, I've been averaging three egg sandwiches every day for the last week. At the next village, a bike mechanic burns a patch onto the tire while I eat fried rice his wife has cooked. For the rest of the afternoon, I alternate between hot and cold flashes, but the strange thing is, the harder I push, the better I feel.

The sun is straddling the mountains behind me by the time I squeak into Qui Nhon, dead tired. I've been eating road dirt so long, all these towns, big and small, look the same to me. Some smell worse than others, and they are all filthy. I crisscross Qui Nhon, going from hotel to hotel, looking for a reasonable deal. After an hour, I settle for Dong Hoi Hotel. It is built like a prison, no outfacing windows. Each room is a cell, with bars on the windows. All windows face inward to the hallway. There is a mess hall on the first floor. Sitting on the long benches, you can look up and see four stories of rails and barred windows.

On the way to my room, the woman fetches me my allotment of goodies: a moth-eaten blanket with a stain that might have been a copious amount of blood, a half roll of toilet paper, coarse and spongy like decoration party ribbons, and a tall thermos. She gives me a word of wisdom concerning the two liters of hot water: *"Use some water for bathing and save some for tea."*

"I biked almost two hundred kilometers today," I mention casually, trying not to brag.

"Hmm," she replies without opening her mouth. She puts the sheet and pillowcase on the bed without making them.

"Took me nine hours. The longest distance I've ever ridden a bicycle."

"Hmm . . . This is the toilet." She opens the bathroom door.

"I'm tired but I could use a beer."

"The diner downstairs has beer and food." With that, she leaves. The invitation for a drink dies in my throat.

The room stinks. I want to celebrate with somebody. Anybody. Cockroaches the size of Medjool dates scamper across the floor. Benevolently, I let them live. The two-inch mattress is covered with parchy linen. I turn on the ceiling fan. It creaks ominously on an unstable axle. Any moment, it can come down on my head like a whirling scythe. I open the window, but this doesn't help much since it looks into the hallway. The woman returns and, standing in the corridor, wordlessly shuts my window from the outside. I am trapped in a puke-green room. The plaster peels off the wall in sheets, revealing cement and bricks.

I go out to start my evening of revelry with tapas of jerked-liver salad in someone's living room turned into a three-table eatery. Perching myself on a footstool, I slug down a 333 Beer, chase it with a Coke. The proprietor, whose two toddlers are playing with my shoelaces, delivers my extra-large plate of julienned green papaya layered with smoked liver, pork jerky, crushed peanuts, and chopped fresh basil, all doused with a vinegary, chili soy sauce. A Vietnamese opera wails from a Sony boom box. Three high school girls cascade around the coffee table next to me, and launch into a series of excited whispers-giggles with glances in my direction. I am still in T-shirt and cycling tights, which must look suspiciously like pantyhose to them.

I feel woozy. With several thousand miles of touring beneath my belt, I know that unless I get something substantial in my stomach, tomorrow will be a very bad day. I bid the proprietor good-bye, and elicit another round of giggles from the girls with my Lycra-clad butt. Downtown at a Buddhist kitchen, I pack in a five-course dinner, hoping a vegetarian meal will help me feel better.

Back at the hotel, I meet up with two British gents, the only other foreigners staying in the hotel, all of us on the same floor. One complains bitterly that a woman working the hotel grabbed his crotch, the other is mortified that a young girl, barely eighteen, has just grabbed his bum. Dead tired, I bid them good night, crawl to my room, and crash onto the bed. Crushed. Totally sapped. Everything aches. The day's exhaustion falls on me like a boulder. The room is stale with mildew. I open the window shutters to let in some air, then go into the bathroom to mix a bath with the complimentary thermos of hot water. This makes about two gallons of tepid water. A rat pokes its head up the floor drain. I put a bucket over it.

It feels like a maniac is tenderizing my gut with an ice pick. I get on the toilet just in time as my gut empties itself. It keeps coming. My insides turn inside out. I'm being eviscerated. I look down and watch my heart emptying into the toilet bowl. I am feverish but covered in gooseflesh. My head throbs. Few things will put the fear of God into me as effectively as seeing blood gushing out where it shouldn't.

I wash up, towel off, bundle up, and snivel to the only chair in the room. The windows are shut again. That sweet front-desk woman. I wonder if I ought to go look for a doctor. It is nearing midnight and any effort to get medical attention at this hour is going to be exorbitant, something my funds can't handle if I am to make it back to Saigon. As I deliberate between life and money, a faint scratching noise comes from the other side of my door. The doorknob turns slowly. The door is pushed inward. It creaks and stops against the dead bolt I'd slid in place. I hear whispers. Silently, without getting up, I reach through the iron grill and latch the window shutters. Again, someone tries the door with no better result. More whispering. Silence. Metallic noises. Whispering. The shutters are tried. Finally, a soft knock on my door. A female voice, low and seductive: "Yoohooo. Hello. Please open. Hello. Please open. Yoohooo."

I half hope they will go away and half wish I had the strength to answer them. It is the rumor I heard among the tourists that worries me: a prostitute sneaks into a foreigner's room and insists that he engage her services. If he refuses, she strips and yells. A policeman conveniently happens to be in the vicinity of the hallway. He barges into the room and arrests the foreigner for consorting with a prostitute. The only alternative to a night in jail is a stiff fine, anywhere from fifty dollars to three hundred dollars, payable immediately.

"Yoo-hoo. Open. You open please. Yoo-hoo."

I want to at least open the shutters and talk to them, but I can barely stand. After a few minutes of "Yoo-hoo," door rattling, and window prying, they must have thought me dead asleep. Footsteps recede from my door. I hear them trying the same tactic on the other rooms. Ten minutes later, they are back at my door, whining. "Please, mister, open. We friend. Yoo-hoo, please open. We cheap, very cheap."

This morning is worse than the last. I sweat in my sleeping bag, unable to move. The rooster—the damnable omnipotent rooster—is nothing but an edible snooze alarm. I vow to eat one first chance I get. When I manage to throw my feet onto the floor, I go directly to the toilet and enjoy another bout of bloody diarrhea. The water in the toilet bowl is so dark with blood I can't see whether there are maggots in my stool. I fall back in bed. I am going to die. Perhaps something is eating me from the inside.

Two hours later, I clomp downstairs. The receptionist directs me to the closest pharmacist. There is always a long wait at the nurse's station, she explains; besides, the pharmacist is very good and can probably fix any digestive problem. The instant I step outside, a cyclo driver peels away from the pack scamming the street and tails me down the sidewalk.

"Oy, oy, Brother. Can I take you somewhere? See some sights? Go to the beach? Restaurant? Shopping?"

"No, thank you. I'm just going around the corner."

"Where?"

"The pharmacy."

"You want to ride in my cyclo?"

"No, thank you."

"Are you sick?"

I wish he would vanish. It is enough merely to keep my bowels in check as I walk. *"No,"* I blurt, rude enough for anyone but him. When I enter the one-counter pharmacy, he invites himself in as well, crowding over my shoulder.

"This Viet-kieu is sick," he proclaims to the woman at the counter.

I turn around and look him in the eyes. *"Please, I can take care of this myself. Do you need some medicine? You can go first. I'll wait."*

"No, no. You go right ahead."

The woman asks me what I need and I tell her that I have a severe stomachache and a fever.

"You have blood in your stool?" he asks me.

"Please!" I snap at him. *"Do you mind? I am talking to her. I don't want to discuss my problem with you. Could you please go outside?"*

He looks at me with incomprehension. I stare him down. He turns to the pharmacist, who regards both of us with mild amusement. She intervenes on my behalf: *"He means that he would like to talk to me in private. Please wait in the street with your cyclo."*

He drags his feet out, a child sent to his room, looking back over his shoulder in case either one of us has a change of heart.

I sigh and, in a whisper, relay my symptoms to the pharmacist. She asks about the shape and size of my stool. I look over my shoulder. The cyclo driver is lurking six feet behind, ears trained on our conversation.

"It's dysentery, I tell you," he says, directing his advice to the pharmacist.

She gives me a fistful of multicolored pills—a four-day course of medication, twice a day, seven different pills each time. I have no idea what they are. She tells me to stay away from rice and meat. The cyclo driver shouts from the sidewalk, *"Tell him to drink young coconut milk."* The entire course of medication, including the cyclo man's advice, is three dollars.

I take the medication. Because I am angry, angry at the weakness of my body, angry at everything, I get on my bike and leave town. To hell with dysentery and fever. I am a survivor.

Fallen-Leaves

A piney smell of plywood, baked by a desert sun. Heat waving down like mist. A steamy wetness of sweat trapped indoors. Flies lazing through the air, dodging the sweep of the electric fan.

An counted the dark eyes and whorls in the plywood, imagining monkeys and monsters. The hotness made his head thick. It was barely past noon, but he had already drunk three Coca-Colas. His mother had weaned him from his bottles of imported baby formula with Cokes. Maybe, she thought, these American things made him plump and troublesome. When he was three, he ate so much she rushed him to the hospital to have his stomach pumped. Last week when she left him at home with the maid, he set a chair on fire. Yesterday, he opened doors and upset clients. The day before, the new girl found him in her room, under her table. Today Anh locked him in the chain-link cage with her. She had the cook bring him the new item on the menu, a big favorite with the GIs.

Women came to the window of the cage, chatted with his mother through the wire mesh, and waved at him, smiling. They gave his mother money—rent, they called it. Anh put the rent on the table next to the bar-cash, the restaurant-cash, and the cabaret-cash, mounting, heaping great big blocks of bills like bricks—a mason laying a foundation. The swiveling fan feathered the bills, exhaling a greasy paper smell into the cubicle.

Tallying cash with the ease of shuffling cards, Anh asked her first son why he didn't like his pizza, an imported delicacy. He made a face and said it was too sour.

An wanted to know whose mountain of paper it was. She told him it was theirs. He wanted to know what she was going to do with it.

Anh said, My son, this money will take you abroad to study. In America you will become a great engineer.

Coca-Cola

In eight months of biking, I drink two or three cans of Coke a day, enough to carbonate my blood for the rest of my life. The caffeine picks me up and keeps me from succumbing to the midday low. The sugar gives me just enough energy to boost the heavy bike over the big hills. The carbonation burns the road grit off the back of my throat. The familiar flavor keeps me anchored in strange locales. The wavy red-and-white logo tells me America has been here.

Coke banners have displaced the Vietnamese flag. You can buy a Coke every five miles from Hanoi to Ho Chi Minh City. It's everywhere, sold by the case in markets as well as by the can in shacks with a six-pack inventory. At sixty cents a can, it is as dear as a third of a laborer's daily wage. Coke—or Koh-ka as Vietnamese pronounce it—is a special refreshment, reserved for special events such as first dates and wedding banquets.

Somewhere along an arid, scrubby stretch of land, I spot a thatched hut with a faded Pepsi flag out front, and a case of Cokes displayed on the windowsill. The noon sun has licked me dry. My mouth is a dusty crack. I pull over, lean my bike against a post, and waddle into the hut.

On a packed-earth floor, three soldiers in olive uniforms with red stripes are crouching on footstools around a coffee table. Their conversation breaks and they look up at me with liquor-shot eyes, their chopsticks hovering above plates of boiled gizzards curly like cashews, pig hearts sliced like truffles, intestines chopped up like rigatoni. The centerpiece is a basket of herbs sided by a pile of ivory garlic cloves. One man who is eating from a bowl of raw, coagulated blood pudding glares at me, the blood dribbling from his scruffy mustache. The still tobacco air pulsates with the sweet bite of raw spices, boiled innards, and home-brewed rice wine the men have burped up over hours of drinking. Hands braced on the table, they sit with their knees up near their ribs, three hyenas tearing into the ruptured belly of a deer.

Instinctively I nod, showing respect for their uniforms. A man growls something unintelligible into his cup.

In the far corner, a woman squats on her haunches, slicing boiled cow tongue on a wooden plank. She stops, alert at the abrupt silence, and, seeing me, tenses. *"What do you want?"* she asks by way of greeting.

"Hello, Older Sister. How are you?"

"Well. What do you want?"

"May I have a cold Coca-Cola?"

"We don't have cold ones. I can give you ice."

I couldn't drink their ice. *"Could you put a can in the ice cooler for me? I'll rest a bit first, then I'll drink it."*

She looks me over, pauses, then nods without a word. Relieved that she didn't take my request as an insult, I beat a hasty retreat to a seat outside. One of the men mumbles that the fucker at the door is a Viet-kieu. Can't drink our ice, says another, too dirty for him. I groan inwardly, wondering if this pit stop is such a good idea after all. They begin to grouse about Viet-kieu in general. Dread settles in my stomach as I remember the mob that nearly lynched me in Ham Tan.

While I debate with my thirst whether to leave, a dust devil kicks up across the street and scares a skinny dog. It whimpers and scoots inside the hut. A drinker flings it a piece of organ meat. The mutt noses the morsel then curls up at the other end of the room, leaving the scrap uneaten. A revelatory silence washes the hut. A humiliating moment. They see me witnessing their shame. The woman hurriedly resumes her chopping, contriving a screen for us all.

"Goddamn dog!" the man with the bloody mustache hisses at the dog, but looks at me.

Another man puts down his chopsticks and leans back away from the food, trying to hide his embarrassment. Glances shoot back and forth. Colors deepen on their faces. Having invaded their world and witnessed their disgrace, I avert my eyes as casually as I can. But, too late, I almost hear their minds shifting gear.

"Three cans of Coca-Cola," Bloody-Mustache shouts to the woman. I feel sick. It has come down to this.

"Fuck! Bring us the Coca-Cola now!" another voice seconds.

The proprietor is firm. *"You can't afford it. How about more rice wine?"*

"Shut up, sister. If we want your advice, we'll ask. Just bring the Coca-Cola."

"With ice," another man adds.

"Please, no," she replies, not yielding ground. *"You owe me 22,000 dong for this session already and you haven't paid your tab this month. No money, no Coca-Cola."*

The man wails, *"I get paid next week! You know I'm good for it!"*

"You already owe me most of it." Army grunts earn $120 a year, and most of their earnings go to rice wine.

"Fuck this place. Fuck you, Sister. Fuck you for serving a Viet-kieu a Coca-Cola and not us. Fuck you!" the man brays.

They rattle the hut with gusts of *"FUCK YOU!"* and *"FUCK YOUR MOTHER!"* and *"BITCH!"*

"Let's get out of here. We don't have to take this crap from her," Bloody-Mustache shouts to his companions and they stagger out of the hut.

My thought of hightailing out of the joint perishes with the sound of their stools clattering on the dirt. What a gamble: my neck for a soda, one measly Coke, which I drank all my life without thinking. The one American thing touted throughout Vietnam. The only token of America the commoner can almost afford.

In an instant, they surround me, each one a goner, tomato-faced and intoxicated to the hilt. Two weave uncertainly on their feet. I avoid their eyes, oddly noting the state of the Vietnamese army: threadbare uniforms and cheap brown army–issue plastic sandals. They have dark bony chicken feet.

"You think you're better than us, don't you," spits Bloody-Mustache.

The roughest and tallest of the bunch, Cross-eyed, is about my height. He sneers, *"Fucking traitor. Fucking Viet-kieu. You raped the country, then you fled to America. You . . . you American pet. Now you come back rich. America pays off traitors well, don't they?"*

I stifle an urge to knock his teeth in. I don't reply. It doesn't matter, they are going to give me what they think I deserve anyway. This Viet-kieu is going to pay for all his treasonous privileges. What the soldiers say aren't mere drunken words. They carry weight, seemingly steeped in the sentiment of too many Vietnamese, things I've heard obliquely in conversations, between the pauses where people reevaluate their words before uttering them.

I watch them looming over me, coiling myself for the inevitable. I could take any one of them if I strike first, maybe two given their drunken state. But three against one are terrible odds, not to mention the trouble I'll get from the local cops, win or lose.

"Speak up, bastard! You think you're too good to talk to us?"

I raise a placating hand. *"I'm just thirsty. I don't want any trouble."*

My reassurance is lost on them. It seems the fight had been started a long time ago by someone else. Two decades ago. But slights, real or imagined, between brothers are not easily forgotten. Now, with alcohol to wash away civility and reason, the undercurrent is clear on the breath of these men, who may have been my classmates in our schoolboy days.

"I could have gone to America, too," blurts the soldier to my left, a string bean of a man who I figure is the least dangerous of the lot. *"My sister went with her husband, but I stayed because of my parents. Because this is my country! My country, not yours!"*

Cross-eyed spits the words at me: *"Go home, Viet-kieu! You don't belong here."*

Bloody-Mustache lurches forward. I jump aside, fists cocked for a swing. The man crumbles to his knees and vomits, splattering the ground with bits of boiled intestines and liver and flecks of green herbs, whole sprigs of cilantro and mint leaves barely chewed. The hot ground steams his gastric juices. He retches, wetting his chest, tries to stand up, slips and falls on his own puke. His friends lift him off the dirt.

A voice rings with disgust from across the street: *"Indulge to one's capacity, not to one's greed."* An old proverb.

Bloody-Mustache spins on the speaker, a soldier in uniform: *"Shut your mouth!"*

The soldier snickers. Two more men come out of the diner across the street. The three of them chortle at the drunks. The first man wags a finger at Bloody-Mustache. *"You should shut your own mouth or you'll vomit up your wages."*

"Fuck your mother!"

Cross-eyed jumps into the exchange: *"Mind your own business, fool."*

The man chuckles. *"Mind yourself. Look at you all. You're a disgrace to your uniforms."*

"You shut up or I'll break your head!" howls Bloody-Mustache, at the limit of his tolerance.

"Vomit-face, you break my head? Ha! What a bunch of losers."

Cross-eyed shrieks, the cords jumping out of his neck, *"Coward, come here and say it to my face!"*

The solider shrugs and saunters across the street, his two buddies closing behind. The drunks charge and a six-man brawl erupts in the middle of the national highway. Fists fly, thudding into faces. They kick each other sloppily, looking absurd in their plastic flip-flops.

With a nod to the shopkeeper, I hop on my bike. *"Thank you, Sister, but I won't need that Coca-Cola."*

She bobs her head vigorously. *"Go. Go quickly, Brother."*

I pour everything I have into the pedals, then summon more. One, two. One, two. Steady hammering strokes. Something hot burns in the pit of me and keeps the chain humming on the highest gear. The asphalt blurs by, and within a few breaths I fly beyond the village, cutting across the cornfields, heading home, wherever that is.

Brother-Brother

"An, I called Huy in Berkeley yesterday to tell him to come home for Thanksgiving," Mom told me in her high-pitched catastrophic voice. "That Laura girl answer the phone! You know, that punk-rock girl with the nose ring and purple hair. She's living there in his apartment! You tell him I don't want him involve with her. You tell him, he should not live with her!"

"Mom, Huy is not sleeping with her," I said gently. "He's sleeping with Sean."

"WHAT?! What you mean?"

"He's gay . . . likes boys."

"You shut up! Don't talk ridiculous!"

"I'm serious. He's gay."

We were standing in her kitchen next to the fridge. I could tell the news startled her badly so I decided not to venture on to Hien's homosexuality. We all had discussed at length how to break the news to the folks. The family was still grieving Minh's suicide and each one of us was dealing with it in his own way. Tired of his closet, Huy wanted to come clean with our parents. Mom wrung the hand cloth, looking at the wall. She didn't say a word for minutes. I could hear chopsticks rattling in her head, calculating, gauging the omens, scheming.

"An, you tell him Laura is a nice girl. I like her. He should date her. Bring her home for dinner."

Huy showed up for Thanksgiving dinner with Sean. They looked so similar it was almost incestuous. They were both tall, lanky with preppy-boy buzz cuts: blue jeans, white T-shirts, and suede shoes. Four-eyed all around. Mom and Father received Sean warmly, treating him just like another one in the long succession of guy "friends" Huy dragged home on vacation from college.

Mom and Father gave up on the turkey they could never get right. Thanksgiving at the folks' had degenerated to an international pot-luck. Huy and Sean brought Chinese honeyed walnut prawns and chive dumplings. Kay's boyfriend, Trinh, brought Vietnamese yam-and-shrimp fritters with fishsauce. Father made his classic split-pea-and-ham soup, another hideous newspaper recipe. I made a pot roast. Hien showed up with fruit tarts and ice cream. He didn't invite his boyfriend because they weren't at *that* stage yet. Tien brought antipasto and wine. His girlfriend, Ann, provided half a pound of French pâté. As always, Mom steamed a pot of rice.

Father had stopped saying grace over Thanksgiving dinner a long time ago. We all knew he was an atheist who on his best days might venture to admit he had agnostic inclinations. Eventually, the table conversation turned to each of our personal lives. Mom wanted to know about mine and Huy's marriage prospects.

"I'm very different from An and Tien," Huy said, piling his plate with food. Hien just looked on, nowhere near coming out to his family.

"How's your nice friend Laura?" Mom asked Huy, switching to Vietnamese because she was serious but trying not to let it show.

"She's fine. She's not at my apartment anymore. She was just staying until she found her own place."

"Ah," Mom murmured, clearly disappointed. Father concentrated on his food. He could be very deaf when he wanted.

Tien, Kay, and I were grinning tightly, trying not to laugh. Poor Sean began to sweat.

"How did you boys become friends?" Mom probed with a straight face.

Huy and Sean exchanged glances. Sean replied, *"We met at a party."*
"You play sports together? Huy likes tennis."
"Oh, yes, Huy and I play tennis."
"Ah, you and Huy are good friends," Mom concluded, not wanting a confirmation. *"Best school buddies. Tennis partners. That's good."*

Huy had told me he was gay a couple of months before Thanksgiving. It was right after his college graduation. He took me out to lunch, steak fajitas at a local cantina. At Huy's instruction, the waitress kept the margaritas coming. I was fairly toasted by the time he hit me with: "An, I'm gay."

I looked at him, trying to reconcile what he was saying. Huy was a great practical joker, but something about his demeanor, a touch of fear maybe, told me he wasn't kidding. Because I didn't know what else to say, I patted him on the shoulder and said, "Okay, Huy. I'm okay with it."

He looked so relieved I had no idea he had been that worried about how I would react. He heaved a big sigh and we sat there measuring each other over the salt-crusted rims of our goblets. It was brave of him. Minh's death had given him that. I realized Huy was making his peace with everyone.

We began to talk haltingly, the conversation forced. I asked him whether he had ever been with a woman. He said he was never interested. Not even once? Never. But all those girls hanging around you, Huy. All those opportunities. They were crazy about your starving-artist looks and your dimples. He shrugged and said girls didn't turn him on. Why don't you just try? I asked. He smiled knowingly at me: Why don't you try a guy?

I was discovering my brother for the first time. His life came out one secret at a time.

"I've been gay all my life, Mister An. Ever since I was a kid. As long as I can remember."

I saw him all over again: the four-eyed boy who ate his Froot Loops cereal with a toothpick; the fifth-grader addicted to Chinese salty-sour dried plums, who saved the pits so he could suck on them later; the straight-A high school senior who, on a Friday night, wept at his desk, tear-smearing his SAT course work, because Father forbade him to go to the biggest seniors' party of the semester—*Why, the SAT exam is only two months away, you must study! I won't let you ruin your education like your brother An, who couldn't even get into UC Berkeley! He got only one lousy scholarship.*

"You know, Huy, I'm sorry I screwed things up for you guys. Father came down hard on you."

"It's okay," Huy said generously. "Dad meant well. I'm successful. I had my fun in college."

We talked a long time. We settled the bill and tipped our waitress so she could go home, then started another bar tab. He walked me through his "gay history." He lectured me on his community's terminology. Gay sex. Anal sex. Top. Bottom. Rice queens. Potato queens. The joy of oral sex. He even offered to give me the number of a famous gay practitioner of this art—reciprocation not expected. *No woman could possibly know more about a penis than a man. Just close your eyes.*

"You know, my roommate is gay," Huy said.

"Ray? Good looking, Speedo model, *GQ* cover-boy Ray?"

"Ultragay. He thinks you're decent looking."

"Oh, yeah?" Oddly, I was somewhat flattered. "Really. Cool."

Huy rolled his eyes and snorted, "Well, don't get a big head, Mr. An."

"I could take that three ways."

We laughed. It felt very good talking plainly to each other.

Father-Son

"Prostitutes," Father said to me. "I should have taken Huy and Hien to prostitutes. Your uncles urged me but I didn't listen. Now it's too late; they're gay."

His favorite adage had come to haunt him: *When you're young, you go looking for trouble. When you're old, trouble comes looking for you.* He was forever mulling over his thousand woes, whipping himself for every wrong turn he'd made, wondering how he could have changed each of our lives for the better. A long time after Chi had died, Father was facing retirement and was petrified of it. He confessed to me: "I don't think I can retire. I must work, be busy until the day I die. My mind cannot rest, because I am a man of regrets."

We were sitting in the living room at 2 a.m. in the months immediately before I left on my bicycle. Warm milk for him. A beer for me. The television on mute, splashing our faces blue. The world asleep, everything silent. These were the parameters of our father-son communication, for there had never been father-son moments and we had never learned how to talk. Our love and resentments went both ways; him loathing the way I squandered the opportunities he had secured for me with his sacrifices; me hating his indirect urgings and silent expectations. Of course, these were things we never broached facing each other.

"Your mother wants me to retire, but I'm afraid to retire. What will I think about? My mind cannot rest."

He didn't say it but the words hung there between us: It's my punishment for my punishing Chi. He seemed suddenly old and rotting with doubts, doomed like a worm-eaten clipper banished from all harbors in its shortening days. Condemned to die at sea. Disconcerted, I tried to humor him. "Oh, Father. What is there to regret? Look at yourself. Look at your children. You've done well. You've lived a full life and now is the time to enjoy your golden years."

He turned from me and I caught his awful sadness in profile. "I should have been a better father to you boys. I should have been more like an American father. They know how to cherish their children. I should have taken you camping . . . or something."

An emptiness waited between us as I fumbled to find something to say as he tried to utter what was really at his core.

"Chi," he said at last. "I shouldn't have beaten her like that. I was wrong."

"It was a long time ago, Father."

"I didn't know better. It is the Vietnamese way. You beat your children if you love them. You beat them to show them the right way to live. You beat them to let them know they are important to you."

"I know, Father."

There lurked something else in him. I could feel it.

"My father beat me. I didn't know any other way," Father said, averting his eyes. Shoulders heaving, he was fighting his face, shocked at himself over his sudden confession.

"I know you meant well, Father." I wanted to tell him I forgave him, but he did not ask. And I could not presume. "The rest of us turned out decent."

We did, Father, we really did. Huy and Hien are gay, but not because you beat them. They are gay, not because you forced them to study and forbade them to have girlfriends. They are happy now, handsome successful men. Tien inherited your mind. He is kind, brilliant, and thoughtful, as you are at your best. Kay has all the best parts of us. And I have caged my beast, have not struck in anger since Hien pulled the knife—the best thing Hien could have done for me.

"My father was violent. I was an abused child," Father said. "He was abusive. And . . . I was abusive."

I wished with all my might that he hadn't said it. For him, it was too much. He was a man of the old world, given to the old ways, the harsher values. He wasn't American, not like me. With this conception of his having been an "abused child"—this American definition—he could not survive, for all his guilt, real and imagined, came crashing down on his age-brittle shoulders. Where was his survival instinct—the one that refused to understand victimization—when he needed it most?

I knew his father—my grandfather, the opium addict who was doomed in his delusions of lost grandeur. I knew his son, Uncle Hien, also an addict. The way Grandpa Pham chained his son to a post like a dog to cure Uncle Hien of what he could not cure himself. Once, Uncle Hien's street gang visited him at the house and slipped him a mini-saw in a baguette, something they must have read in a spy novel. Grandpa chased them into the street with a machete. My father was my grandfather's sort of man, only he was cursed with a dose of sensitivity that surfaced in his old days. He was a giver, a ready sacrifice for his family.

He was a worrier, a planner, a schemer, his brain an algorithm with too many variables which frequently crashed and never yielded the optimal solution. But, again, that was the best thing about him. He was a man of logic, a programmer with a program that could be rewritten and continually updated. He was an intellectual, the quintessential Vietnamese, a man given to passion and mountainous determination. He was a poet, a tireless, award-winning translator of French verse. He was enamored with classical guitar music. And although I never knew it during my school years when he was discouraging me from becoming a painter, he was himself a fair artist. All this in a man whose life was a mad saga: the first son of an abusive aristocrat, a teenager who lost his mother, a war and famine survivor, a refugee from the North Vietnamese Communists, a ditchdigger, a star academic, a disobedient son who wedded his beloved, a civic official, a soldier, an officer in the

Nationalist Army, a government propagandist, a teacher of mathematics, a successful businessman, a prisoner in the labor and reeducation camp, an escapee from Communist Vietnam, a penniless refugee in America, a janitor, a college student, a programmer, a software engineer. Amid his travails, his daughter ran away, became a man, came home fourteen years later, and, at last, committed suicide.

He was forever forced to rewrite his paradigm, even if only to survive. Now, looking down the road of his dwindling years, he found that his shifted philosophy—from the Vietnamese to the American way—laid the blame of what he interpreted as our collective misfortunes squarely on his shoulders. The easiest lesson had always eluded him. A survivor does not have the luxury of counting his blessings.

After Grandpa Pham passed away, Father clipped a short newspaper article, hardly more than a blurb, taped it to the lampshade in the living room, and left it there for ten years. It was written by a man who, after his father's death, regretted never having said *I love you, Dad.*

Viet-Kieu

44 The closer I come to Nha Trang the more frequently I see group tours busing to local points of interest. The locals are familiar with the tourist traffic and don't shout *"Oy! Oy!"* at foreigners. The main road loops around a mountain and enters the outskirts of the city from the south side. There is a shortcut, some high school kids point out to me, up the mountain and along the cliff. It's a good sporting ride, they say. I'm about to bag 120 miles today and have no wish to climb a mountain. I come into the city the easy way.

Although the outlying area is a mirror image of all the other dusty little towns, the city center is far more developed than anything I've seen. I limp the battered bike through town, heading toward the water where the locals have told me there is lodging. Shady lanes unroll between banks of sprawling buildings set back behind brick fences. There's a nice flavor here predating the Liberation of '75. I was just a kid then, but I remember Mom being very hip with her bell-bottoms and buggy sunglasses. She must have wasted scores of film rolls in Nha Trang, her favorite city. The breeze is fresh, sweet, not salty like Phan Thiet. Out on the beachfront boulevard, I am suddenly in Waikiki! Someone has ripped it out of Hawaii and dropped it in downtown Nha Trang. A colossal skeleton of the Outrigger

Hotel is being framed on the beach practically in the surf line. Tall, gleaming towers of glass and steel are already taking residence a stone's throw from the water. The sandy stretch of beach is jammed with fancy restaurants, bars hopping with modern rock, jazz, and Vietnamese pop. Aromas of grilled food turn heads and sharpen appetites. Along the avenue, fat Europeans and Australians pad about in thong bikinis, sheer sarongs, and Lycra shorts, dropping wads of dollars for seashells, corals, lacquered jewelry boxes, and bad paintings, loot, mementos, evidence.

I take the cheapest room available to a Viet-kieu at a government-run hotel (for some reason, Danes and Germans get lower rates), jump through a cold shower, then get back on my bike to head to the Vietnamese part of Nha Trang, where the food is cheaper and better. I am ravenous. Diarrhea be damned. Tonight I'm going to eat anything I want. After nearly three months of sporadic intestinal troubles, I'm still hoping that my system will acclimatize. I'm Vietnamese after all, and these microorganisms once thrived in my gut as thoroughly as in any Vietnamese here.

I eat dinner at an alley diner, nine tables crammed between two buildings lit with a couple of bare light bulbs. The family running the place says they are happy to have me, although they generally don't like foreigners. Eat too little, drink too little, but talk too much, they complain. Foreigners like to sit and sit and talk. Vietnamese eat and get out. Lounging is done in coffeehouses and beer halls. No problem. I prove to them I'm Vietnamese. I down two large bottles of Chinese beer and gorge myself on a monstrous meal of grilled meat served with a soy-and-pork-fat gravy, wrapping the meat in rice paper, cucumber, mint, pickled daikon, sour carrot, fresh basil, lettuce, chili pepper, cilantro, and rice vermicelli. Then I clear out quickly. I go to a hotel to check on a friend who might be in town. As a tour guide, he is a regular at the hotel. The concierge confirms that my friend Cuong and his tour are in town. I leave him a note and wait for him at an ice-cream parlor down the street.

"Hello! Andrew!"

"Cuong!"

I met him a few weeks after I arrived in Saigon. We bummed around the city several times with his girlfriends. I like him. We both agreed to check on each other when in Nha Trang or Vung Tau, both major cities on his itinerary.

He skips across the street, penny-loafing around the dog shit as he dodges motorbikes. Cuong doesn't wear sandals. No more. Not ever again. He told me, You can tell a Vietnamese by the way he wears his sandals. Is the stem firmly held between the toes? Or does the ball of the heel drag beyond the sandal? Do the sandals flap like loose tongues when he walks? Does he know there is mud between his toes? All this from a man who—in his own words—*"dribbled away [his] youth as a roadside petrol-boy selling gasoline out of glass bottles, wiping down motorbikes, hustling for dimes, and playing barefoot soccer in the dirt."*

He smoothes his shirt, fingers the ironed pleats of his gray slacks, straightens his pin-striped blue tie with red polka dots. Then, grinning, he steps closer and pumps my hand enthusiastically. "Calvin," he corrects me. "I'm sticking with your suggestion: Calvin. It's easier for the foreigners to pronounce." I'd come up with the name at his request. He wanted something that started with a "C" and was short and sharp and American.

"You made it! You're not hurt? No?" he says, patting me on the arm and looking me over. "A little thinner and darker, yes. Incredible. You biked all that way? Yes, yes, of course you did."

"You got my message?"

"Of course. May I join you?" he queries, forever the Vietnamese gentleman. I fill him in on all that happened since I last saw him nearly two months ago. When a waitress brings him his chilled Coke—no ice, just like the way foreigners drink their soda—he thanks her. She looks at him, a little startled to hear a Vietnamese man uttering platitudes like Westerners. Calvin has picked up the habit because he finds it more genteel and civilized.

I first made his acquaintance at a sidewalk café. He took me for a Japanese and wanted to practice his English. When I told him I was a Vietnamese from California, he was very uncomfortable using the term Viet-kieu, explaining that people said it with too many connotations. Sometimes, it was just a word, other times an insult or a term of segregation. *"Vietnamese are Vietnamese if they believe they are,"* he had said by way of explanation, and I liked him on the instant.

By Saigon standards, Calvin is a yuppie who came into his own by the most romantic way possible—by the compulsion of a promise made to his mother on her deathbed. One afternoon, when we were touring the outer districts of Saigon on his motorbike, Calvin pointed to a pack of greyhound-lean young men, shirtless, volleying a plastic bird back and forth with their feet. *"That was me. That's how I was until I was twenty-two. Can you believe it? I threw away all my young years, working odd jobs and messing around. I just didn't care."* His mother bequeathed him, her only child, a small sum, which he spent on English classes, not bothering to finish up high school. With what little remained, he bribed his way into a job as a hotel bellhop and worked his way up. He entered a special school for tour guides. After three years of intense training, he makes four hundred dollars a month plus two hundred in tips. Now, twenty-nine, single, and rich even by Saigon standards, he fares better than college grads who are blessed if they can command two hundred dollars a month. His biggest regret: *"I wish my mother could see me now."*

Calvin sips his Coke and plucks a pack of Marlboros from his shirt pocket, the American cigarette one of his main props for marking himself one of the upwardly mobile. "I'm down to half a pack a day," he mumbles apologetically, offering me a smoke. I decline. He puts his cigarette down saying: "Dirty, dirty Vietnamese habit." Calvin keeps a list of "dirty Vietnamese habits" and steels himself against them.

I tell him that Americans used to call cigarettes "white slavers." He considers that for a moment then smirks. *"That has a double meaning for us, doesn't it."* He counts the cigarettes remaining in the pack. *"Last one today,"* he announces. He seems to want my approval so I nod. Vindicated, he ignites the last of his daily nicotine allowance. He sighs the smoke downwind. *"Tell me. Tell me everything about your trip."*

As I recount the events since I last saw him, Calvin grows increasingly excited, digging me more for the details of Vietnam than for the actual mechanics of bike touring. How did the police treat you?

Hanoi people are more formal than Southerners, aren't they? You think Uncle Ho's body is a hoax? What's the countryside like? Is it pretty like the Southern country? He flames another cigarette and orders us a round of beer. By our third round, he has chain-smoked into a second pack of Marlboros.

Late in the night, when I am sapped of tales from the road, Calvin, who is beer-fogged, leans back in his chair and asks, *"America is like a dream, isn't it?"*

After all I've seen, I agree. *"Sure."*

We contemplate the beer in our glasses. I ask him, *"Do you want to go there?"* I don't know why I ask him this. Maybe, believing that he is my equivalent in Vietnam, I want him to say he really loves the country and that it is magical, wonderful in ways I have yet to imagine. More powerful, more potent than the West.

Calvin sounds annoyed. *"Of course. Who wouldn't?"* He pauses, taking long, pensive drags on his cigarette. *"But perhaps only to visit. To see, understand-no?"*

"Why?"

"Simple. Here . . . here, I am a king." He leans over the table, shaking the cigarette at me. *"In America you, I mean all you Viet-kieu, are guests. And guests don't have the same rights as hosts."* He sits back, legs crossed at the knees, and throws a proprietary arm over the city. *"At least, here, I am king. I belong. I am better than most Vietnamese."*

"No, we're not guests. We're citizens. Permanent. Ideally we are all equal. Equal rights," I insert lamely, the words, recalled from elementary school history lessons, sounding hollow.

"Right, but do you FEEL like an American? Do you?"

Yes! Yes! Yes, I do. I really do, I want to shout it in his face. Already, the urge leaves a bad taste in my mouth. *"Sometimes, I do. Sometimes, I feel like I am a real American."*

I wish I could tell him. I don't mind forgetting who I am, but I know he wouldn't understand. I don't mind being looked at or treated just like another American, a white American. No, I don't mind at all. I want it. I like it. Yet every so often when I become really good at tricking myself, there is always that inevitable slap that shocks me out of my shell and prompts me to reassess everything.

How could I tell him my shame? How could I tell him about the drive-bys where some red-faced white would stick his head out of his truck, giving me the finger and screaming, "Go home, Chink!" Could I tell him it chilled me to wonder what would happen if my protagonist knew I was Vietnamese? What if his father had died in Vietnam? What if he was a Vietnam vet? Could I tell Calvin about the time my Vietnamese friends and I dined in a posh restaurant in Laguna Beach in Southern California? A white man at the next table, glaring at us, grumbled to his wife, "They took over Santa Ana. And now they're here. This whole state is going to hell." They was us Vietnamese. Santa Ana was now America's Little Saigon.

Could I tell Calvin I was initiated into the American heaven during my first week Stateside by eight black kids who pulverized me in the restroom, calling me Viet Cong? No. I grew up fighting blacks, whites, and Chicanos. The whites beat up the blacks. The blacks beat up the Chicanos. And everybody beat up the Chinaman whether or not he was really an ethnic Chinese. These new Vietnamese kids were easy pickings, small, bookish, passive, and not fluent in English.

So, we congregate in Little Saigons, we hide out in Chinatowns and Japantowns, blending in. We huddle together, surrounding ourselves with the material wealth of America, and wave our star-spangled banners, shouting: "We're Americans. We love America."

I cannot bring myself to confront my antagonists. Cannot always claim my rights as a naturalized citizen. Cannot, for the same reason, resist the veterans' pleas for money outside grocery stores. Cannot armor myself against the pangs of guilt at every homeless man wearing army fatigues. Sown deep in me is a seed of discomfort. Maybe shame. I see that we Vietnamese Americans don't talk about our history. Although we often pretend to be modest and humble as we preen our successful immigrant stories, we rarely admit even to ourselves the circumstances and the cost of our being here. We elude it all like a petty theft committed ages ago. When convenient, we take it as restitution for what happened to Vietnam.

Calvin senses my discomfort. It is his talent, a marked skill of his trade. He looks away, reaching for yet another cigarette to cover the silence I opened. He asks me the one question that Vietnamese throughout Vietnam have tried to broach obliquely: *"Do they look down on Vietnamese in America? Do they hate you?"*

I don't want to dwell on that. Vietnamese believe that white Americans are to Viet-kieu as Viet-kieu are to Vietnamese, each one a level above the next, respectively. And, somehow, this shames me, maybe because I cannot convince myself that it is entirely true or false. I divert the thrust and ask him, *"You are Westernized. You know how different foreigners are from Vietnamese. How do you feel showing them around the country?"*

"I like the work. Many of them are very nice. Curious about our culture. I like the Australians most. Rowdy and lots of trouble, but they respect Vietnamese."

"But don't you see the reactions on their faces when they see our squalor? Don't you hear the things they say about us? Don't tell me you've never heard it."

He looks uncomfortable, drawing deep from his nicotine stick, sighing the smoke to the stars. Then to his credit and my everlasting respect for him, he says quietly, facing the sky, *"I do. I can't help it but I do. I take them out on the Saigon streets, you know, the poor parts because they ask me. They want pictures. I see them flinch at the beggars, the poverty of Vietnamese. The chicken-shacks we live in."*

A wordless lull falls between us. We're both drunk. I am irritated at having to delve into a subject I avoid, and feeling mean-spirited I have goaded him onto equally disconcerting ground.

"It's very hard being a tour guide. Sometimes I feel like a pimp." He switches into his tour-guide English: "Here, look at this, sir. Yes, ma'am, these are the average Vietnamese. Yes, they are poor. Yes, sir. Here is our national monument. Very big. Very important to Vietnamese. You impressed? No, not so big?" He shrugs, saying, *"I know they've got bigger monuments in their countries. Older, more important. What do our little things mean to them?"*

The silence tells me we are moving too far into no-man's-land. One more cigarette. More beer. Tusking the smoke out of his nostrils, he seems to brace himself, gathering force like a wave, building before cresting white. As his beliefs come barreling out, I know the crushing impact of his words will stay with me, for in them I catch a glimpse of myself and of the true Cuong, the Cuong that came before and is deeper than the suave Calvin facing me. *"Vietnamese aren't ashamed of our own poverty. We're not ashamed of squatting in mud huts and sleeping on rags. There is no shame in being poor. We were born into it just as Westerners are born white. The Westerners are white as we are yellow. There is already a difference between us. Our poverty is minor in the chasm that already exists. A small detail. The real damning thing is the fact that there are Viet-kieu, our own brothers, skin of our skin, blood of our blood, who look better than us, more civilized, more educated, more wealthy, more genteel. Viet-kieu look kingly next to the average Vietnamese. Look at you, look at me. You're wearing old jeans and I'm wearing a suit, but it's obvious who . . . who is superior. Can't you see? We look like monkeys because you make us look like monkeys just by your existence."*

"Is this truly how Vietnamese see us Viet-kieu?"

"Some call you the lost brothers. Look at you. Living in America has lightened your skin, made you forget your language. You have tasted Western women and you're probably not as attracted to Vietnamese women anymore. You eat nutritious Western food and you are bigger and stronger than us. You know better than to smoke and drink like Vietnamese. You know exercise is good so you don't waste your time sitting in cafés and smoking your hard-earned money away. Someday, your blood will mix so well with Western blood that there will be no difference between you and them. You are already lost to us."

I listen with dismay as his observations fall on me like a sentence, but I can tell in the back of his mind he is saying: And I want to be more like you because that's where the future is. He must suspect I am doubting what he has told me the first time our paths crossed: *"Vietnamese are Vietnamese if they believe they are."*

Calvin and I bid each other good night, each going his own way. He has to resolve a fracas of intoxicated Australians in his charge back at the hotel. In our drunkenness, our conversation crossed forbidden boundaries and we are both depressed. Maybe it is just the beer wearing off. I pedal down to the beach for some sea air. As I coast along the ocean boulevard, a gorgeous girl, unusually tall for a Vietnamese, dressed in the traditional *ao dai* like a college student, tails me on her expensive motorbike, a Honda Dream, the Vietnamese Cadillac. Hello, she says in English. Hello, I smile. She thinks I'm Japanese or Korean. How are you, she asks me. Good, I say—always glad to talk to students eager to practice their English. And you, I say to keep the conversation going, how are you? You are very pretty, she tells me. No, I chuckle, standing now with her on the dark sidewalk, you are pretty. Very pretty. Pretty enough, I fancy silently to myself, for me to fall madly in love with. My heart dances ahead of me with improbable possibilities. Wild schemes streak through my head ratting out ways for me to stay in Nha Trang longer to make her acquaintance. Maybe get a job here. There are so many foreign companies, it should be easy. And on and on. Hopeful. I am smiling.

Then she says, "You go with me?"

"Yes, sure. Where? Anywhere! Let's go!"

"You go with me very cheap. You go. Me very cheap, very good. You go with me very cheap. Very, very cheap. I make you happy."

My smile feels waxy. I turn away, looking at the surf rolling on the white sand, the moon pearling us all. She parrots it over and over.

No, yes, maybe, later, I must meet a friend now, see you soon, bye, I blurt for the sake of blurting and I ride away from the tourist boardwalk with my money, my opportunities, my privileges, my life. I look back once and see her glossy cherry lips mouthing those words to me, a red wound in the neon night of Nha Trang.

Chi-Me

 It was dark.

Christmas lights winked merry in the neighborhood.

But we felt no cheer.

It was only Chi-Minh and me, our final moment.
We were ambling down broken sidewalks in the cold.

I said something. Hard times, he said, hard times. Dead leaves crunched beneath our feet. Wood smoke trapped the night but there was no fireplace warmth in the air. You all right? I asked, trying to catch his eyes in the gloom.

Slow, heavy steps. Sighs. Silence. Our hands deep in our empty pockets. Big dark trees blotting out the stars.

Minh, you remember the star fruits we used to eat on the roof? —Yeah. —Me, too. I thought I caught him smiling. But it was dark. —Star fruit and chili-salt, good wasn't it? he said. —Yes, pretty good. You know, they're importing star fruits: you can buy them in any supermarket now. —But, he shook his head, not as good as the star fruits from Grandma's tree. —No, I admitted, never that good.

You, okay? —Yeah. —You sure? —Hard times, just figuring things out.

We came to an intersection. The streetlamp had burnt out. Winter leaves piled the gutters like old letters from forgotten seasons. Headlights swept across us. Abruptly, we felt naked. We should have made the crossing, or we should have turned the corner. But we didn't. We stood there uncertain. I should have placed a hand on his shoulder.

Lonely, he said.

Your ex . . . ?

Just figuring things out.

Take care of yourself, okay?

Yeah.

We gotta hang out together more. Soon, okay?

———

Yeah, sure.

It was my season of unraveling. And his as well. I couldn't remember all, what it was he said. Nor what I said. Maybe he wished I'd said something. And I him. Perhaps we should have shared our troubled hearts. But in the end—my long-staying memory—I heard only the wavering catch in his voice.

Some nights I lie in moonlit fields, thinking of him, star fruits, and dying angels.

Blue-Peace

 46 The road goes on and on before me and there is nothing to do but to get on it and push the pedals round and round. The days march at me single file. I have grown accustomed to the pocked asphalt rolling beneath my worn tires. Dysentery has left me on a lasting high, a feeling of someone whose fever has just broken and is taking his first breath of fresh air. It seems I have gone through all the colors, through all the land I knew.

After Nha Trang, the land dries up. The sky hurts with a whispering blue. The air chafes, a marine tinge, rough on its hot grainy edge. Down by the strung-out coast, the sea lies open, three shades deeper than the bright above. The road is black and broad, curving round sandstone mountains and cutting straight through the flat beige stretches. *Suong rong*—dragon bones, squatty Vietnamese cacti—cast the vast empty into a shallow prickly graveyard. They say dragons came here to die. The land scorched itself in sorrow over the great beasts' passing.

Somewhere near Ca Na, I duck into the thatched shade of a roadside café perched on stone pilings by the water. A waitress brings me an espresso—Vietnamese chicory-roasted coffee, a gift, a legacy of the colonial French. *A tool of subjugation, a crutch in the Vietnamese progress,* Calvin had fumed at me, hating the image of idle, jobless Vietnamese men lounging in white plastic chairs, espresso presses before them, the black drops oozing down painstakingly. He had forsworn this rite of his countrymen, opting for the teas of the older ways. I sip the mud, preferring it without the sweetened condensed milk Vietnamese adore. It is good, bitter, but wholesome like this desert shore.

There is magic in this place: I could be anywhere. The turquoise idyll, the tittering waves. On the mustard sand, coils of bleached rope lace broken seashells and bamboo crab cages. A skinny sand-colored dog woofs, warning the boys against sticking their heads in the traps. Way out, a one-man fishing boat sputters, zippering white on blue.

For some unexplainable reason, I leave my bike and belongings at the café without concern and run down to the beach, my backpack heavy with beer, candies, and cupcakes I bought from bus-stop vendors. I stroll along the chewed-up coast, boulder-hopping from one beach to the next for the sheer joy of it. Chi and I had done this long ago during one of our family vacations. We scrabbled along the rocky shore and climbed up a cliff where we looked down on the hulking wreck of a mighty freighter jutting out of the jade water. The waves frothed white around it, and, in the westering sun, the rusted hull had this bright coppery color that looked like cheap orange soda held against light. Chi said it was the most beautiful color she had ever seen.

The crab-cage kids find me napping in the sun. I hand out candies and cakes. One of the boys grabs two cupcakes and runs off chattering. Soon he comes back, a watermelon balanced on his shoulder. A girl uses a sharp stone to open the melon. We eat it in gobs, scooping out the red foam with our fingers, sticky juice running down our necks. I hold a watermelon-seed-spitting contest, awarding prizes to all contenders.

They spit the black seeds, they shoot them in sprays of saliva. They swallow their ammo, giggling and reminding me of the first time I won a watermelon-seed-spitting contest. Decades ago at a Christian summer camp, I flew a seed a magical thirty-two feet, five inches to claim a gold medal—my bursting joy made from the cap of a baby-food jar. After two years in the States, I had learned that I could earn

forbearance, if not acceptance, from my peers if I made myself unob-
trusive. Mediocre grades, adequate athletics. A moderate disappointment to the teachers. So it was special for me—the only nonwhite kid
at a camp of three hundred—to receive their applause. I remember
thinking then that maybe this America wasn't so bad after all. And
that the last time I had seen a crowd of Asian faces I was in Vietnam.

But now, I miss the white, the black, the red, the brown faces of
America. I miss their varied shapes, their tumultuous diversity, their
idealistic search for racial equality, their bumbling but wonderful pioneering spirit. I miss English words in my ears, miss the way the language rolled off my tongue so naturally. I miss its poetry. Somewhere
along the way, my search for roots has become my search for home—
a place I know best even though there are those who would have me
believe otherwise.

Phan Thiet, the town of my birth, the end of my journey, lies only
a few hours' ride away, but the marching drums that have driven me
onward for a year now have abruptly quieted. An unexpected lull.
The finish line seems unimportant, secondary, symbolic. So when the
sun is setting behind the desert, I do as I did—it seems now—so long
ago: I lay out my bedroll on the sand and wait for the stars to wake.
First time in Vietnam no one invades my camp. I am alone.

A year ago, in the days immediately before I met Tyle, I had found
myself camping on a deserted beach in Baja. One morning, I woke
on that sandy rim of the Pacific with a sea tanginess upon my lips and
the chill of the northerly in my bones. I opened my eyes and it struck
me a silent-thunderous blow: the solidity of the sand, the futile passion of the surf, the pensive vastness of the sea, the swollen anger of
the sky, all a chaos of gray.

A powerful melancholy clamped over me and cheated away my
warmth. I curled in my blanket, staring at the fisting sky. In a fleeting
moment, a rhythm paced through, the reason for all the reasons I had
been searching. Like turning to catch a movement seen out of the
corner of my eye, I reached for that sublime. But it was gone, fleeing
through my fingers like shiny flecks of sand in a receding tide. I stood
on the shore secure, comforted by an unwordable glimpse that was
already fading into a hunch.

This feeling is with me now. Three nights and days, I sleep and play by the ocean. During the day, I look out on the water and let the memories roll over me. I swim in the ocean of morning gray and wade in the surf of evening gold. The blue here is so vast, no war could ever measurably sap it, not even the one in me. My faults, all my shortcomings, my wrongs against Chi-Minh, pale away, disintegrating, in this desert-ocean-peace. I remember the joy of our being near each other. I know my love for her now, refelt my love for her then and all the love I felt for her in the between years. It isn't forgiveness I seek. All my sins, my sorrows but a drop of ink in this blue vastness.

And my standing here and all the roads opening before me are not my tribute to Chi but her gifts to me.

I know now Crazy Ronnie was right. Hugging herself in the premature August chill, she stood at the foot of the stairwell of her urban hovel, bidding me farewell: "The perfection of intention. In the end, it is all that matters." Just then the sun burned through the trees and baked the stucco facade of the apartment, and she was engulfed in this lustrous glow that I knew would be how I shall always remember her. And although I did not understand it then, I knew that what she said chimed with significance.

I wade into a blue-green pool, the warm water lolls soft and clean against me. I swim, rejoicing in my aloneness. Someone cries from the beach. A-lo! A-lo! An old woman laughs at me. I grin. She shucks her rubber sandals, stumbles in fully clothed, fat arms jiggling above her head, waving greetings. A-lo! Okay! Okay! she yells, exuberant.

I laugh at the sight of her, a portly grandmother splashing like a child, her white peasant shirt billowing in the water. We stand on flat stones, chest deep across from each other, beaming. She says something in English, but I can't understand her, so I keep smiling and nodding. She laughs, I laugh with her. She tries a phrase in French. I shake my head. Never thinking I could understand her, she prattles in Vietnamese, It is beautiful, no? Very beautiful, very peaceful here, isn't it?

I smile.

I smile at her from my anonymity, refusing to answer in our common tongue. I don't want her to leave. I don't want to disappoint her with my commonality, to remind her of our shared history. So, I let her interpret my half-truths. At this I am good, for I am a mover of betweens. I slip among classifications like water in cupped palms, leaving bits of myself behind. I am quick and deft, for there is no greater fear than the fear of being caught wanting to belong. I am a chameleon. And the best chameleon has no center, no truer sense of self than what he is in the instant.

No guilt. I realize suddenly, looking into her joy-gushing face. We stand on separate islands, nothing between us except our designs. And the perfection of our intention is enough. We: friends sharing a sea bath. Our skein of history casts no shade on this moment. I wish at once Tyle were here in my shoes under this sky. Maybe he would understand that his past wrongs can be mended with the totality of his regrets, a pure desire that things might have been different, a wish of wellness for the survivors. Forgiveness is a hollow gift when there is no mountain to move as compensation for the wrongs. For our truths change with time. There is nothing else. No mitigating circumstances and no power to undo the sins. No was. Only is. Between us, there is but a thin line of intention.

Epilogue

"You-me: one. Not two. One. No difference," Son shouts at me in his best English, driving his imperative into my soul with the sheer force of his conviction.

And I shout back at him: "Yes, Brother! Yes! Yes, no difference!"

We are mad-drunk. Hung is looking on, smiling, sweating beer. At our feet, three milk crates of empty Tiger bottles clutter the sidewalk. Traffic whizzing by, riders lying on the horn as always. I have made it back to Saigon penniless and Son and Hung are giving me the best farewell party a guy can wish for. The girls—Son's girls—dropped by earlier and knocked off a couple of Tigers apiece, all four of them, before going back to work.

"Come on, you have time. Just an hour, eh?" Son is begging to give me a parting present: a roll in the sheets with one of his girls—my pick. My plane leaves in ninety minutes.

"Thanks Son, but I've got to go. I'm too drunk, my friend."

"Shit! Fuck! Shit!" Son sputters. Then he apologizes as though he is responsible for my inebriated state.

Hung, grinning like the Kitchen God, is mopping his face with a roll of toilet paper that doubles as napkin dispenser in his beerhouse. Hung tambourines his hand and croons, *"Unbearable."* He laughs merrily, all game. *"Don't worry, I'll get you to the airport on time. Let's go see our little sisters. They like you a lot. They think you are one sick, crazy guy."*

The alcohol has uncaged my lust, made me dangerous. I know if I ever step into that massage parlor again, if I ever set eyes on Son's harem again, I'll stay in Vietnam and drink and whore my days away with Hung and Son because it is too easy. I like them too much. I could burn up a decade here as easily as flaming a whole matchbook at once.

I shake my head.

"What will you do in America?" Son asks, reverting back to English as he usually does when he is serious.

The answer falls on me, a drop of water from a blue sky: "Be a better American."

Son just looks at me, his face unreadable, and after a moment I find myself grinning, feeling inexplicably good. I struggle to my feet and clasp Son's hands in mine. His hands are dark, soft like an old woman's; the fight—the iron of the Green Beret—has gone out of them. I will probably never see him again. U.S. Immigration approved his papers because he spent five years in a labor camp for being a Green Beret, but the Vietnamese bureaucrats won't let him go. They say once he arrives in America they have no guarantee he will support his nine illegitimate children stranded in Vietnam. His old nemesis has a chain around his neck and he knows it. Son accepts his lot, a lover of life.

"So long, Son."

"Do not say good-bye, my friend Andrew." Son stalls me with a raised hand. "You are not gone from me. I have you in my heart."

I straddle the Vespa behind Hung, who insists on taking me to the airport. Son doesn't budge an inch. I doubt he could. He slouches in the low beach chair, his legs splayed out on the concrete before him like an overturned frog, his massive hands dangling from his wrists dripping over the plastic armrests. Impotent. His vitality seems to have ebbed suddenly from him. Then he smiles this half-grin which I have come to adore greatly, and I know all the wickedness, the mislaid idealism, the precocious humor are alive within that withered shell of history. We pull away and I look around. Son is not getting smaller. He is still grinning with half of his face. My waylaid Buddha.

It takes the Boeing 747 twenty-two hours to bring me back to where I had started running a year ago. Our captain announces our arrival in San Francisco and the cabin begins to boil with the nervous energy of nearly a hundred immigrating Vietnamese. They have come under a U.S.–sanctioned program for those who had served America during the war and had been imprisoned for three years or more by Communist Vietnam. Out of concern for these first-time fliers, the flight attendants seated them in the center seats far from the windows, which might make them nauseous. They are jumpy, anxious, like caged animals smelling freedom, in a panic to get a glimpse of the promised land. The FASTEN SEAT BELT sign is on, but they scoot up and down the aisle like children jostling for a look at the Christmas tree, clambering into empty seats and leaning over other passengers to get to the windows. One older Vietnamese man, whose seat is across the aisle from mine, is practically in my lap. I insist he take my window seat. We peer through the Plexiglas together.

Below, the curling headland of Point Reyes, just north of San Francisco, comes into view. It is late February, the hills lush, almost tropical if it weren't for the chill. I remember that finger of land and the punishing, dangerous road that climbs along that enchanting coast. The nights I slept on the side of the road. The hundred friends I made along the way, the Vietnam vets, the hippies, the housewives, the fading retirees. All the ordinary, the extraordinary people who took me into their homes, their lives even, for an evening. I can taste again my stifling fears, my irrepressible joys of struggling up this coast. Below me, all my sweetest memories of America.

"This is America?" the man asks me in a reverent tone, eyes never leaving the window, nose pressed to the glass like a child wishing himself into a baker's shop.

"Yes, Brother," I smile. *"Welcome home."*

Acknowledgments

Where do our stories end and others' begin? Are the borders negotiable?

My eternal gratitude to my parents, Thong and Anh Pham, for their sacrifices, their perseverance, their love, their good intentions. And may they forgive me for writing this book.

For letting me tell our stories, my thanks to my aunt Hai Dung, my sister Kay, and my brothers Huy, Tien, and Hien.

I am deeply indebted to Stephanie D. Stephens, who was there when I penned the first as well as the last sentence of *Catfish and Mandala*. She single-handedly edited the manuscript—the only person to have read the entire work before I sent it out to literary agents. Her encouragement, enthusiasm, and faith in this project sustained me through some difficult passages.

For their friendships, I thank Deborah Hansen and Lisa McKenzie. Because we had agreed on it, thank you, Jessa Vartanian. To my devoted friend Pamela Andreatta, all my best wishes, my fondest affection.

My humble gratitude to the Nguyen family for everything, and to all the wonderful people I met on the road who opened their hearts and homes to me: Patty Smythe, Sasha Kaufman, Jim Faulkner,

Dianna Hoffman, Marty Nelson, Donna Bronson, Son, Calvin Luong, Tam Nguyen, and Uncle Tu. And to yet countless others whose names I have lost, forgotten along the way.

I am grateful to my friend and longtime newspaper editor, Lorraine Gengo, who gave me my first chance at freelance writing, and her successor, Sharan Street, for being a friend.

Many thanks to my beautiful agent, Jandy Nelson, for her unwavering faith and all the beers we drank together, and my editor, John Glusman, for his sensitivity.